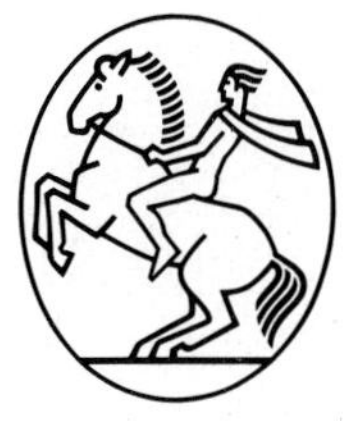

Journal of Neural Transmission

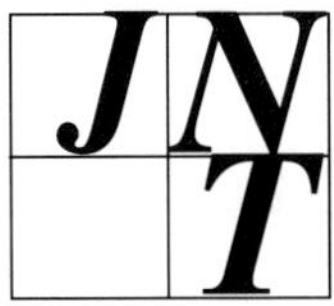

Supplement 45

U. Bonuccelli and J. M. Rabey (eds.)

Old and New Dopamine Agonists in Parkinson's Disease

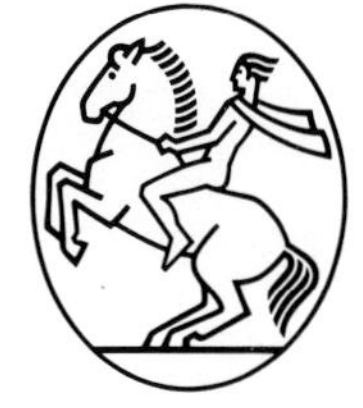

Springer-Verlag   *Wien New York*

Prof. Dr. U. Bonuccelli
Institute of Clinical Neurology, University of Pisa, Pisa, Italy

Prof. Dr. J. M. Rabey
Department of Neurology, Assaf Harofe Medical Center, Zerifin, Israel

Printed in Austria

Product Liability: The publisher can give no guarantee for information about drug dosage and application thereof contained in this book. In every individual case the respective user must check its accuracy by consulting other pharmaceutical literature. The use of registered names, trademarks, etc. in this publication does not imply, even in the absence of a specific statement, that such names are exempt from the relevant protective laws and regulations and therefore free for general use.

Typesetting: Best-set Typesetter Ltd, Hong Kong
Printing: A. Holzhausens Nfg., A-1070 Wien
Printed on acid-free and chlorine-free bleached paper

With 73 Figures

Library of Congress Cataloging-in-Publication Data

Old and new dopamine agonists in Parkinson's disease/U. Bonuccelli and J. M. Rabey (eds.).
p. cm. – (Journal of neural transmission. Supplement, ISSN 0303-6995; 45)
Includes bibliographical references and index.
ISBN 3-211-82717-X (alk. paper). – ISBN 0-387-82717-X (alk. paper)
1. Parkinsonism – Chemotherapy. 2. Dopamine – Antagonists – Therapeutic use. I. Bonuccelli, U. (Ubaldo), 1949–. II. Rabey, J. M. (Jose Martin), 1945–. III. Series: Journal of neural transmission. Supplementum; 45.
[DNLM: 1. Parkinson Disease – physiopathology – congresses. 2. Parkinson Disease – drug therapy – congresses. 3. Dopamine Agonists – therapeutic use – congresses. 4. Receptors, Dopamine – drug therapy – congresses. W1 J0781A no. 45 1995/WL 359 044 1995]
RC382.0475 1995
616.8'33061 – dc20

ISSN 0303-6995
ISBN 3-211-82717-X Springer-Verlag Wien New York

Foreword

Nulla dies sine linea
Plinius Major

It is a great honour for me to introduce this volume, edited by one of my most distinguished associates at the Institute of Clinical Neurology of Pisa, Ubaldo Bonuccelli, and by the internationally recognised neurologist of the Israeli school, Jose M. Rabey. The work collects the papers presented at the 1st International Congress on dopamine agonists held in Pisa in December 1993 on the occasion of the 650th anniversary of the founding of the University of Pisa. The difficulties inherent in the pharmacological treatment of Parkinson's disease (PD) provided the main clinical impetus for our organising the meeting.

Dopamine agonists are a heterogeneous group of drugs which share the ability to exert antiparkinsonian effects through the activation of dopamine receptors. The first dopamine agonist, bromocriptine, was developed in the early 1970s with the aim of reducing the inevitable side effects of long-term levodopa therapy, such as motor performance fluctuations, abnormal movements and psychiatric complications. To date, many other dopamine agonists have been developed and are currently available in clinical practice, but none has proved to be as effective as levodopa. Many clinical studies have, however, demonstrated the effectiveness of dopamine agonists as adjuncts to reduce motor fluctuations in levodopa-treated PD patients, as well as their power to decrease the incidence of response oscillations when administered in the disease's early stages. These are the main reasons why development of new dopamine agonists has continued over the last few years. The papers in this supplement will focus on the role of "classic" dopamine agonists in the management of early and advanced PD; they also cover recent advances in the pathophysiology of dopaminergic systems and the neurobiology of dopamine receptors.

You will not find it surprising, now at the height of "the decade of brain", to hear me assert that only major advances in basic neuroscience will bring about the parallel development of new therapeutic strategies. Recently, neuropharmacological and neurobiological research has led to the identification of new dopamine-receptor subtypes (beyond the classic D1 and D2 ones), whose functional role has yet to be completely uncovered. Moreover, we have gained new insights into the functional neuroanatomy of basal ganglia pathways and the interaction between dopamine and other neurotransmitter systems. Particularly, we are now aware of the relevance of glutamatergic dysfunction in the pathophysiology of PD; the way which glutamate receptor blockade exerts its antiparkinsonian effect in animal models may be traced to specific interactions with dopamine at D1-like or D2-like receptors.

For all these reasons, the supplement has been designed as a multidisciplinary effort, ranging from basic neuroscience on the neurophysiology and neurobiology of dopaminergic systems in PD to the clinical pharmacology of dopamine agonists.

A special section is devoted to recent advances in the understanding of the mechanisms underlying nigral neuronal death and the exciting concept of neuroprotection. Some papers, in fact, focus on dopamine agonists' ability to reduce potential free-radical species in experimental models. Today, however, it has not yet proved possible to exploit any of these discoveries to provide unequivocal clinical therapeutic benefits, but neuroprotective use of dopamine agonists needs to be considered in perspective.

While efforts should be made to search for new therapeutic strategies, it is also imperative that we continue to explore the most judicious use of existing treatments; take apomorphine, for example – it was rediscovered in the late 1980s and introduced for the treatment of advanced PD patients and is the best example I know of the value of "old drugs" in modern therapy.

It is hoped that the content of this supplement will illustrate the potential of old dopamine agonists, as well as the new drugs currently under clinical investigation. We also aim to underscore how important it is that the work of the neurologist be bolstered by basic neuroscience. In this respect, I trust our meeting will be a "seminar" in its truest sense – that it will plant the seeds for the growth of new therapeutic strategies in PD.

Pisa, October 1995

A. Muratorio
Professor and Chairman
Institute of Clinical Neurology
University of Pisa, Italy

Contents

Neurodegeneration and neuroprotection

J Neural Transm (1995) [Suppl] 45: 1–9

Differential diagnosis of parkinsonism

M. Manfredi[1,2], **F. Stocchi**[1,2], and **L. Vacca**[1]

[1] Department of Neuroscience, University "La Sapienza", Roma, and
[2] Mediterranean Institute of Neuroscience "Sanatrix", Pozzilli(is), Italy

Summary. The diagnosis of idiopathic Parkinson's disease (PD) is essentially clinical and is reached by exclusion. An akinetic rigid syndrome frequently means PD, although a number of other neurodegenerative diseases can share bradykinesia, rigidity, postural instability, and sometimes tremor. Parkinsonism can be classified as follows: degenerative, metabolic, vascular, iatrogenic, toxic, infectious, traumatic, and secondary to mass effect. The diagnostic approach are discussed.

Introduction

A number of diseases, globally called parkinsonism, may share the akinetic rigid syndrome of idiopathic Parkinson's disease (PD) (Denny-Brown, 1968). For a correct diagnosis of parkinsonism, at least two of the following signs have to be observed: tremor, rigidity, akinesia, and posture instability, but a precise differential diagnosis is of peculiar complexity (Marsden, 1984). At present, careful clinical examination, neuroradiological and neuropsychological assessment, response to oral and intravenous levodopa and autonomic function test are to be considered the best parameters for diagnostic purposes. A number of classifications of parkinsonism have been suggested by different authors. This comprehensive clinical entity might be divided, for practical purpose, into eight groups (Table 1). Of all this impressive list of syndromes, we will discuss here only the most important ones for the clinician.

Postencephalitic parkinsonism

Encephalitis lethargica, or Von Economo's encephalitis, is at present the only viral infection recognized as a cause of persistent parkinsonism (Mijasaki and Fujita, 1977). Today such patients are limited to sporadic cases after an encephalitis-like disease (Howard and Lees, 1987), but a great number of them has been described in the thirties after the viral epidemic that spread over Europe and the U.S.A. between 1914 and 1918 (Von Economo, 1931). Although the presence of oculogyric crises and early age of onset are highly

Table 1. Parkinsonian syndromes

Degenerative
— Parkinson's disease
— multiple system atrophy
— progressive sopranuclear palsy
— corticobasal degeneration
— diffuse Lewy's bodies disease
— Huntington's disease (rigid variant)
— essential tremor

Metabolic
— Wilson's disease
— basal ganglia calcification
— Hallervorden-Spatz's disease
— Alexander's disease (adult variant)
— bilateral striatal necrosis (Leigh's
  disease)
— neuroacantocytosis
— perinatal anoxia

Vascular
— multi-infarct syndrome
— Binswanger's disease

Iatrogenic
— neuroleptics
— flunarizine, cinnarizine
— metoclopramide
— reserpine

Toxic
— manganese
— CO
— MPTP

Infectious
— Creutzfeldt-Jakob's disease
— encephalitis letargica
— viral, rickettsial encephalitis
— syphilis
— AIDS
— van Bogaert's disease
— disseminated encephalomyelitis

Traumatic
— dementia pugilistica

Mass effect
— low pressure hydrocephalus
— high pressure hydrocephalus, tumours

characteristic of postencephalitic parkinsonism, it has to be reminded that some cases with post-mortem diagnosis do not present these signs, and that other patients with idiopathic PD may have a history of encephalitis and oculogyric crises (Duvoisin and Yahr, 1965). Diagnosis may be facilitated by the presence of ocular movement disturbance, dystonias, and stabilization of the disease after an initial rapid worsening. Post-mortem examination of subjects who had been affected by postencephalitic parkinsonism shows bilateral diffuse degeneration and gliosis of the substantia nigra and locus coeruleus, without Lewy bodies but with neurofibrillary filaments in the brainstem, substantia nigra, locus coeruleus, mesencephalic tegmentum, hypothalamus, and hippocampus (Alvord, 1965). These patients do not respond consistently to levodopa, while positive results are obtained with anticholinergic drugs.

Drug-induced parkinsonism

It is widespread affection whose incidence increases with aging, as is the case with PD. A large number of neuroleptics and major tranquillizers may induce a parkinsonian syndrome (Table 2). The onset is generally rapid and patients show rigidity, tremor, and a slight bradykinesia. Akathisia and neurodysleptic crises may complete the picture. Patients usually recover within 6 to 24 months after drug withdrawal. Some cases of parkinsonism are also due to calcium-entry blocker compounds (flunarizine and cinnarizine), as has recently been reported especially in elderly patients given long-term treatments with these drugs.

Progressive Sopranuclear Palsy or Steele-Richardson-Olszewski disease (PSP)

This entity was first described by Richardson and his colleagues in 1963. According to the authors, this is a progressive, non familial disease, with onset during the 5th-6th decade of life, marked by supranuclear ocular paralysis and by at least two the following primary symptoms: axial dystonia and rigidity; pseudobulbar palsy; bradykinesia and rigidity; signs of frontal lobe lesion; postural instability with retropulsion (Lees, 1987). The PSP syndrome differs from PD in that it has bilateral symmetric onset with frequent gait disorder; tremor is extremely rare while extensive stiffness may be present. As the

Table 2. Pharmacologic causes of parkinsonism

— Neuroleptics	phenotiazines
	butyrophenones
	thioxanthines
	benzamides
— Reserpine, tetrabenazine	
— Calcium-entry blockers	flunarizine
	cinnarizine
— Miscellaneos agents	alpha-methyldopa
	lithium

disease progresses, the pseudobulbar signs become more evident with difficulties in swallowing and phonation. There are no signs of autonomic nervous system impairment and little or no response to L-dopa therapy. Life expectancy is 4–6 years from the onset (Jackson et al., 1983). The patology is characterized by neurofibrillary degeneration, neuronal loss and gliosis of brainstem structures, subthalamic nucleus of Luys, pallidum, substantia nigra, periaqueductal gray, superior colliculus, locus coeruleus, dentate and raphe nuclei (Alvord, 1965). A substantial damage in the projections directed from the brainstem to the frontal cortex seems to be common in these subjects (Whitehouse et al., 1983). A percentage of patients do not show gaze abnormalities. CT, PET and SPECT may be helpful for the diagnosis (Brusa and Peloso, 1993).

Multiple System Atrophy (MSA)

MSA includes a number of disorders associating the akinetic-rigid syndrome with other neurological and disautonomic signs. Classically, three entities are grouped under the MSA label: the striato-nigral degeneration (Takei and Mirra, 1973); the Shy-Drager syndrome (Shy and Drager, 1960) and the sporadic forms of olivopontocerebellar atrophy (Duvoisin, 1987). MSA may account for up to 10% of patients with parkinsonism, Most MSA patients show pyramidal and cerebellar signs associated with stiffness and akinesia, and sometimes ocular voluntary motion palsy. Signs of autonomic nervous system failure are typical (Oppenheimer, 1983). However, in a considerable number of cases, MSA patients are thought to be truly affected by PD, MSA reproducing the exact clinical picture of idiopathic PD, expecially during the early years of disease. A mild of poor response to oral or, better, intravenous L-dopa administration should arise suspicions as to the nature of the disease, even in absence of gross autonomic failure (Table 3). CT scan or MRI examination show sometimes a marked atrophy at the level of the brainstem or cerebellum, but a negative neuroradiological picture does not necessarily exclude MSA. EMG of anal sphincter and urodynamic study may be very helpful. EMG usually shows a denervation while urodynamic evaluation shows hypereflexia with dyssynergia, and may be indicative even in the early stages of the disease (Stocchi et al., 1994). Cardiovascular tests are less specific. Pathologically, MSA is characterised by cell loss and gliosis occurring in some or all of the following "at risk" structures: substantia nigra, caudate, putamen (especially pars externa), inferior olives, pontine nuclei, cerebellar Purkinje cells, intermediolateral cell columns of the spinal cord and Onuf's nucleus. Locus coeruleus, dorsal motor nucleus of vagus, vestibular nuclei, pyramidal tracts and anterior horns may also be involved. Together with the distribution of cell loss, the absence of Lewy body distinguishes MSA from idiophatic Parkinson's disease; the lack of neurofibrillary tangles separates it from Steele-Richardson-Olszewski disease and post-encephalitic Parkinsonism (Quinn, 1989). The degeneration may involve other neural structures in the case of additional clinical complications (Forno et al., 1986).

Table 3. Multiple system atrophy (diagnostic criteria)

Striatonigral type (predominantly parkinsonism		Olivopontocerebellar atrophy type (predominantly cerebellar)
sporadic adult-onset non or poorly levodopa responsive parkinsonism*	Possible	sporadic adult-onset cerebellar syndrome with parkinsonism
above, plus severe symptomatic autonomic failure[#] or cerebellar signs or pyramidal signs or pathological sphincter EMG	Probable	sporadic adult-onset cerebellar syndrome* (with or without parkinsonism or pyramidal signs), plus severe symptomatic autonomic failure[#] or pathological sphincter EMG
post-mortem confirmed	Definite	post-mortem confirmed

*Without dementia or generalized tendon areflexia, prominent supranuclear palsy for downgaze or other identifiable cause
[#] Postural syncope and/or marked urinary incontinence or retention not due to other causes (Wenning et al., 1994)

Wilson's disease (hepatolenticular degeneration)

The classic description of "progressive lenticular degeneration: a familial neurologic disease associated with cirrhosis of the liver" was made by Wilson in 1912. The disease is an autosomal disorder and its incidence is of about 1/200,000. The first clinical signs, consisting of hepatosplenomegaly, thrombocytopenia and consequent haemorrhages, become usually evident during the second or third decade of life. Early neurological signs may be tremor, bradykinesia, dysarthria, dysphagia, choreic-athetosic movements, dystonic postures, and cerebellar ataxia. Occasionally, psychiatric disturbances, such as behavioural disorders, depression and intellectual impairment can be present from the beginning of the illness. The Kayser-Fleisher ring is another important clinical sign, but it becomes evident in only about 25% of patients in the hepatic stage. Serum ceruloplasmin values are low (less than 20 mg/dl) in about 95% of the patients, with consequent low bound copper serum values (below 60 pg/dl). Urinary copper excretion is significantly increased (more than 100 pg/24 h). Total copper content may be normal due to the large quantity of free circulating copper. Hepatic copper concentration in liver biopsy is generally in excess (more than 250 ug/g of dry tissue), but this may not always be the case even for patients with neurological symptoms. Notably, in some cases, hepatic copper content may be reduced to as little as 100 ug/g, since copper tends to be accumulated in the brain tissue. Consequently, values below 250 ug/g do not allow to exclude definitely Wilson's disease. On the other hand, it has to be underlined that high copper content in liver tissue, with normal serum ceruloplasmin, is not indicative of Wilson's disease even in the presence of a Kayser-Fleisher ring. In this respect, a test with labelled Cu might be helpful. CT scan and MRI examination show alterations in the basal ganglia, cerebellar nuclei, brainstem, and white matter. It is quite rare to observe the loss of matter in the basal ganglia as described by Wilson, while it is common to find atrophy and a light brown pigmentation of these nuclei. There may also be a loss of neurons and white matter in the putamen, substantia nigra, and caudate. Tipically, a diffuse gliosis (with type I and II Alzheimer cells) in the cortex, basal ganglia, brainstem nuclei and cerebellum is observed (Walshe, 1976). Treatment consist in removing the excess copper from brain and liver. This can be done by administering 1 g/day of penicillamine. In resistant cases dimercaprol (BAL) (3 g/day), or trie-thylenetetramine (1 g/day) should be tried. Recent reports show that the daily administration of zinc (100–200 mg) inhibits the absortion of copper from the gastrointestinal tract.

Idiopathic calcification of the basal ganglia (Fahr's disease)

These patients present calcifications of the basal ganglia associated with evidence of a parkinsonian syndrome with choreic-athetosic movements proceding or following it. The age of onset is generally the fifth decade. Serum calcium levels are usually normal. A familial form with onset during adolescence is also known, mainly characterized by ataxia and dementia. Serum calcium level are low in this form. Serum calcium level and CT scan findings are mandatory for diagnosis.

Pick's disease

This is a cerebral degenerative syndrome in which atrophy is confined mainly to the frontal and temporal lobes and involves both the gray and the white matter. The caudate nucleus, thalamus, subthalamic nucleus, substantia nigra, and globus pallidus may be affected. Clinically, the symptoms of frontal deficit prevail: apathy, abulia, gait impairment, urinary incontinence, extrapyramidal signs, and cortical liberation reflexes (Brown and Marsden, 1984). The histologic features consist of loss of neurons, mainly in the first three cortical layers, and of neuronal swelling in the surviving cells with argentophilic bodies in the cytoplasm (Alvord, 1965). Problem of differential diagnosis with Pick's disease may occur in the early stages of this affection. A cerebral CT scan may prove helpful.

Cerebrovascular diseases (Pseudobulbar palsy; Binswanger's disease; arteriopathic parkinsonism)

Pseudobulbar palsy is caused by multiple lacunar infarcts of both corticospinal tracts. Parkinsonism is associated with pyramidal signs and sopranuclear impairment of inferior cranial nerves. Patients also present progressive dementia, spasmodic crying and laughing, and a mixed rigid-spastic hypertonia.

Binswanger's subcortical encephalopathy is caused by demyelinization and multiple infarcts in the periventricular white matter. Cortex and basal ganglia are unaffected. Symptoms are both of pyramidal and extrapyramidal origin: gait apraxia, urinary incontinence, and dementia are the most notable (Boller et al., 1980; Parkes et al., 1974). CT scan is crucial for an accurate diagnosis. MRI shows typical periventricular luminescence.

Arteriopathic parkinsonism is not entirely accepted. Histological studies on brain from presumed idiopathic PD patients claim that about 6% of them presented serious vascular damage with a mild degeneration of the substantia nigra (Alvord, 1965). However, in arteriopatic parkinsonism damage of striatal functions is produced by multiple lacunar infarcts of the basal ganglia. Clinical elements to be considered are the age of onset, the presence of vascular risk factors, additional the presence of asymmetrical pyramidal signs and intellectual impairment of subcortical type. Obviously, MRI can be quite useful.

Huntington's chorea

This affection may cause, in addition to the well known dementing chorea, an akinetic-rigid syndrome, known as the Westphal rigid form. It usually occurs during the second decade of life, but also, rarely, in adults (Marsden, 1984). Differential diagnosis is possible considering behavioural disorders, dementia, and autosomal dominant inheritance with expanded triplet in chromosome 4.

Essential tremor

Although quite different in clinical presentation, the most common condition misdiagnosed as PD is essential tremor, in a proportion varying from 4 to 6% of patients. However, the positive family history, the type of tremor (postural-kinetic, 5–9 Hz), the extent to which head and voice are affected, the absence of bradykinesia, rigidity and postural instability, the slowly progressive course of the disease, the benefit from alcohol, provide sufficient elements to make a correct diagnosis of essential tremor.

Diffuse Lewy body disease (DLBD)

It is a clinopathologic entity that shares features with both Parkinson's disease and Alzheimer's disease, but differs from them by the presence of Lewy bodies in small cells of widespread areas of the neocortex, as well as brainstem and diencephalic neurons (Gibb et al., 1989). Most patients with DLBD have gait impairment concurrent with mild to moderate dementia. Abnormalities of tone or resting tremor, hallucinations, and delusions also are prominent early symptoms (Crystal et al., 1990). It is difficult to make a certain diagnosis of DLBD during life time and a neurophatological post-mortem demonstration is generally necessary.

Corticalbasal degeneration

Cortical-basal ganglionic degeneration combines an asymmetrical akinetic-rigid syndrome with cortical sensory deficits and/or apraxia (Rebeiz et al., 1968). Additional features may include action tremor, dystonia, oculomotor disturbance, pyramidal tract signs, orthostatic imbalance, and focal myoclonus. The distinctive pathological finding is that of widespread cortical neuronal achromasia.

References

Alvord EC (1965) The pathology of parkinsonism: etiologic, pathogenetic and prognostic implications. Trans Am Neurol Assoc 90: 167–168

Boller F, Mizutami R, Roessmann U, Gambetti F (1980) Parkinson's disease, dementia and Alzheimer's disease: clinicopathological correlations. Ann Neurol 1: 329–335

Brown RG, Marsden CD (1984) How common is dementia in Parkinson's disease? Lancet i: 1262–1265

Bursa A, Peloso PF (1993) An introduction to progressive sopranuclear palsy. Steele-Richardson-Olszeski syndrome. John Libbey CIC, Roma

Crystal HA, Dickson DW, Lizardi JE, Davies P, Wolfson LI (1990) Antemortem diagnosis of diffuse Lewy body disease. Neurology 40: 1523–1528

Denny-Brown D (1968) Clinical symptomatology of disease of the basal ganglia. In: Vinken PJ, Bruyn GJ (eds) Handbook of clinical neurology, vol 6. Diseases of the basal ganglia. North-Holland, Amsterdam, pp 133–211

Duvoisin RC (1987) The olivopontocerebellar atrophies. In: Marsden CD, Fahn S (eds) Movement disorders, 2nd edn. Butterworths Scientific, London, pp 249–271

Duvoisin RC, Yahr MD (1965) Encephalitis and parkinsonism. Arch Neurol 12: 227–239

Forno LS, Langston JY, Delanney LE, Irwin I, Ricaurte GA (1986) Locus coeruleus lesions and eosinophilic inclusions in MPTP-treated monkeys. Ann Neurol 20: 449–455

Gibb WRG, Mountjoy CQ, Mann DMA, Lees AJ (1989) A pathological study of the association between Lewy body disease and Alzheimer's disease. J Neurol Neurosurg Psychiatry 52: 701–708

Howard RS, Lees AJ (1987) Encephalitis lethargica. A report of four recent cases. Brain 110: 19–33

Jackson JA, Jankovic J, Ford J (1983) Progressive supranuclear palsy: clincal features and response to treatment in 16 patients. Ann Neurol 13: 273–278

Langston JW, Ballard PA (1983) Parkinson's disease in a chemist working with 1-methyl-4-phenyl-1,2,3,5,6 tetrahydropyridine (MPTP). N Engl J Med 309: 310

Lees AJ (1987) The Steele-Richardson-Olszewski syndrome (progressive supranuclear palsy). In: Marsden CD, Fahn S (eds) Movement disorders, 2nd edn. Butterworths Scientific, London, pp 272–287

Marsden CD (1984) Motor disorders in basal ganglia disease. Hum Neurobiol 2: 245–250

Mijasaki K, Fujita T (1977) Parkinsonism following encephalitis of unknown etiology. J Neuropathol Exp Neurol 34: 1–8

Oppenheimer DR (1983) Neuropathology of progressive autonomic failure. In: Bannister R (ed) Autonomic failure. Oxford University Press, New York, pp 267–283

Parkes JD, Marsden CD, Rees JE, Carjon M (1974) Parkinson disease, cerebral arteriosclerosis and senile dementia. Q J Med 43: 49–61

Quinn N (1989) Multiple system atrophy: the nature of the beast. J Neurol Neurosurg Psychiatry [Suppl] 78: 89

Rebeiz JJ, Kolodny EH, Richardson EP (1968) Corticodentatonigral degeneration with neuronal achromasia. Arch Neurol 18: 20–33

Richardson JC, Steele J, Olszewski J (1963) Supranuclear ophtalmoplegia, pseudobulbar palsy, dystonia and dementia. Trans Am Neurol Assoc 88: 25–27

Shy GM, Drager GA (1960) A neurological syndrome associated with orthostatic hypotension. Arch Neurol 2: 511–527

Stocchi F, Barbato L, Carbone A, Fabbrini G, Ruggieri S, Bonamartini A, Baffigo G, Agnoli A (1993) Urodynamic study in the differential diagnosis between Multiple System Atrophy and Parkinson's disease. Arch Neurol 60: 434–437

Takei Y, Mirra SS (1973) Striato-nigral degeneration: a form of multiple system atrphy with clinical parkinsonism. Prog Neuropathol 21: 26–32

Von Economo C (1931) Encephalitis lethargica. Its sequelae and treatment. Newman KO (transl). Oxford University, London

Walshe JM (1976) Wilson's disease (Hepatolenticular degeneration). In: Vinken PJ, Bruyn GW, Klawans HL (eds) Handbook of clinical neurology, vol 27. Metabolic and deficiency disease of the nervous system, part 1. Elsevier, New York, pp 379–414

Wenning GK, Ben Shlomo Y, Magalhaes M, Daniel SE, Quinn NP (1994) Clinical features and natural history of multiple system atrophy, an analysis of 100 cases. Brain 117: 835–845

Whitehouse P, Hedreen JC, White C, DeLong M, Price DL (1983) Basal forebrain neurons in dementia of Parkinson's disease. Ann Neurol 13: 243–248

Wilson SAK (1912) Progressive lenticular degeneration. A familial nervous disease associated with cirrhosis of the liver. Brain 34: 295–309

Authors' address: Dr. F. Stocchi, Department of Neuroscience, Viale dell'Universita 30, I-00185 Roma, Italy.

J Neural Transm (1995) [Suppl] 45: 11–19

Autonomic disorders in Parkinson's disease

E. Martignoni, C. Pacchetti, L. Godi, G. Micieli, and **G. Nappi**

Department of Neurology, Parkinson's Disease Centre, IRCCS — C. Mondino,
University of Pavia, Italy

Summary. Patients with idiopatic Parkinson's disease (IPD) often show signs and symptoms of autonomic involvement, related to the disease itself or to its progression. The more frequently disturbances reported are connected with loss of extrapyramidal motor control, i.e. dysphagia, gastric emptying and the most common constipation. They concern about 73% of the patients. A high frequency of urinary symptoms, ranging from 37% to 71%, is also reported in IPD, in particular detrusor hyperreflexia causing urgency, frequency of micturing or urgency incontinence. Another autonomic groups of symptoms are related to the failure of cardiopressor adaptability which involve 15% of the subjects and are more typical of late onset cases or forms bordering with the Multiple System Atrophy, finally resulting in orthostatic hypotension (OH).

Introduction

Parkinson's disease is primarily a disorder of the motor system as a result of a degenerative process affecting the specific dopaminergic nigro-striatal system. However, due to the extension of the lesions out of the basal ganglia, also mood, cognitive, sensory and vegetative disturbances could be, to a varying extent, an integral part of the clinical picture.

Autonomic dysfunction in IPD has already been described in a number of reports, including James Parkinson's original monograph (Parkinson, 1817), but very few report its prevalence. In association with parkinsonism, it may be part of more complex diseases than IPD, as striato-nigral degeneration (SND) (Adams et al., 1961), olivo-ponto-cerebellar atrophy (OPCA) (Déjerine and Thomas, 1900), Shy-Drager syndrome (SD) (Shy and Drager, 1960), clinical conditions which are today classified as multiple system atrophy (MSA) (Graham and Oppenheimer, 1969; Bannister and Oppenheimer, 1972; Quinn, 1989). Other than parkinsonism, all these entities may show a combination of cerebellar and pyramidal signs and symptoms, as well as of autonomic failure (AF) (Bannister, 1984; McLeod and Tuck, 1987; Chokroverty, 1984; Adams and Salam-Adams, 1986), due to the loss of preganglionic sympathetic cells (intermediolateral column cells) from the thoracic cord (Spokes et al., 1979; Oppenheimer, 1988). This clinical involvement is not always observed in SND or OPCA and, if it occurs, it is usually milder than in SD (Chokroverty, 1984; Adams and Salam-Adams, 1986) in which it is considered the "key" manifestation of the disease, so that SD is also called MSA + AF (Bannister, 1988).

Autonomic involvement in IPD (Parkinson, 1817; Appenzeller and Goss, 1971; Martignoni et al., 1986; Korczyn, 1990) can be related to the disease "per se" or to the progression of the degenerative process towards other areas of the central and/or peripheral nervous system, i.e. posterior hypothalamus, locus coeruleus, n. dorsalis vagi, sympathetic ganglia and adrenal medulla (Rajput and Rozdilsky, 1976; Langston and Forno, 1978; Tomonaga, 1986) or, finally, to the various therapies applied (Calne, 1970; Markham et al., 1970; Leibowitz and Lieberman, 1975; Murdock et al., 1975; Yen et al., 1979; Quinn et al., 1981). The exact definition of widespread and sometimes severe autonomic imbalance in IPD, with particular regard to the presence of OH and genito-bladder dysfunction, plays an important role in the differential diagnosis with SD. In a retrospective study we carried out on 215 consecutive IPD cases we found that the incidence of almost all the symptoms of autonomic dysfunction like seborrhea, constipation, impotence, sialorrhea, bladder dysfunction, dysphagia, sweating and orthostatic hypotension was greater among treated patients (Martignoni et al., 1986). The finding was probably related to the more advanced age and longer duration of the disease seen in the treated patients than in the "de novo" ones (Pacchetti et al., 1990). Another more recent clinical study on 130 IPD and 10 SD out-patients controlled in our Section for Parkinson's disease was designed to ascertain the frequency, extent, severity, clinical correlations and outcome of autonomic disturbances. Table 1 shows the frequency of autonomic disturbances in IPD patients. From the analysis of the data it emerged that autonomic disturbances were distributed in more than 90% of our IPD. The little group of IPD patients without autonomic involvement was characterized by a very short duration of disease, slight motor impairment and absence of pharmacological treatment. This high incidence of signs and symptoms of autonomic dysfunction in the patients suggests these to be an integral part, even if to a different extent, in the clinical picture of IPD (Martignoni et al., 1994).

Autonomic symptoms

In general, IPD patients showed prominent *gastrointestinal manifestations* (Table 1) linked to the severity of the disease as showed by their positive correlation with motor examination score (Columbia University Rating Scale) and duration of illness (Martignoni et al., 1986; Pacchetti et al., 1990). *Dysphagia* (9%) and *sialorrhea* with disabling drooling (54%) prevailed in patients with the akinetic-rigid type and in the advanced stages (Martignoni et al., 1986). The initial manifestations were the increase of mealtimes and difficulty of mastication. Later on, there was evidence of episodic choking despite a soft diet. Radiological investigation reported varying degrees of esophageal dilatation in parkinsonian patients, from light to severe (Gibberd

Table 1. Frequency of autonomic disturbances in 130
patients with Parkinson's disease

Symptoms	% of frequency
Orthostatic hypotension	15.38
Urgency	13.85
Urinary incontinence	2.31
Sialorrea	54.62
Dysphagia	9.33
Constipation	72.31
Seborrhea	60.77
Sweating	13.08
Heat/cold intolerance	22.00
Impotence	20.00

et al., 1974). Other observations revealed defective esophageal peristalsis, especially in the lower third of the esophagus. In addition to defective esophageal motility, abnormalities in all stages of swallowing were reported by other authors. The passage of food to the back of the mouth by tongue movement, and the transit through the pharynx, are slowed with vallecular stasis. While L-dopa may be of benefit, anticholinergic agents could induce an increase in nonperistaltic swallows thus possibly worsening dysphagia (Eadie and Tyrer, 1965).

Constipation is another gastro-intestinal common problem in IPD, widly distributed (73%). It is probably the result of many different factors, including decreased motor activity, reduced forcefulness of abdominal muscle contractions, and insufficient intake of food and water. Although specific abnormalities of intestinal motilities are assumed, these have not been conclusively demonstrated.

Sialorrhea was seen in IPD patients to a lesser or greater extent (54%); when it was severe, drooling occured with obvious implications for the patient's social life. Some authors mantain that this is the result of an excessive secretion of saliva due to cholinergic overstimulation. while others suggest the involvement of involuntary mechanisms of swallowing (Eadie and Tyrer, 1965).

Seborrhea (61%) was prominent in males, according to the hypothesis of hormonal dysregulation (Shuster et al., 1983), rather than of a pure autonomic disorder, and its frequency related to the duration of disease (Martignoni et al., 1986). Also a recent study by our group suggested a dysregulation of the androgenic control of sebum secretion in male parkinsonian patients (Godi et al., 1994).

Excessive sweating (Table 2) was observed above all in fluctuating patients (13%) and hyperhidrosis was related to the "off" phases, especially if tremor was also present (Martignoni et al., 1986). A high frequency of *urinary symptoms* (Table 3) in IPD was first reported by Langworthy in 1936, while subsequent studies mentioned the incidence of bladder dysfunction ranging from 37% to 71% of cases (Murnagham, 1961; Porter and Bors, 1971). In our study

Table 2

— Gastrointestinal disturbances in Parkinson's disease
   • Sialorrhea
   • Gastric emptying
   • Dysphagia
      increase of mealtimes
      difficulty of mastication
      episodic choking
      ab ingestis pneumonia
      nasogastric tube use
   • Constipation
      increase dietary bulk
      laxative use
      enema
      megacolon
      pseudoobstruction
      true sigmoid volvulus
      acute intestinal ostruction
— Thermoregulatory disturbances in Parkinson's disease
   • Sweating
      Hyperidrosis
      Hypoidrosis
      Abnormal sensation of heat or warm

---

bladder dysfunctions and thermoregulatory disorders (sweating and heat/cold intolerance) were unrelated to any clinical variables (Martignoni et al., 1986).

The most frequent micturition disturbance in IPD patients was urgency (14%), and only a few cases showed urinary incontinence (3 patients) one of whom also had retention; urodynamic studies in these patients have revealed a high incidence of involuntary detrusor contraction which occur in response to bladder filling. In fact by using urodynamic testing equipment it has been revealed that the most frequent neurogenic bladder abnormality in IPD is hyperreflexia (Murdock et al., 1975; Pavlakis et al., 1983). Detrusor hyperreflexia causes urgency, frequency of micturition or urgency incontinence; these irritative symptoms are treatable with anticholinergic drugs, which, however, may be responsible for bladder disturbance of an obstructive type. In patients treated with anticholinergics, bladder areflexia or hypercontractility may occur, together with a failure of perineal muscle relaxation; the sustained contraction of perineal and abdominal muscles could represent the attempt to induce micturition without bladder contraction (Pavlakis et al., 1983). Neverthless, L-dopa may also induce an obstructive syndrome (like difficulty in initiating micturition) due to increased sympathetic outflow which is described as internal sphincter dyssynergia (Yalla et al., 1977). In fact L-dopa and its metabolites cause either alpha-adrenergic activity which contracts bladder neck or beta-adrenergic activity which relaxes the detrusor muscle (Murdock et al., 1975). Moreover, the obstructive micturition syndrome due to L-dopa therapy has been described (Quinn et al., 1981) together with so-called sphinteric bradykinesia (Pavlakis et al., 1983). This is characterized by delayed onset or micturition due to a typical extrapyramidal hypertonia involving the perineal muscles which in normal conditions relax just before the reflex of detrusor muscle occurs (Ravasi et al., 1984). IPD patients also rarely show bladder retention which necessitates catheterization. These patients usually suffer from coexistent prostatic obstruction that is precipitated by the use of anticholinergic drugs.

Finally, the prevalence of *orthostatic hypotension* (Table 3) in IPD was similar to that found by our group in a previous retrospective analysis (15%) (Martignoni et al., 1986; Pacchetti et al., 1990). Orthostatic hypotension is a severe dysautonomic symptom which may lead to a transient loss of consciousness, caused by an inadequate cerebral blood flow. Usually, the symptoms are significantly worse in the morning, after meals (post-prandial hypotension) (Seyer-Hansen, 1977), in hot weather and after exercise; in fact all these situations can cause an unfavorable redistribution of blood volume. In many cases the postural blood pressure falls may remain asymptomatic, probably because of an adaptive resetting of cerebral blood flow regulation mechanisms. Even if asymptomatic, IPD patients frequently exhibit instrumental findings of post-prandial (or post-cibal) hypotension (Micieli et al., 1987), as do SD subjects (Mathias et al., 1988). Post-prandial hypotension may occur 10 to 15 minutes after ingestion, and reaches its peak around 60 minutes (Bannister, 1984). On the basis of our instrumental findings of post-prandial hypotension in IPD and SD patients, we believe that such changes may be a first step towards widespread derangement in cardiopressor adaptive response (Micieli et al., 1989). It may be followed by symptomatic orthostatic hypotension, a development which is influenced, to a lesser or greater extent, by the involvement of cardiopressor adaptive changes, and by the natural evolution of the illness. In some cases, orthostatic hypotension has appeared only alongside the intake of drugs (i.e. dopaminergic drugs), but in a few cases, it has become an integral symptom of the disease itself. Widespread neuronal abnormalities and Lewy bodies can be found in the autonomic nervous system of IPD patients, both in central and peripheral autonomic areas (Tomonaga, 1986). But, despite these pathological findings, the anatomical site of dysfunction which may be responsible for the orthostatic

Table 3

— Urinary disturbances in Parkinson's disease
  - Frequency of micturing
  - Urgency of micturing
  - Urgency incontinence
  - Retention
— Cardiovascular disturbances in Parkinson's disease
  - Orthostatic hypotension
      dizziness
      sense of visual blurring
      asthenia
      syncope

---

hypotension in IPD is still unknown. Instead, in SD patients, there is strong evidence for looking at the loss of neurons in the intermediolateral column of the spinal cord, as the anatomic substrate of autonomic failure (Spokes et al., 1979; Oppenheimer, 1988).

In some patients, the postural hypotension is preceded by hypertension for several years. This disturbance will continue thereafter as recumbent hypertension. This curious condition could be due to a partial denervation supersensitivity as a first phase, which is followed by loss of baroreflex control and probably also by the supersensitization of peripheral receptors to the neurotransmitter noradrenaline (Bannister, 1988). Although the clinical symptomatology occurs at various drops in blood pressure levels, according to clinical test investigations hypotension is defined as certain when a fall of more than 20 mmHg in systolic pressure is found by repeated measurements made at 60° using the head-up tilt position test (Bannister, 1988).

In our study, when orthostatic hypotension occurred for the first time the patient's age ranged from 54 to 80 years. The median age of the subjects with pre-fainting symptoms was 62 years, while the group which also experienced syncopes had a median age of 72 years. In general, the prevalence of orthostatic hypotension was higher in IPD patients over 65 years and its severity had a positive correlation with age. None of the patients had ever had such symptoms before the onset of the disease (Pacchetti et al., 1986). In the present sample, patients with orthostatic hypotension were found to be older than other IPD subjects, and autonomic failure occurred several years after the onset of the disease with no relation to the severity of the disease itself.

Comment

In conclusion, in IPD it is possible to distinguish two different patterns of autonomic disturbances: the first, e.g. gastrointestinal symptomatology, as stated also by other authors (Korczyn, 1989), is widely encountered and is presumably connected with slowness or dysfunction of extrapyramidal motor control, related to the evolution of motor disturbances, and thus typical of IPD; the second has been observed in a small number of patients, about the 15% of the subjects we tested, and is characterized by the failure of cardiopressor adaptability. This latter pattern resembles, with the exclusion of genito-urinary dysfunctions, the autonomic imbalance found in SD subjects, although to a lesser extent. This group can be differentiated from the general parkinsonian population because of its older age; OH may be due to an age-related decline in the neural and endocrine controls of homeostatic regulation. It could be viewed as a possible indicator of a pivotal role of aging processes in the alteration of the cardiopressor homeostatic mechanism, as suggested by several reports which point to a higher incidence of orthostatic hypotension in the elderly (Caird et al., 1973; Robbins and Rubenstein, 1984; Korczyn, 1989). On the other hand, IPD itself could imply a predisposition to cardiopressor dysfunction which, in concomitance with old age, may cause postural hypotension to develop.

By another standpoint these IPD subjects could be considered cases on the borderline of SD, but their older age and earlier development of autonomic failure in the course of illness, distinguish them as having a distinct clinical condition, in which it is not possible to exclude a central role for an age related decline of homeostatic regulation (Pacchetti et al., 1990).

Another important facet of the autonomic dysfunction relates to drug-induced changes (Korczyn and Rubenstein, 1982). It is yet an open question whether the effects of the medication are "normal", i.e. whether the same alterations would be produced in non-Parkinsonian subjects when these drugs are given, or wheather specific changes predispose patients with Parkinson's disease to develop these side effects. Be this as it may, recognition of these side effects would allow selection of appropriate drugs for the treatment of individual patients with Parkinson's disease.

References

Adams RD, Salam-Adams M (1986) Striatonigral degeneration. In: Vinken PJ, Bruyn CW, Klawans HL (eds) Handbook of clinical neurology, vol 5 (49). Extrapyramidal disorders. Elseviers Science Publishers BV, Amsterdam, pp 205–212

Adams RD, van Bogaert L, van der Eecken H (1961) Dégénérescenses nigro-striées, et cerebello-nigro-striées. Psychiat Neurol 142: 219–259

Appenzeller O, Goss JE (1971) Autonomic deficits in Parkinson's syndrome. Arch Neurol 24: 50–57

Bannister R (1984) Disease of autonomic nervous system. In: Matthews WB, Glaser H (eds) Recent advances in clinical neurology. Churchill Livingstone, London, pp 67–85

Bannister R (1988) Clinical features of autonomic failure. Symptoms, signs and special investigations. In: Bannister R (ed) Autonomic failure. A textbook of clinical disorders of the autonomic nervous system, 2nd ed. Oxford University Press, Oxford, pp 267–288

Bannister R, Oppenheimer DR (1972) Degenerative diseases of the nervous system associated with autonomic failure. Brain 95: 457–474

Bannister R, Mathias C (1988) Management of postural hypotension. In: Bannister R (ed) Autonomic failure. A textbook of clinical disorders of the autonomic nervous system, 2nd ed. Oxford University Press, Oxford, pp 569–595

Bannister R, Mathias C (1988) Testing autonomic reflexes. In: Bannister R (ed) Autonomic failure. A textbook of clinical disorders of the autonomic nervous system, 2nd ed. Oxford University Press, Oxford, pp 289–307

Bannister R, Christensen NJ, da Costa DF, Mathias CJ, Wright H, Ukachii-lois J (1984) Mechanisms of post-prandial hypotension in autonomic failure. J Physiol (London) 349: 367

Calne DB, Brennan J, Spiers ASD, Stern GM (1970) Hypotension caused by L-dopa. Br Med J 1: 474–475

Caird FI, Andrews GR, Kennedy RD (1973) Effect of posture on blood pressure in the elderly. Br Heart J 35: 527–530

Chokroverty S (1984) Autonomic dysfunction in olivopontocerebellar atrophy. Adv Neurol 41: 105–141

Déjerine J, Thomas AA (1900) L'atrophie olivo-ponto-cerebelleuse. Nouv Iconog de le Salpetrière 13: 330–370

Den Hartog Jager WA, Bethlem J (1969) The distribution of Lewy bodies in the central and autonomic nervous system in idiopathic paralysis agitans. J Neurol Neurosurg Psychiatry 23: 283–290

Eadie MJ, Tyrer JH (1965) Radiological abnormalities of the upper part of the alimentary tract in parkinsonism. Australas Ann Med 14: 23–27

Gibberd FB, Gleeson JA, Gossage AAR, Wilson RSE (1974) Oesophagel dilatation in Parkinson's disease. J Neurol Neurosurg Psychiatry 37: 938

Godi L, Pacchetti C, Berardesca E, Vignoli GP, Gabba P, Martignoni E, Nappi G (1993) Valutazione della seborrea nella malattia di Parkinson. Atti XX Riunione L.I.M.P.E. Varese, October 21–23, 1993, pp 343–355

Graham JG, Oppenheimer DR (1969) Orthostatic hypotension and nicotine sensitivity in a case of multiple system atrophy. J Neurol Neurosurg Psychiatry 32: 28–34

Korczyn AD (1989) Autonomic nervous system screening in patients with early Parkinson's disease. In: Przuntek H, Riederer P (eds) Early diagnosis and preventive therapy in Parkinson's disease. Springer, Wien New York, pp 41–48

Korczyn DA (1989) Autonomic nervous system dysfunction in Parkinson's disease. In: Calne DB, Crippa D, Trabucchi M, Comi G, Horowski R (eds) Parkinsonism and aging. Raven Press, New York, pp 211–219

Korczyn A (1990) Autonomic nervous system disturbances in Parkinson's disease. In: Streifler MB, Korczyn AD, Melamed E (eds) Advances in neurology, vol 53. Parkinson's disease: anatomy, pathology and therapy. Raven Press, New York, pp 463–468

Korczyn A, Rubenstein AE (1982) Autonomic nervous system complications of therapy. In: Silverstein A (ed) Neurological complications of therapy. Futura, New York

Langston JW, Forno LS (1978) Hypothalamus in Parkinson's disease. Ann Neurol 3: 129–133

Langworthy OR, Lewis LS, Dees Je, Hesser FH (1936) Clinical study of control of bladder by central nervous system. Bull John Hopkins Hosp 58: 59

Leibowitz M, Lieberman A (1975) Comparison of dopadecarboxilase inhibitor (carbidopa) combined with L-dopa and L-dopa alone on the cardiovascular system of patients with Parkinson's disease. Neurol 25: 917–921

Markham CH, Treciokas L, Acesel LD (1970) Blood pressure in parkinsonian patients receiving L-dopa. In: Barbeau A, McDowell FH (eds) L-dopa and parkinsonism. Davis, Philadelphia, pp 225–230

Martignoni E, Micieli G, Cavallini A, Pacchetti C, Magri M, Nappi G (1986) Autonomic disorders in idiopathic parkinsonism. J Neural Transm 22 [Suppl]: 149–161

Martignoni E, Pacchetti C, Micieli G, Nappi G (1995) Autonomic disturbances in Parkinson's disease and Shy-Drager syndrome. In: Korczyn A (ed) Marcel Dekker, New York Basel Hong Kong, pp 235–252

Mathias CJ, da Costa DF, Fosbraey P, Bannister R, Christensen NJ (1988) Post-cibal hypotension in autonomic failure. In: The sympathoadrenal system (Alfred Benzon Symposium, 23). Munksgaard, Copenhagen, pp 402–413

McLeod JG, Tuck RR (1987) Disorders of autonomic nervous system: pathophysiology and clinical features. Ann Neurol 21: 419–430

Micieli G, Martignoni E, Cavallini A, Sandrini G, Nappi G (1987) Postprandial and orthostatic hypotension in Parkinson's disease. Neurol 37: 386–393

Micieli G, Martignoni E, Congedo M, Pacchetti C, Cavallini A, Sibilla L, Nappi G (1989) Parkinson's disease and cardiopressor adaptive disturbances: neurochemical and hemodynamic correlates. In: Nappi G, Caraceni T (eds) Parkinsonism: diagnosis and treatment. Laurel House Publishing Co, Yorktown, pp 129–142

Murdock MI, Olsson CA, Sax DS, Krane RJ (1975) Effects of levodopa on the bladder outlet. J Urol 113: 803–805

Murnagham GF (1961) Neurogenic disorders of the bladder in parkinsonism. Br J Urol 33: 403

Oppenheimer D (1988) Neuropathology and neurochemistry of autonomic failure. Neuropathology of autonomic failure. In: Bannister R (ed) Autonomic failure. A textbook of clinical disorders of the autonomic nervous system, 2nd ed. Oxford University Press, Oxford, pp 451–483

Pacchetti C, Sibilla L, Bruggi P, Cavallini A, Micieli G, Martignoni E, Nappi G (1990) Autonomic disturbances in Parkinson's disease and Multisystem Atrophy: clinical aspects. Funct Neurol vol V [Suppl] 4: 49–56

Parkinson J (1817) An essay on the shaking palsy. Neely A, Jones D (eds) Sherwood, London

Pavlakis AJ, Siroky MB, Goldstein I, Krane RJ (1983) Neurologic finding in Parkinson's disease. J Urol 129: 80

Porter RW, Bors E (1971) Neurogenic bladder in parkinsonism: effect of thalamotomy. J Neurosurg 34: 27

Quinn N (1989) Multiple system atrophy — the nature of the beast. J Neurol Neurosurg Psychiatry [Spec Suppl]: 78–89

Quinn N, Illas A, Lhermitte F, Agid Y (1981) Bromocriptine in Parkinson's disease: a study of cardiovascular effects. J Neurol Neurosurg Psychiatry 44: 426–429

Rajput AH, Rozdilsky B (1976) Dysautonomia Parkinsonism: a clinicopathological study. J Neurol Neurosurg Psychiatry 39: 1092–1110

Ravasi S, Pacchetti C, Mensi M, Micieli G, Ghezzi M, Martignoni E, Scoppetta FP (1984) Sui disordini vescicali della malattia di Parkinson. In: Agnoli A, Bertolani G (eds) Atti X Riunione LIMPE Pavia, pp 48–61

Robbins AS, Rubenstein LZ (1984) Postural hypotension in the elderly. J Am Geriatr Soc 32: 769–774

Seyer-Hansen K (1977) Post-prandial hypotension. Br Med J 2: 1262

Shuster S, Thody AJ, Goolamali SK, Burton JL, Plummer N, Beats D (1983) Melanocyte stimulating hormone and parkinsonism. Lancet 1: 463–464

Shy GM, Drager GA (1960) A neurologic syndrome associated with orthostatic hypotension. Arch Neurol 2: 511–527

Spokes GSE, Bannister R, Oppenheimer DR (1979) Multiple System Atrophy with autonomic failure. J Neurol Sci 43: 59–82

Tomonaga M (1986) Neuropathology of autonomic dysfunction in Parkinson's disease. Auton Nerv Syst [Suppl]: 441–446

Yalla SY, Bunt KY, Fam BA, Costantinople NL, Gittes RF (1977) Detrusor-urethal sphincter dyssynergia. J Urol 118: 1026–1029

Yen TT, Stamm NB, Clemens JA (1979) Pergolide: a potent dopaminergic antihypertensive. Life Sci 25: 209–216

Authors' address: Dr. E. Martignoni, Istituto Neurologico "C. Mondino", via Palestro, 3, I-27100 Pavia, Italy.

J Neural Transm (1995) [Suppl] 45: 21–25

A genetic study of Parkinson's disease

**G. De Michele[1], A. Filla[1], R. Marconi[2], G. Volpe[1], A. D'Alessio[1], R. Scala[1],
G. Ambrosio[1], and G. Campanella[1]**

[1] Department of Neurology, Federico II University, Naples, and [2] "Sanatrix"
Neurological Institute, Pozzilli (IS), Italy

Summary. We performed a case-control study on 100 patients with Parkinson's disease, their spouses and the same number of sex- and age-matched neurological controls to clarify if family history of Parkinson's disease or essential tremor may increase the risk for the disease. We included in the study 68 male and 32 female parkinsonian patients with a mean age $\pm$ SD of 62.0 $\pm$ 9.9 years and a mean disease duration of 7.5 $\pm$ 5.7. The odds ratio for familial Parkinson's disease was 13.4 (95% confidence limits = 6.5–27.7) and for familial essential tremor 3.1 (95% confidence limits = 1.5–6.3). We also reviewed the genetic features of 122 parkinsonian patients with at least one affected relative. The presence of secondary cases among both first-degree (n = 83) and less close relatives (n = 72) suggests that sharing environmental factors does not explain the familial aggregation of the disease. Secondary cases were significantly more frequent in the paternal than in the maternal line (70 vs. 39). The presence of secondary cases among both siblings (46) and parents (37) and the unilateral distribution of ancestral secondary cases suggest an autosomal dominant inheritance with incomplete penetrance.

Introduction

Gowers (1888) reported a 15% familial occurrence of Parkinson's disease (PD) and first suggested a possible genetic origin of the disease. Mjönes (1949) found a familial occurrence of 38% and proposed an autosomal dominant inheritance with incomplete penetrance. On the other hand, Duvoisin et al. (1969) reported a low proportion of familial cases of PD (2.5%) in a study conducted in New York City. Differences in diagnostic criteria with inclusion of atypical cases, and methodological differences may account for these conflicting results. It has been suggested that idiopathic PD is not homogeneous and that in familial cases there are two main patterns of genetic transmission: dominant with prevalence of tremor and recessive with prevalence of akinesia and rigidity (Barbeau and Pourcher, 1982; Roy et al., 1983; Barbeau and Roy, 1984). According to these authors family history of essential tremor (ET) might increase the susceptibility to PD.

Table 1. Twin studies in Parkinson's disease

		Pairs	
		Total	Concordant
Ward et al.	MZ	43 (48*)	1 (4*)
(1983)	DZ	19	0 (1*)
Marsden	MZ	11	1
(1987)	DZ	11	1
Marttila et al.	MZ	18	0
(1988)	DZ	14	1
Total		116 (121*)	4 (8*)

*Including possible and atypical cases (Johnson et al., 1990).
MZ monozygotic twin; *DZ* dizygotic twin

Twin studies have shown a low concordance for PD between monozygotic twins, not higher than that found among dizygotic (Table 1). These studies established that the major factors in the etiology of PD are nongenetic. However, Johnson et al. (1990) reexamined the results of the twin study by Ward et al. (1983) and concluded that the data could not disprove the genetic hypothesis. Furthermore, a PET study by Burn et al. (1992) showed that some unaffected twins had subclinical PD.

Aim of this study is to investigate whether family history of PD or ET are relevant risk factors for the development of PD. We report the results of a case control study on 100 PD patients and the genetic analysis of a large series of patients with familial PD.

Patients and methods

For the case-control study the index cases were 100 consecutive PD patients (68 males, 32 females) examined at the Department of Neurology of the Federico II University of Naples. The control groups were constituted by the same number of patient's spouses and neurological controls, matched by sex and age (± 2 years).

Requirements for the diagnosis of PD were the presence of at least two of bradykinesia, rigidity and rest tremor, a chronic progressive course, a good response to levodopa, and the absence of atypical features (gaze palsy, autonomic dysfunction, etc), of possible causes of secondary parkinsonism and of significant cognitive impairment. The diagnoses among neurological controls were cerebrovascular diseases, neurosis and depression, neuromuscular diseases, multiple sclerosis, myelopathies, epilepsy and vertigo.

All patients and controls were asked about two genetic risk factors: family history of PD or of ET.

We considered the diagnosis of PD in the familial cases *definite* when we could personally observe the secondary case or examine absolutely reliable medical records; *probable* when it was made by a neurologist; *possible* when it was made on the basis of information given by relatives.

We evaluated the number of subjects exposed to the risk factor, the chi-square value (df = 1) and the odds ratio according to Mantel-Haenszel.

Results

Case-control study

Mean age of the cases and of the controls, mean onset age and disease duration of the cases are shown in Table 2.

The analysis of the genetic risk factors is shown in Table 3. All the odds ratios were significantly higher than 1, showing positive association between the risk factors and PD. Positive family history for PD was found in 20 male and 15 female cases (35% of the total cases). Their mean age of onset $\pm$ SD was 54.1 $\pm$ 12.8 years. Positive family history increased the risk of about 13 times, including all the diagnoses of PD. The inclusion of the definite and probable diagnoses only or of the definite diagnoses only increased the risk furtherly. Individuals with familial ET had a risk of about 3.

Analysis of familial cases

We reviewed the genetic features of 122 PD patients with at least one affected relative. Thirty-five of them partecipated in the case-control study and the other 87 were found reviewing the records of 412 PD patients observed at our

Table 2. Case-control study on 100 triplets

	Parkinsonian patients	Spouses	Neurological controls
Sex	68 M–32 F	32 M–68 F	68 M–32 F
Age (M $\pm$ SD)	62.0 $\pm$ 9.9	60.7 $\pm$ 11.1	61.8 $\pm$ 10.2
Disease duration (M $\pm$ SD)	7.5 $\pm$ 5.7		
Onset age (M $\pm$ SD)	54.6 $\pm$ 10.6		

Table 3. Genetic risk factors in Parkinson's disease

Risk factor	Positive family history Patients	Spouses	Controls	Odds ratio (95% C.L.)	Chi square	p value
	(No. of triplets = 100)					
Parkinson's disease						
Total diagnoses	35	2	6	13.4 (6.5–27.7)	55.05	$<10^{-6}$
Definite diagnoses	8	1	0	not calculable	14.06	$<10^{-3}$
Definite or probable diagnoses	21	2	3	19.5 (6.9–55.4)	31.11	$<10^{-6}$
Essential tremor	17	5	6	3.1 (1.5–6.3)	9.45	0.002

Table 4. Distribution of ancestral secondary cases of Parkinson's disease

	Secondary cases			Combinations of pairs		
Proband	Paternal	Maternal	Total	Pat-pat	Pat-mat	Mat-mat
4		2	2			1
25	2		2	1		
27		2	2			1
48	2		2	1		
79	4		4	6		
86		2	2			1
102		4	4			6
111	2		2	1		
Totals	10	10	20	9		9

*The number of possible combinations of pairs of n affected relatives is n(n − 1)/2

Department. The overall frequency of cases with familial PD was 24% (122:512). In 18 cases two relatives were affected, in four cases three, in one four and in one five. The total number of secondary cases was 155, with 83 cases among first-degree relatives (46 siblings, 37 parents). Secondary cases were more frequent in the paternal than in the maternal line (70 to 39; chi square = 8.26; p < 0.01).

Table 4 shows the distribution of ancestral secondary cases in eight cases with at least two affected relatives among ascendants (excluding parents). In a dominant disorder the ratio of unilateral (paternal or maternal) to bilateral (paternal and maternal) pairs should be higher than 2:1 (Young et al., 1977). A lower ratio is in favour of a multifactorial inheritance. In all our eight kindred ancestral secondary cases were unilaterally distributed.

Discussion

The results of our study show that family history of PD strongly increases the risk for the disease. Family history of PD was more frequent among cases than both among spouses and neurological controls. The frequency of familial PD was 24% considering all the PD patients and 35% considering only the patients from the case control study. We believe that a thorough interview is required to detect the secondary cases. Familial aggregation of PD could be due either to genetic or to shared environmental factors (Calne et al., 1987). First-degree relatives are likely to share the same environment. We found high prevalence of secondary cases also among less close relatives. These data suggest that heredity plays a major role in the etiology of PD.

The preponderance of secondary cases in the paternal line confirms previous results (Campanella et al., 1984; Maraganore et al., 1991) and is not in favour of X-linked or mitochondrial inheritance. Since both siblings and ascendants are affected, an autosomal dominant inheritance of a mutant gene or genes with reduced penetrance appears the most likely. This hypothesis is supported by the report of two large, probably related, kindreds with autopsy-confirmed PD, apparently inherited in autosomal dominant fashion (Golbe et al., 1990). The distribution of ancestral secondary cases is also in favour of an autosomal dominant inheritance.

Our data show that a positive family history for ET significantly increases the risk of developing PD. Barbeau suggested that some environmental factors could transform a dominantly inherited ET into full-blown PD (Roy et al., 1983). Another explanation is that PD might present with a phenotype mimicking ET in some patients.

References

Barbeau A, Pourcher E (1982) New data on the genetics of Parkinson's disease. Can J Neurol Sci 9: 53–60

Barbeau A, Roy M (1984) Familial subsets in idiopathic Parkinson's disease. Can J Neurol Sci 11: 144–150

Burn DJ, Mark MH, Playford ED, et al (1992) Parkinson's disease in twins studied with ^{18}F-dopa and positron emission tomography. Neurology 42: 1894–1900

Calne S, Shoenberg BS, Martin W, Uitti RJ, Spencer P, Calne DB (1987) Familial Parkinson's disease: possible role of environmental factors. Can J Neurol Sci 14: 303–305

Campanella G, Idone M, De Michele G, Filla A (1984) Paternal preponderance in familial Parkinson's disease. Neurology 34: 1398–1399

Duvoisin RC, Gearling PR, Schwerger MP (1969) A family study of parkinsonism. In: Barbeau A, Brunette JR (eds) Progress in neurogenetics. Excerpta Medica, Amsterdam, pp 492–496

Golbe LI, Di Iorio G, Bonavita V, Miller DC, Duvoisin RC (1990) A large kindred with autosomal dominant Parkinson's disease. Ann Neurol 27: 276–282

Gowers WR (1888) A manual of diseases of the nervous system. Blakiston and Sons, Philadelphia, pp 636–657

Johnson WG, Hodge SE, Duvoisin RC (1990) Twin studies and the genetics of Parkinson's disease — a reappraisal. Mov Dis 5: 187–194

Maraganore DM, Harding AE, Marsden CD (1991) A clinical and genetic study of familial Parkinson's disease. Mov Disord 6: 205–211

Marsden CD (1987) Parkinson's disease in twins. J Neurol Neurosurg Psychiatry 50: 105–106

Marttila RJ (1988) Parkinson's disease in a nationwide twin cohort. Neurology 38: 1217–1219

Mjönes H (1949) Paralysis agitans: a clinical and genetic study. Acta Psychiatr Scand [Suppl] 54: 1–195

Roy M, Boyer L, Barbeau A (1983) A prospective study of 50 cases of familial Parkinson's disease. Can J Neurol Sci 10: 37–42

Ward CD, Duvoisin RC, Ince SE, Nutt J, Eldridge R, Calne DB (1983) Parkinson's disease in 65 pairs of twins and in a set of quadruplets. Neurology 33: 815–824

Young WI, Martin WE, Anderson VE (1977) The distribution of ancestral secondary cases in Parkinson's disease. Clin Genet 11: 189–92

Authors' address: Dr. G. De Michele, Clinica Neurologica, Università Federico II, via S. Pansini 5, I-80131 Napoli, Italy.

J Neural Transm (1995) [Suppl] 45: 27–34

Do cognitive changes of Parkinson's disease result from dopamine depletion?

B. Dubois and **B. Pillon**

Fédération de Neurologie and INSERM U 289, Hopital de la Salpêtrière,
Paris, France

Summary.   Cognitive changes have long been observed in patients with Parkinson's disease: visuo-spatial deficits, memory disorders, dysexecutive syndrome. Given the modulatory role of the basal ganglia and related structures, these deficits might result from more fundamental disorders concerning the allocation of attentional resources, the temporal organization of behavior, the maintenance of representations in working memory or the self-elaboration of internal strategy, all of which resemble dysfunctions of processes that are commonly considered to be controlled by the frontal lobes. This suggests a functional continuity between the basal ganglia and association areas of the prefrontal cortex. The recent description in primates of parallel, segregated loops that interconnect well defined subregions of the basal ganglia to discrete areas of the prefrontal cortex via the thalamus may give some support to this hypothesis.

In Parkinson's disease (PD), a true dementia is unfrequent, about 15 to 20% of the cases (Pillon et al., 1991). The cause of this dementia is a matter of discussion but there is a trend to consider that it results, at least in part, from additional cortical lesions such as Alzheimer's like changes and cortical Lewy bodies that have been recently reported post-mortem in the brain of PD patients. In contrast, certain cognitive deficits are observed very frequently in these patients, which may be related to the subcortical pathology of the disease for at least two main reasons: firstly, these disorders are observed in almost all of the patients; secondly, they are observed even at the early stages of the disease, i.e. at a time when the lesions are considered to be restricted to the nigrostriatal dopaminergic pathway. These disorders are usually referred as "specific" for these reasons and they mainly affect visuo-spatial, memory, and executive functions.

What are the specific cognitive changes of Parkinson's disease?

There is multiple evidence for a *visuo-spatial and visuo-motor dysfunction* in PD, the nature of which remains, however, under debate. Although some authors believe that there is a genuine visuo-spatial deficit in PD, most attribute impaired performance to the motor component or to the high cognitive demand usually required by these tasks. Indeed, except for difficulties in discriminating line orientation, the deficits are observed in complex visuo-spatial paradigms requiring planning and sequencing, mental flexibility, and self-generation of strategies in the absence of external cues (Brown and Marsden, 1986; Ransmayr et al., 1987), and result rather from a more generalized dysfunction or a decrease in central processing resources than from a specific alteration of visuo-spatial functions.

Several *memnonic functions* are impaired in PD (Dubois et al., 1991): 1) *working memory*, as shown by defective short-term recall in the Sternberg paradigm and in the digit ordering test or in situations where the manipulation of interfering stimuli is required, as in the Brown and Peterson procedure; 2) *long-term memory*, where the deficit in verbal and visual free recall is severe, whereas cued recall and recognition are normal; 3) *procedural learning*, as suggested by recent evidence that remains to be confirmed. As for visuo-spatial functions, the performance of patients on explicit memory tests is dramatically dependent on the nature of the task, the most difficult being those which require organization of the to-be-remembered material, such as recency discrimination (Taylor et al., 1986), temporal ordering (Sagar et al., 1988), and conditional associative learning tasks (Gotham et al., 1988), or the activation of search strategies needed for retrieval of stored information, as recently demonstrated (Pillon et al., 1993). In the latter study, explicit memory was assessed with several tasks, including the Grober and Buschke procedure which controls for the effective encoding of the verbal items. Although demented PD patients exhibited a marked deficit in free recall in all memory tasks, their performance was dramatically improved by the semantic cueing which triggered efficient retrieval processes. Under these conditions, total recall scores approached those of normal elderly subjects, suggesting that recall deficit is not primarily due to a memory disruption, since the ability to register, store and consolidate information is preserved, but rather to difficulties in activating the neuronal processes involved in the functional use of memory stores. Two arguments favor the role of a frontal dysfunction in the defective activation of memory processes. First, in the previous study, correlation analyses showed that memory scores are strongly related to performance on tests of executive functions. Second, the recall deficit is always more severe in PD patients when the to-be-learned material is not semantically organized, as in word-list acquisition (Weingartner et al., 1984), the Rey Auditory Verbal Learning Test (Taylor et al., 1986) or the Buschke Selective Reminding Test (Helkala et al., 1989), i.e., in situations which require sustained effort and self elaboration of internal strategies to organize the material. Thus, in PD, memory processes requiring functional integrity of the frontal lobes seem to be impaired, particularly the ability to spontaneously generate efficient encoding and retrieval strategies.

Executive functions are altered in PD. This cognitive domain refers to the mental processes involved in adaptive behaviors generated in response to new challenging environmental situations: generation of new concepts, shifting or maintenance of a mental set, problem-solving and planning. These processes are disturbed after damage of the frontal lobes. They can be investigated with several tasks which all require cognitive flexibility or internally-guided behavior: 1) concept formation and rule finding tasks (Wisconsin card and Delis sorting tests; delayed response tasks); 2) set-shifting tasks (Trail Making and Odd Man Out tests); 3) set-maintenance (word fluency; Stroop test); 4) problem-solving (tower tasks). Interestingly, each of these tasks has been shown in one or more studies to be impaired in PD (Dubois et al., 1993).

The underlying mechanism: a frontal lobe dysfunction

Thus, besides the apparent diversity of cognitive disorders reported in several domains, there is a trend to consider that these deficits may result from some fundamental or more generalized dysfunction: *a difficulty in behavioral control and regulation* (Bowen et al., 1975) responsible for the inability to change or to maintain mental sets or to perform complex visuo-spatial tasks; *an inability to elaborate efficient strategies* and to use internally-guided behaviors (Taylor et al., 1986) which may account for recall and problem-solving deficits; *a decrease in processing resources and in internal control of attention* (Brown and Marsden, 1988) which penalizes PD patients in tasks heavily loaded in cognitive demands. Whatever the relevance and validity of these hypotheses, they all implicate functions under the control of the frontal lobes, and there is now general agreement that the specific cognitive changes encountered in non-demented PD patients result from a frontal lobe dysfunction. How is this possible?

It is well known that degeneration of nigrostriatal dopaminergic neurons is the major lesion in PD. Can such a lesion, by itself, cause a frontal lobe dysfunction? Some evidence can be drawn from the study of the cognitive changes associated with intoxication by 1-methyl-4-phenyl-1,2,3,6, tetrahydropyridine (MPTP), a drug which selectively destroys the nigrostriatal dopaminergic neurons both in animals, following experimental injection, or in humans, after accidental administration. Stern and Langston (1985) have shown that patients with MPTP-induced lesions have cognitive deficits similar to those of patients with idiopathic PD, such as reduced verbal fluency and impaired Stroop test performance. In line with this finding is the fact that MPTP-exposed monkeys exhibit difficulty solving a detour-reaching problem in an object retrieval task that tests planning ability (Taylor et al., 1990), and perform poorly in a delayed response task (Schneider and Kovelowski, 1990) known to be specifically dependent on frontal function. The fact that patients with PD experience difficulties in performing the Wisconsin card sorting and Stroop tests, even at the earliest stages of the disease (Pillon et al., 1991), when the neuronal damage is thought to be restricted to the nigro-striatal dopaminergic system, is consistent with this statement.

How does the lesion of the nigrostriatal dopaminergic neurons produce frontal lobe deficits? Recent descriptions of striatofrontal circuits in primates

(Alexander et al., 1986) may provide a coherent explanation. Five independent, parallel, and recurrent loops have been postulated, each of which interconnecting specific areas of the prefrontal cortex to restricted, well-defined sub-regions of the basal ganglia. The functional role of these striato-frontal circuits is more or less established for the "motor loop" and the "oculo-motor" loop. This is not the case, however, for the three remaining circuits which are, consequently, labelled by their cortical components, respectively "dorsolateral", "orbitofrontal" and "anterior cingulate". Given the cortical targets, it is reasonable to assume that these loops are involved in complex cognitive, behavioral or motivational functions. Thus, the frontal dysfunction observed in nondemented PD patients may result from the disruption of the complex loops either at the level of the striatum, resulting from the lesion of the nigro-stiatal dopaminergic pathway, or at the level of the prefrontal cortex, resulting from the lesion of the meso-cortical system. According to this hypothesis, cognitive changes in nondemented PD patients should be alleviated after the reestablishment of dopaminergic transmission following levodopa therapy. There is some evidence for such fluctuations in cognitive performance in relation to levodopa status, as shown by the study of PD patients cognitively assessed in both ON and OFF states. Delayed recall, verbal fluency, and working memory are the main cognitive processes that are sensitive to such a dopaminergic modulation. As a matter of fact, the positive effect of levodopa is rather noticed on more basic processes such as cognitive speed, temporal discrimination, and information processing.

The involvement of the striatum in sensory integration has been demonstrated by Artieda et al. (1992), who showed that PD patients displayed abnormal temporal discrimination ability, characterized by an increase of the time interval needed to perceive two stimuli as separate. The striatum can therefore no longer be considered as having a purely motor function, but should rather be thought of as focusing attention on a single event while "suppressing" all others, as postulated by Hassler (1978). The deficit observed in sensory integration would result from decreased selectivity to sensory stimuli of the neurons in the striato-pallidal complex. An alternative explanation would be a disturbance of an internal clock in PD, lengthening the time interval necessary for discriminating between paired stimuli. The latter hypothesis is supported by the finding that time estimation is modified following striatal lesions in rats (Meck, 1994) or in patients with PD (Pastor et al., 1992; Malapani et al., 1993) who tend to underestimate the duration of time intervals and have difficulty in reproducing time intervals, both deficits that are reversed by levodopa treatment. The fact that sensory discrimination and time estimation improved significantly, although not entirely, when levodopa treatment was resumed, suggests that these functions, modulated by dopaminergic transmission, may be supported by a striatofrontal circuit.

The role of the striatum in simultaneous cognitive processing has been recently showed by Malapani et al. (1994). In this study, the ability to process two simultaneous informations was significantly impaired in patients who were in a state of striatal dopaminergic depletion. The experimental procedure consisted of two different tasks: 1) a choice reaction time (CRT) to visual stimuli (squares of different colors appearing on a screen) with a right hand response to the red square; and 2) a CRT to auditory stimuli (high or low frequency sounds) with a left hand response to the high frequence tone. The tasks were presented first separately and, then, simultaneously. In the simultaneous condition, the inter-response interval — the difference between the first and the second response times — reflects the ability to process concurrent sensory informations in parallel. Compared to controls, treated PD patients performed normally. De novo patients, although they had shorter disease duration than that of the treated PD group (1.7 ± 0.3 versus 8.1 ± 1.1 years), showed a significant increase in the inter-response interval. Such an increase of the inter-response interval wa also observed in another group of PD patients assessed in the "OFF" state — after a short withdrawal of levodopa treatment — compared to their performance in the "ON" state — at the maximal effect of treatment. Taken together, these results illustrate the role of the striatum in information processing and sensori-motor integration, both of which are modulated by dopaminergic transmission.

The role of non dopaminergic and cortical lesions

The dopamine hypothesis is attractive because it takes into account the most severe lesion reported in PD, Indeed, dopamine depletion, which is the first biochemical deficiency to appear, probably plays a primary role in the genesis of the frontal dysfunction observed in the early stages of the disease. It remains to be explained, however, why the restauration of central dopaminergic transmission with levodopa does not improve the cognitive changes to the same extent as dopamine-dependent motor signs. This may be interpreted in two ways: 1) cognitive changes are mediated by a dopaminergic mechanism, but are unresponsive to levodopa for pharmacodynamic reasons that are not yet understood; 2) cognitive changes are mediated, at least in part, by lesions of non-dopaminergic neuronal systems; in this case, levodopa would not be expected to be fully effective.

Indeed, during the course of the disease, patients become increasingly handicapped as motor symptoms unresponsive to levodopa — gait disorders or dysarthria — appear, or cognitive disorders worsen (Pillon et al., 1989). These symptoms may correspond to the development of non-dopaminergic lesions which have been reported, post-mortem, such as in the ascending cholinergic, noradrenergic and serotoninergic systems (Dubois and Pillon, 1992). Each of these ascending systems has been shown, on the basis of pharmacological, pathological or experimental evidence, to have an effect on cognition. For example, blockade of cholinergic transmission with anticholinergic drugs consistently results in learning and memory deficits, and in frontal lobe-like dysfunction in patients with PD (Dubois et al., 1990). Lesions of the locus coeruleus, the site of origin of cortical and limbic noradrenergic innervation, reduce selective attention and impair learning and memory in animals, and may contribute to cognitive slowing in PD patients (Stern and Mayeux,

1984). The respective role of each of these additional neuronal lesions remains, however, difficult to establish. It is noteworthy that in PD, blockade of cholinergic transmission induces an impairment on tasks relying on internal control of attention or on self elaboration of strategies, as did dopaminergic deficiency. Thus, both cholinergic and dopaminergic deficiencies may produce the same kind of frontal lobe dysfunction. We do not know whether one or the other neuronal lesion (or both) is responsible for the frontal syndrom of PD patients. What is clear is that the functional consequence of the neuronal lesions is determined rather by the cortical target of these neuronal systems than by the nature of the systems themselves. In other words, these systems are thought to regulate neuronal cell activity in regions of projection involved in specific functions, rather than transmitting function-specific information. Thus, cognitive changes in PD may result from the deactivation of cognitive programs distributed along specific neuronal networks. Deactivation may occur beyond a certain threshold of neuronal degeneration. For example, degeneration of cholinergic neurons, which is severe in demented PD patients, is present in all patients even in the absence of intellectual impairment or memory disorders. If so, intellectual impairment will occur when synaptic adjustments (hyperactivity of the remaining neurons or supersensitivity of muscarinic receptors) can no longer compensate for neuronal loss. Age of onset of the disease may influence the threshold at which neuronal lesions become symptomatic. The compounding effect of aging on cognitive disturbances has been demonstrated by comparing the neuropsychological performance of early-onset and late-onset PD patients to age-matched controls (Dubois et al., 1990). Additional age-related brain lesions may decrease the efficacy of normal compensatory mechanisms. This might account for the high frequency of cognitive disorders and dementia in PD patients whose disease began later in life.

Cortical changes must also be taken into account to explain cognitive disorders in PD. Neuronal loss, Alzheimer's disease-like histological changes and Lewy bodies in the cerebral cortex may play a crucial role in the intellectual deterioration, in addition to subcortical lesions. The role of cortical lesions in PD is not, however, clearly established. Some cases of dementia, defined according to the DSM III criteria, have been reported in the absence of apparent cortical lesions, suggesting that subcortical lesions may be sufficiently severe to cause overt dementia, at least in some patients. Thus, the respective roles of two contingents of lesions (cortical and subcortical) remain to be determined, even if there are strong arguments to believe that the subcortical lesions are responsible for the preponderance of frontal dysfunction observed in PD patients, even in those who are demented. For this reason, it is probably inaccurate to label the cognitive changes associated with PD as subcortical dementia. On the other hand, the concept of subcortical dementia has some heuristic value, because it underlines the importance of the anatomical and biochemical relationships between the cerebral cortex and subcortical structures, paticularly the basal ganglia. We wish to propose that the disruption of the connections between these structures is the initial basis of cognitive impairment of PD.

References

Alexander GE, Delong M, Strick P (1986) Parallel organization of functionally segregated circuits linking basal ganglia and cortex. Ann Rev Neurosci 9: 357–381

Artieda J, Pastor MA, Lacruz F, Obeso JA (1992) Temporal discrimination is abnormal in Parkinson's disease. Brain 115: 190–210

Bowen FP, Kamieny RS, Burns MM, Yahr MD (1975) Parkinsonism: effects of levodopa on concept formation. Neurology 25: 701–704

Brown RG, Marden CD (1986) Visuospatial function in Parkinson's disease. Brain 109: 987–1002

Brown RG, Marsden CD (1988) Internal versus external cues and the control of attention in Parkinson's disease. Brain 111: 323–345

Dubois B, Pillon B (1992) Biochemical correlates of cognitive changes and dementia in Parkinson's disease. In: Huber SJ, Cummings JL (eds) Parkinson's disease: neurobehavioral aspects. Oxford University Press, Oxford, pp 178–198

Dubois B, Pillon B, Lhermitte F, Agid Y (1990) Cholinergic deficiency and frontal dysfunction in Parkinson's disease. Ann Neurol 28: 117–121

Dubois B, Boller F, Pillon B, Agid Y (1991) Cognitive deficits in Parkinsons' disease. In: Boller F, Grafman J (eds) Handbook of neuropsychology, vol 5. Elsevier Science Publishers, Amsterdam, pp 195–240

Dubois B, Pillon B, Sternic N, Lhermitte F, Agid Y (1990) Age-induced cognitive disturbances in Parkinson's disease. Neurology 40: 38–41

Dubois B, Pillon B, Malapani C, Deweer B, Verin M, Partiot A, Défontaines B, Sirigu A, Texeira C, Agid Y (1993) Subcortical dementia and Parkinson's disease: what are the cognitive functions of the basal ganglia? In: Wolters Ch, Scheltens P (eds) Mental dysfunction in Parkinson's disease. Vrije Universiteit, Amsterdam, pp 195–210

Gotham AM, Brown RG, Marsden CD (1988) "Frontal" cognitive functions in patients with Parkinson's disease "on" and "off" levodopa. Brain 111: 299–321

Hassler R (1978) Striatal control of locomotion, intentional actions and of integrating and perceptive activity. J Neurol Sci 36: 187–224

Helkala EL, Laulumaa U, Soininen H, Riekkinen PJ (1989) Different error pattern of episodic and semantic memory in Alzheimer's disease and Parkinson's disease with dementia. Neuropsychologia 27: 1241–1248

Malapani C, Deweer B, Pillon B, Dubois B, Agid Y, Rakitin B, Penney T, Hinton S, Gibbon J, Meck W (1993) Impaired time perception in Parkinson's disease is reversed with Apomorphine. 1993 Annual Meeting of Neurosciences. Washington DC, November 7–12

Malapani C, Pillon B, Dubois B, Agid Y (1994) Impaired simultaneous cognitive task performance in Parkinson's disease: a dopamine related dysfunction. Neurology 44: 319–326

Meck WH (1994) Neuroanatomical localization of an internal clock: a functional link between mesolimbic-mesocortical and nigrostriatal dopaminergic systems. Behav Brain Res (in press)

Pastor MA, Artieda J, Jahanshani M, Obeso JA (1992) Time estimation and reproduction is abnormal in Parkinson's disease. Brain 115: 211–225

Pillon B, Dubois B, Cusimano G, Bonnet AM, Lhermitte F, Agid Y (1989) Does cognitive impairment in Parkinson's disease result from non-dopaminergic lesions? J Neurol Neurosurg Psychiatry 52: 201–206

Pillon B, Dubois B, Ploska A, Agid Y (1991) Severity and specificity of cognitive impairment in Alzheimer's, Huntington's, and Parkinson's diseases and progressive supranuclear palsy. Neurology 41: 634–643

Pillon B, Deweer B, Agid Y, Dubois B (1993) Explicit memory in Alzheimer's, Huntington's, and Parkinson's diseases. Arch Neurol 50: 374–379

Ransmayr G, Schmidhuber-Eiler B, Karamat E, Engler-Ploer S, Poewe W, Leidlmair K (1987) Visuoperception and visuospatial and visuorotational performance in Parkinson's disease. J Neurol 235: 99–101

Sagar HJ, Sullivan EV, Gabriel JD, Corkin S, Growdon JH (1988) Temporal ordering and short-term memory deficits in Parkinson's disease. Brain 111: 525–535

Schneider JS, Kovelowski C (1990) Chronic exposure to low doses of MPTP: cognitive deficits in motor asymptomatic monkeys. Brain Res 519: 122–128

Stern Y, Langston JW (1985) Intellectual changes in patients with MPTP-induced Parkinsonism. Neurology 35: 1506–1509

Stern Y, Mayeux R, Cote L (1984) Reaction time and vigilance in Parkinson's disease: possible role of norepinephrine metabolism. Arch Neurol 41: 1086–1089

Taylor JR, Elsworth JD, Roth RH, Sladek JR, Redmond DE (1990) Cognitive and motor deficits in the acquisition of an object retrieval/detour task in MPTP-treated monkeys. Brain 113: 617–637

Taylor AE, Saint-Cyr JA, Lang AE (1986) Frontal lobe dysfunction in Parkinson's disease. Brain 109: 845–883

Weingartner H, Burns S, Diebel R, Lewitt PA (1984) Cognitive impairment in Parkinson's disease: distinguishing between effort-demanding and automatic cognitive processes. Psychiatry Res 11: 223–235

Authors' address: Prof. B. Dubois, INSERM U 289 et Fédération de Neurologie, Hôpital de la Salpêtrière, 47 Boulevard de L'Hôpital, F-75651 Paris cedex 13, France.

J Neural Transm (1995) [Suppl] 45: 35–45

The role of monoamine oxidase and catechol O-methyltransferase in dopaminergic neurotransmission

A. Napolitano, A. M. Cesura, and **M. Da Prada**[†]

Pharma Division, Preclinical Research, F. Hoffmann-La Roche Ltd, Basel, Switzerland

Summary. The action of dopamine (DA) released in the synaptic cleft is mainly terminated by its reuptake and catabolism by the enzymes monoamine oxidase (MAO) and catechol O-methyltransferase (COMT). Preclinical data show that the reduction of the catabolism of DA elicited by MAO and COMT inhibitors leads to an enhancement of DA neurotransmission. Moreover, there is evidence suggesting that MAO-B inhibition might protect DA neurons from oxidative stress. Nevertheless, due to differences in enzyme localization and activity between man and rodents, results obtained in experimental animals might not reflect the actual situation in humans. Today the availability of potent and selective MAO and COMT inhibitors makes it feasible for the clinician to test whether the blockade of catabolic enzymes would result in a symptomatic improvement in Parkinsonian patients, and whether MAO-B inhibition might additionally exert a neuro-protective effect.

Introduction

Parkinson's disease (PD) is characterized by a loss of nigrostriatal dopaminer-gic neurons, resulting in massive depletion ($\geq 80\%$) of striatal dopamine (DA) (Hornykiewicz, 1982).

Several pharmacological tools are currently available to restore the dopaminergic neurotransmission in PD patients. Substitution therapy with the DA-precursor amino acid L-DOPA combined with a peripheral aromatic amino acid decarboxylase (E.C 4.1.1.28, AADC) inhibitor, e.g. benserazide in Madopar® and carbidopa in Sinemet®, remains the standard treatment. After the administration of L-DOPA, the amino acid is actively transported into the brain and is eventually decarboxylated to DA in dopaminergic as well as non-dopaminergic neurons. As an alternative therapy, the activity of DA on post-synaptic receptors may be mimicked by the administration of DA-agonists, which preferentially stimulate D2 receptors. In the past, little attention has been given to the possibility of enhancing DA neurotransmission by reducing

---

[†] Deceased

the catabolism of DA, i.e. by inhibiting monoamine oxidase (MAO, EC 1.4.3.4) and/or catechol O-methyltransferase (COMT, EC 2.1.1.6).

In this survey we discuss the enzymes involved in the catabolism of DA, namely MAO and COMT, focusing on recently discovered potent and specific inhibitors and on their potential impact in the therapy of PD.

Main characteristics of monoamine oxidase and catechol O-methyltransferase

MAO, an enzyme located on the outer mitochondrial membrane, is present in two subtypes, namely MAO-A and MAO-B (Bach et al., 1988), which differ in their primary structure, tissue localization and specificity of substrate. These isoenzymes are encoded by two different genes located on the short arm of the human chromosome X (Kochersperger et al., 1986). In Table 1, the substrate specificity for both isotypes are summarized (Dostert et al., 1989). Brain noradrenergic neurons contain MAO-A, whereas MAO-B is mainly located in serotonergic and histaminergic neurons; both isoenzymes have been consistently found in glial cells (Table 2) (Arai et al., 1986; Saura et al., 1992). Although DA shows similar affinities for both MAO isotypes in vitro, it is predominantly deaminated by MAO-A in rats and by MAO-B in humans

Table 1. Preferential substrates of cerebral MAO-A (A) and MAO-B (B)

Substrate	In vivo		In vitro
	Man	Rat	
5-Hydroxytryptamine	A	A	A
Noradrenaline	A(B)	A	A + B
Adrenaline	A	A	A + B
Dopamine	B(A)	A	A + B
2-Phenyletylamine	B	B	B
Tyramine[a]	A + B	A + B	A + B
MPTP	B	B	B

[a] Exogenous tyramine is mainly metabolized by MAO-A in the intestinal tract. See text for references

Table 2. Occurrence of MAO-A and MAO-B in the CNS

		MAO-A	MAO-B
Neurons	Serotonergic	+	+ +
	Noradrenergic	+ +	−
	Dopaminergic	(+)[a]	−
	Histaminergic	−	+ +
Glial cells		(+)	+

+ present, − absent; [a] MAO-A is present only in a minor population of neuromelanin-containing DA neurons in the human substantia nigra. See text for references

(Waldmeier, 1987). Surprisingly enough, rat and human DA-neurons of the substantia nigra contain little if any MAO-A and no MAO-B (Westlund et al., 1988).

COMT is a widely distributed Mg^{2+}-dependent enzyme which catalyzes the transfer of a methyl group from S-adenosyl-L-methionine to a hydroxyl group of a catecholic substrate (Männistö et al., 1992a). This enzyme is largely involved in the catabolism of L-DOPA, catecholamines (DA, noradrenaline, and adrenaline), and their hydroxylated metabolites, e.g. 3,4-dihydroxy-phenylacetic acid (DOPAC). COMT activity is relatively high in peripheral organs, (e.g. liver and kidney) and is present also in CNS neurons and glial cells (Karhunen et al., 1994). It has been recently shown that human dopaminergic nigro-striatal neurons do not contain COMT (Kastner et al., 1994). This is in agreement with previous experiments in rats showing that lesions of the substantia nigra by 6-hydroxydopamine (6-OHDA) do not affect striatal COMT activity (Kaakkola et al., 1987). However, the presence of COMT has been recently observed in medium-size spiny neurons of the human striatum (Kastner et al., 1994), suggesting that the catabolism of DA via COMT might occur not only in glial cells, but also in post-synaptic elements. COMT exists in two forms: a soluble cytoplasmatic form (Guldberg and Marsden, 1975), and a membrane-bound (MB) form (Roth, 1992), located on the rough endoplasmic reticulum (Tilgmann et al., 1992). The MB isoform differs from the soluble form by a N-terminal stretch of 50 (human) or 43 (rat) amino acids containing the membrane anchor domain. Both COMT isoforms are encoded by the same gene (human chromosome 22q11.2) and are thought to derive from initiation of transcription at two alternative sites (Salminen et al., 1990; Bertocci et al., 1991; Lundström et al., 1991). The MB-COMT displays a higher affinity for catechol substrates than the soluble form (Jeffery and Roth, 1984) and is thought to be prevalent in neurons, whereas soluble COMT is mainly localized in glial cells and in peripheral organs (Roth, 1992).

On the metabolism of dopamine in the CNS

After release, the main catabolic processes terminating the effect of DA include uptake into nerve terminals (uptake 1) or into non-neuronal cells (uptake 2) and subsequent deamination by MAO and/or O-methylation by COMT (Fig. 1) (Kopin, 1985).

DOPAC is produced, after DA deamination, via the formation of an aldehyde intermediate, which in turn is enzymatically oxidized to the acid. It has been proposed that DOPAC levels reflect the intraneuronal DA metabolism, and these levels are therefore generally used as a biochemical index of the rate of DA synthesis and turnover (Westerink, 1985). However, due to the apparent absence of MAO in dopaminergic neurons (see above), the exact compartment in which DA deamination occurs is still a matter of debate.

DA can also be converted by COMT into 3-methoxytyramine (3-MT). Since COMT is absent in dopaminergic terminals, 3-MT levels are believed to be an accurate index of extraneuronal DA metabolism and therefore of DA release (Wood and Altar, 1988). The proportion of DA which is directly

A. Napolitano et al.

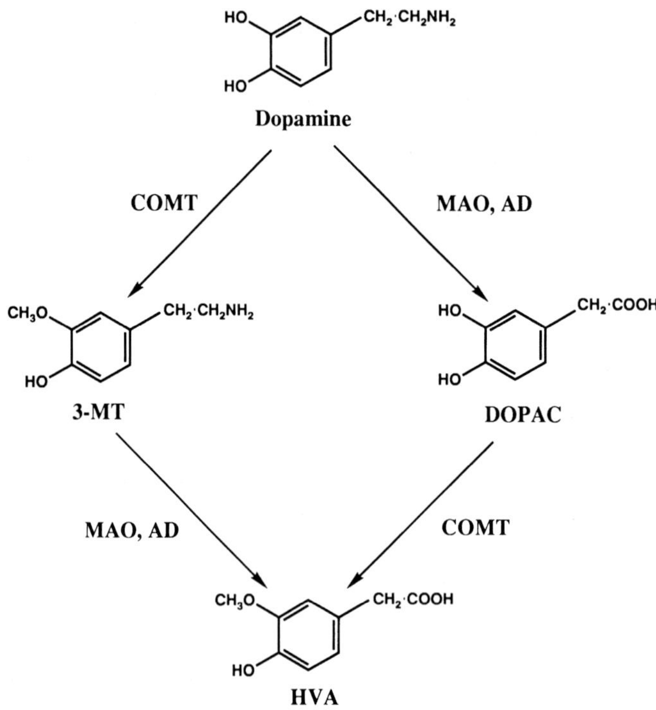

Dopamine

3-MT

DOPAC

HVA

Fig. 1. Dopamine catabolic pathway. *AD* aldehyde dehydrogenase; *COMT* catechol-O-methyltransferase; *DOPAC* 3,4-dihydroxyphenylacetic acid; *HVA* homovanillic acid; *3-MT* 3-methoxytyramine. The structures of the intermediate aldehyde products of monoamino oxidase activity are not shown

O-methylated into 3-MT varies in different dopaminergic areas of the rat brain, accounting for about 15% of released DA in the striatum and in the nucleus accumbens, and for more than 60% in the frontal cortex (Karoum et al., 1994). DOPAC and 3-MT can be then converted into homovanillic acid (HVA) by the action of COMT and MAO, respectively. HVA and dopac are finally actively transported outside the brain and excreted in the urine as O-glucuronated and/or O-sulphated derivatives (Kopin, 1985).

Effects of selective MAO inhibitors on dopamine metabolism

The development of selective and reversible MAO inhibitors (Cesura and Pletscher, 1992) has renewed interest in these drugs for neuropsychiatry, following several years during which the clinical use of irreversible and non-selective inhibitors has been hampered by the fear of fatal brain haemorrage due to the occurrence of sudden hypertensive crises ("cheese-effect") (Da Prada et al., 1988a), as well as by a risk of hepatotoxicity. For several years, our laboratories have been involved in the discovery, characterisation, and development of selective and reversible inhibitors of MAO-A (moclobemide, Aurorix®) (Da Prada et al., 1989), and of MAO-B (lazabemide) cDa Prada et al., 1988b), which are devoid of the side effects typical of the first generation MAO inhibitors.

Microdialysis experiments in rats have proven that the administration of either irreversible (Kato et al., 1986; Butcher et al., 1990) or reversible (Colzi et al., 1993) MAO-A inhibitors leads to an increase in striatal extracellular levels of DA and to a decrease of DOPAC and HVA, whereas MAO-B inhibitors are devoid of any effect on DA metabolism (Kato et al., 1986; Colzi et al., 1990). Interestingly, it has been demonstrated that the destruction of DA neurons by nigral injections of 6-OHDA abolishes the ability of clorgyline to enhance the DA striatal levels, without increasing its deamination by MAO-B (Wachtel and Abercrombie, 1994). Altogether, these data confirm that in the rat the deamination of DA is accomplished almost exclusively by MAO-A and appears to occur in dopaminergic terminals. However, in contrast to the rat, MAO-B activity of the human brain is higher than that of MAO-A (Dostert et al., 1989). For this reason caution has to be taken in using the results obtained in rats for explaining how DA is actually deaminated in man. In addition, we have found that lazabemide is able to potentiate the turning behaviour induced by L-DOPA in 6-OHDA-lesioned rats (Da Prada et al., 1994), suggesting that the role of MAO-B in DA metabolism might become relevant in this species when non-physiologically high levels of DA are produced in the brain after administration of exogenous L-DOPA.

The use of MAO-B inhibitors in PD can also be supported by other arguments. For example, it is well known that MAO-B plays a pivotal role in the neurotoxicity of 1-methyl-4-phenyl-1,2,3,6-tetrahydropyridine (MPTP), by catalyzing its conversion into the toxic metabolite 1-methyl-4-phenyl-pyridinium (Markey et al., 1984; Da Prada et al., 1985). The administration of selective MAO-B inhibitors completely prevents MPTP-induced toxicity (Heikkila et al., 1984; Da Prada et al., 1986). This finding has raised interest in the possible existence of endogenous or environmental MPTP-like neurotoxins which may be activated by MAO-B in a similar manner (Tanner, 1989). It has also been postulated that MAO-B may participate in the formation of oxygen free radicals (oxidative stress) in the aging processes and in some neurodegenerative disorders (Olanow, 1993). Inhibition of MAO-B might therefore decrease the oxidative stress by reducing the formation of hydrogen peroxide generated during MAO-B-mediated oxidative deamination of DA. For this reason, MAO-B inhibitors have been proposed to be neuroprotective. This is consistent with the observation that $(-)$deprenyl seems to delay the onset of disability, necessitating L-DOPA therapy, in de novo PD patients (Tetrud and Langston, 1989; The Parkinson Study Group, 1989). However, the neuroprotective effect of $(-)$deprenyl in humans has not been fully established, since it has been suggested that this drug might exert a "symptomatic" effect, for example by stimulating DA release after its conversion to $(-)$amphetamine and $(-)$metamphetamine (Reynolds et al., 1978). Since lazabemide is more specific than $(-)$deprenyl as MAO-B inhibitor and is not transformed into pharmacologically active metabolites, this compound now provides an ideal tool for clarifying the role played by MAO-B in the metabolism of DA and its putative neuroprotective effect.

COMT inhibitors and dopamine metabolism

In the late 80's, we and two other research groups discovered a new generation of orally active COMT inhibitors (Bäckstrom et al., 1989; Borgulya et al., 1989; Waldemeier et al., 1990). Two of the novel COMT inhibitors, i.e. tolcapone (Ro 40-7592) and entacapone (OR 611) possess a nitrocatechol moiety and are active in vitro in the low nanomolar range (Männistö et al., 1992a). After oral administration in rats, tolcapone and entacapone are able to block the peripheral formation of 3-O-methyldopa (3-OMD) elicited by the administration of L-DOPA combined with peripheral AADC inhibitors, thereby increasing the bioavailability of L-DOPA in plasma and in brain (Zürcher et al., 1990; Männistö et al., 1992b). Tolcapone is able to cross the blood-brain barrier, and to inhibit COMT activity also in the brain (Zürcher et al., 1991), whereas entacapone behaves mainly as a peripheral COMT inhibitor (Nissinen et al., 1992). The third COMT inhibitor under preclinical investigation is CGP 28014. This pyridine derivative does not inhibit COMT in vitro (IC_{50} in the mM range). However in vivo, following L-DOPA administration, this compound behaves as a preferential central COMT inhibitor, decreasing HVA and 3-MT levels without affecting the 3-OMD formation in plasma (Waldemeier et al., 1990; Männistö et al., 1992b). Whether CGP 28014 actually exerts its pharmacological actions through the inhibition of COMT remains to be established (Männistö et al., 1992b).

The availability of central COMT inhibitors has prompted many investigators to use these drugs to clarify the role of COMT in the metabolism of brain DA. Microdialysis studies have shown that the administration of tolcapone to the rat elicits pronounced changes on the striatal levels of DA metabolites, i.e. a decrease of HVA and 3-MT and a concomitant increase of DOPAC, without affecting the levels of the neurotransmitter (Acquas et al., 1992; Brannan et al., 1992). This effect could be explained by the fact that, even under conditions of COMT blockade, DA can be taken up intraneuronally by an active carrier and then deaminated by MAO. In fact, when the carrier system or MAO-A activity are inhibited by nomifensine or clorgyline, respectively, the administration of tolcapone produces an increase of the extracellular DA levels (Kaakkola and Wurtman, 1992).

We have extensively investigated the effect of central COMT blockade on striatal DA output in rats treated with L-DOPA plus benserazide by means of brain microdialysis (Fig. 2). The addition of tolcapone to L-DOPA plus a peripheral AADC inhibitor is reportedly able to enhance the striatal DA outflow more efficiently than entacapone (Kaakkola and Wurtman, 1993). By comparing the effect of the two COMT inhibitors, we were able to confirm the results quoted above. Moreover, we observed that, when tolcapone was co-administered L-DOPA plus benserazide, the formation of 3-MT was markedly reduced, suggesting that, under L-DOPA therapy, the resulting decrease in O-methylation of DA might contribute to potentiation of dopaminergic neurotransmission.

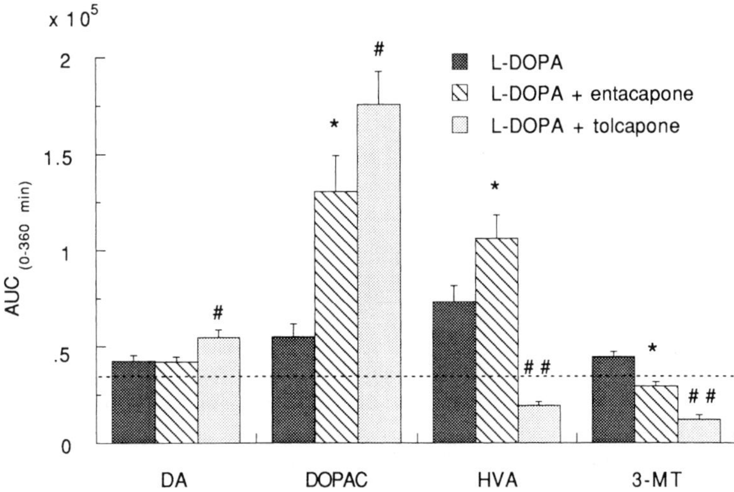

Fig. 2. Comparison of the effect of entacapone (30 mg/kg) and tolcapone (30 mg/kg) on L-DOPA + benserazide (30 + 15 mg/kg)-induced changes in extracellular striatal DA, DOPAC, HVA and 3-MT levels. Data are means ± SEM of 5 rats, expressed as AUC of the percent changes over baseline (= 100). All changes are significant ($p < 0.05$) compared to basal efflux (dashed line). *$p < 0.05$ compared to L-DOPA; [#]$p < 0.05$, [##]$p < 0.01$ compared to L-DOPA and L-DOPA + entacapone (ANOVA for repeated measures followed by Newman-Keuls multiple comparison test)

This conclusion is further supported by behavioural experiments, which demonstrate that tolcapone increases locomotor activity in L-DOPA-treated mice (Maj et al., 1990) and markedly potentiates the turning behaviour in rats unilaterally lesioned with 6-OHDA (Da Prada et al., 1994).

Conclusive remarks

The development of potent and selective inhibitors of the two MAO subtypes and of COMT offers a unique opportunity for the assessment of the actual role played by these enzymes in the metabolism of DA in the CNS of experimental animals, as well as in humans.

The vast preclinical knowledge accumulated in this field has provided the rationale for the use of these drugs in the treatment of PD. The results of the first clinical trials clearly show that COMT inhibitors may represent a breakthrough in the add-on therapy of PD (Limousin et al., 1993; Kaakkola et al., 1994). Ongoing clinical studies with lazabemide in Parkinson's and Alzheimer's patients should clarify the role of MAO-B inhibition in both DA metabolism and neuroprotection.

Finally, the availability of these pharmacological tools should allow the clinician to shape the therapy of PD according to the individual's clinical picture, taking into account other factors such as the presence of concomitant depression.

                         A. Napolitano et al.

Acknowledgement

We would like to thank Dr. D. Hartman for critical reading of the manuscript.

References

Acquas E, Carboni E, de Ree RAH, Da Prada M, Di Chiara G (1992) Extracellular concentrations of dopamine and metabolites in the rat caudate after oral administration of a novel catechol-O-methyl-transferase inhibitor Ro 40-7592. J Neurochem 59: 326–330

Arai R, Kimura H, Maeda T (1986) Topographic atlas of monoamine oxidase-containing neurones in the rat brain studied by an improved histochemical method. Neuroscience 29: 905–925

Bach AJW, Lan NC, Abell CW, Bembenek ME, Kwan SW, Seeburg PH, Shih JC (1988) cDNA cloning of human liver monoamine oxidase A and B: molecular basis for difference in enzymatic properties. Proc Natl Acad Sci USA 85: 4934–4938

Bäckstrom R, Honkanen E, Pippuri A, Kaiarisalo P, Pystynen J, Heinola K, Nissinen E, Linden IB, Männistö PT, Kaakkola S, Pohto P (1989) Synthesis of some novel potent and selective catechol O-methyltransferase inhibitors. J Med Chem 32: 841–846

Bertocci B, Miggiano V, Da Prada M, Dembic Z, Lahm HW, Malherbe P (1991) Human catechol-O-methyltransferase: cloning and expression of the membrane-associated form. Proc Natl Acad Sci USA 88: 1416–1420

Borgulya J, Bruderer H, Bernauer K, Zürcher G, Da Prada M (1989) Catechol-O-methyltransferase-inhibiting pyrocatechol derivatives — synthesis and structure-activity studies. Helv Chim Acta 72: 952–968

Brannan T, Martínez-Tica J, Yahr MD (1992) Catechol-O-methyltransferase inhibition increases striatal L-dopa and dopamine: an in vivo study in rats. Neurology 42: 683–685

Butcher SP, Fairbrother JSK, Arbuthnott GW (1990) Effect of selective monoamine oxidase inhibitors on the in vivo release and metabolism of dopamine in the rat striatum. J Neurochem 55: 981–988

Cesura AM, Pletscher A (1992) The new generation of monoamine oxidase inhibitors. Prog Drug Res 38: 171–297

Colzi A, D'Agostini F, Kettler R, Borroni E, Da Prada M (1990) Effect of selective and reversible MAO inhibitors on dopamine outflow in rat striatum: a microdialysis study. J Neural Transm [Suppl] 32: 79–84

Colzi A, D'Agostini F, Cesura AM, Borroni E, Da Prada M (1993) Monoamine oxidase-A inhibitors and dopamine metabolism in rat caudatus: evidence that an increased cytosolic level of dopamine displaces reversible monoamine oxidase-A inhibitors in vivo. J Pharmacol Exp Ther 265: 103–111

Da Prada M, Cesura A, Kettler R, Zürcher G, Haefely WE (1985) Conversion of the neurotoxic precursor 1-methyl-4-phenyl-1,2,3,6-tetrahydropyridine into its pyridinium metabolite by human platelet monoamine oxidase type B. Neurosci Lett 57: 257–262

Da Prada M, Kettler R, Keller HH, Bonetti P, Imhof R (1986) Ro 16-6491, a new reversible and highly selective MAO-B inhibitor protects mice from the dopaminergic neurotoxicity of MPTP. Adv Neurol 45: 175–178

Da Prada M, Zürcher G, Wüthrich I, Haefely WE (1988a) On tyramine, food, beverages and the reversible MAO inhibitor moclobemide. J Neural Transm [Suppl] 26: 31–56

Da Prada M, Kettler R, Keller HH, Burkard WP (1988b) Ro 19-6327, a reversible highly selective inhibitor of type B monoamine oxidase, completely devoid of tyramine-potentiating effect: comparison with selegiline. In: Dahlström RH, Belmaker RH,

Scholler M (eds) Progress in catecholamine research, part A. Basic aspects and peripheral mechanisms. Alan R Liss, New York, pp 359–363

Da Prada M, Kettler R, Keller HH, Burkard WP, Muggli-Maniglio D, Haefely WE (1989) Neurochemical profile of moclobemide, a short acting and reversible inhibitor of monoamine oxidase type A. J Pharmacol Exp Ther 248: 400–413

Da Prada M, Zürcher G, Kettler R, Dingemanse J, Jorga K, Dubuis R (1994) Remodelling the kinetics and dynamics of levodopa therapy in Parkinson's disease by inhibiting MAO-B with lazabemide and COMT with tolcapone. In: Poewe W, Lees A (eds) Antiparkinson therapy: 20 years of Madopar®. Editiones Roche, Basel, pp 93–111

Dostert PL, Strolin-Benedetti M, Tipton K (1989) Interactions of monoamine oxidases with substrates and inhibitors. Med Res Rev 9: 45–89

Guldberg HC, Marsden CA (1975) Catechol-O-methyl transferase: pharmacological aspects and physiological role. Pharmacol Rev 27: 135–206

Heikkila RE, Manzino L, Cabbat FS, Duvoisin RC (1984) Protection against the dopaminergic neurotoxicity of 1-methyl-4-phenyl-1,2,3,6-tetrahydropyridine by monoamine oxidase inhibitors. Nature 311: 467–469

Hornykiewicz O (1982) Brain neurotransmitter changes in Parkinson's disease. In: Marsden CD, Fahn S (eds) Movement disorders. Butterworth Scientific, London, pp 41–58

Jeffery D, Roth JA (1984) Characterization of membrance-bound and soluble catechol-O-methyltransferase from human frontal cortex. J Neurochem 42: 826–832

Kaakkola S, Wurtman RJ (1992) Effects of catechol-O-methyltransferase inhibitors on striatal dopamine metabolism. Brain Res 587: 241–249

Kaakkola S, Wurtman RJ (1993) Effects of catechol-O-methyltransferase inhibitors and L-3,4-dihydroxyphenylalanine with or without carbidopa on extracellular dopamine in rat striatum. J Neurochem 60: 137–144

Kaakkola S, Männistö PT, Nissinen E (1987) Striatal membrane-bound and soluble catechol-O-methyltransferase after selective neuronal lesions in the rat. J Neural Transm 69: 221–228

Kaakkola S, Teräväinen H, Ahtila S, Rita H, Gordin A (1994) Effect of entacapone, a COMT inhibitor, on clinical disability and levodopa metabolism in parkinsonian patients. Neurology 44: 77–80

Karhunen T, Tilgann C, Ulmanen I, Julkunen I, Panula P (1994) Distribution of catechol-O-methyltransferase enzyme in rat tissues. J Histochem Cytochem 42: 1079–1090

Karoum F, Chrapusta SJ, Egan MF (1994) 3-Methoxytyramine is the major metabolite of released dopamine in the rat frontal cortex: reassessment of the effects of antipsychotics on the dynamics of dopamine release and metabolism in the frontal cortex, nucleus accumbens, and striatum by a simple two pool model. J Neurochem 63: 972–979

Kastner A, Anglade P, Bounaix C, Damier P, Javoy-Agid F, Bromet N, Agid Y, Hirsch EC (1994) Immunohistochemical study of catechol-O-methyltransferase in the human mesostriatal system. Neuroscience (in press)

Kato T, Dong B, Kayoyo I, Kinemuchi H (1986) Brain dialysis: in vivo metabolism of dopamine and serotonin by monoamine oxidase A but not B in the striatum of unrestrained rats. J Neurochem 46: 1277–1282

Kochersperger LM, Parker EL, Siciliano M, Darlinngton GL, Denney RM (1986) Assignement of genes for human monoamine oxidase A and B to the X chromosome. J Neurosci Res 16: 602–616

Kopin IJ (1985) Catecholamine metabolism: basic aspects and clinical significance. Pharmacol Rev 37: 333–364

Limousin P, Pollak P, Gervason-Tournier CL, Hommel M, Perret JE (1993) Ro 40-7592, a COMT inhibitor, plus levodopa in Parkinson's disease. Lancet 341: 1605

Lundström K, Salminen M, Jalanko A, Savolainen R, Ulmanen I (1991) Cloning and characterization of human placental catechol-O-methyltransferase cDNA. DNA Cell Biol 10: 181–189

Maj J, Rogóz Z, Szuka G, Sowinska H, Superata J (1990) Behavioural and neurochemical effects of Ro 40-7592, a new COMT inhibitor with a potential therapeutic activity in Parkinson's disease. J Neural Transm [PD Sect] 2: 101–112

Männistö PT, Ulmanen I, Lundström K, Taskinen J, Tenhunen J, Kaakkola S (1992a) Characteristics of catechol-O-methyltransferase (COMT) and properties of selective inhibitors. Prog Drug Res 39: 291–350

Männistö PT, Tuomainen P, Tuominen RK (1992b) Different in vivo properties of three new inhibitors of catechol-O-methyltransferase in the rat. Br J Pharmacol 105: 569–574

Markey SP, Johannessen CC, Chieu RS, Burns MA, Herkenham MA (1984) Intraneuronal generation of a pyridinium metabolite may induce drug-induced parkinsonism. Nature 311: 464–467

Nissinen E, Linden IB, Schultz E, Pohto P (1992) Biochemical and pharmacological properties of a peripherally acting catechol-O-methyltransferase inhibitor, entacapone. Naunyn Schmiedebergs Arch Pharmacol 346: 262–266

Olanow CW (1993) A rationale for monoamine oxidase inhibition as neuroprotective therapy for Parkinson's disease. Mov Dis 8: S1–S7

Reynolds GP, Elsworth JD, Blau K, Sandler M, Lees AJ, Stern JM (1978) Deprenyl is metabolised to methamphetamine and amphetamine in man. Br J Pharmacol 6: 542–544

Roth JA (1992) Membrane-bound catechol-O-methyltransferase: a re-evaluation of its role in the O-methylation of catecholamine neurotransmitters. Physiol Biochem Pharmacol 120: 1–29

Salminen M, Lundström K, Tilgmann C, Savolainen R, Kalkkinen N, Ulmanen I (1990) Molecular cloning and characterization of rat liver catechol-O-methyltransferase. Gene 93: 241–247

Saura J, Kettler R, Da Prada M, Richards JG (1992) Quantitative enzyme radioautography with (^{3}H)Ro 41-1049 and (^{3}H)Ro 19-6327 in vitro: localization and abundance of MAO-A and MAO-B in rat CNS, peripheral organs and human brain. J Neurosci 12: 1977–1992

Tanner CM (1989) The role of environmental toxins in the etiology of Parkinson's disease. TINS 12: 49–54

Tetrud JW, Langton JW (1989) The effect of deprenyl (selegiline) on the natural history of Parkinson's disease. Science 41: 519–522

The Parkinson Study Group (1989) Effect of deprenyl on the progression of disability in early Parkinson's disease. N Engl J Med 321: 1364–1371

Tilgmann C, Melen K, Lundström K, Jalanko A, Julkunen I, Kalkkinen U, Ulmanen I (1992) Expression of recombinant soluble and membrane-bound catechol O-methyltransferase in eukaryotic cells and identification of the respective enzymes in rat brain. Eur J Biochem 207: 813–821

Wachtel SR, Abercrombie ED (1994) L-3,4-Dihydroxyphenylalanine-induced dopamine release in the striatum of intact and 6-hydroxydopamine-treated rats: differential effects of monoamine oxidase A and B inhibitors. J Neurochem 63: 108–117

Waldemeier PC (1987) Amine oxidases and their endogenous substrates. J Neural Transm [Suppl] 23: 55–72

Waldemeier PC, Baumann PA, Feldtrauer JJ, Hauser K, Bittiger H, Bischoff S, von Sprecher G (1990) CGP 28014, a new inhibitor of cerebral catechol-O-methylation with a non-catechol structure. Naunyn Schmiedebergs Arch Pharmacol 342: 305–311

Westerink BHC (1985) Sequence and significance of dopamine metabolism in the rat brain. Neurochem Int 7: 221–227

Westlund KN, Denney LM, Rose RM, Abell CW (1988) Localization of distinct monoamine oxidase A and monoamine oxidase B cell populations in human brainstem. Neuroscience 26: 791–802

Wood PL, Altar AC (1988) Dopamine release in vivo from nigrostriatal, mesolimbic, and mesocortical neurons: utility of 3-methoxytyramine measurements. Pharmacol Rev 40: 163–187

Zürcher G, Keller HH, Kettler R, Borgulya J, Bonetti EP, Eigenmann R, Da Prada M
  (1990) Ro 40-7592, a novel, very potent, and orally active inhibitor of catechol-O-
  methyltransferase: a pharmacological study in rats. Adv Neurol 53: 497–503
Zürcher G, Dingemanse J, Da Prada M (1991) Ro 40-7592, a potent inhibitor of extracerebral and brain catechol-O-methyltransferase: preclinical and clinical findings. In:
  Agnoli A, Campanella G (eds) New developments in therapy of Parkinson's disease.
  John Libbey CIC, Roma, pp 37–43

Authors' address: Dr. A. M. Cesura, Pharma Division, Preclinical Research, F.
Hoffmann-La Roche Ltd, PRPN 70/308, CH-4002 Basel, Switzerland.

J Neural Transm (1995) [Suppl] 45: 47–55

Basic research in substantia nigra and ventral tegmental area: clinical implications

F. Stratta, A. Bonci, P. Calabresi, A. Stefani, A. Pisani, G. Bernardi,
and **N. B. Mercuri**

Clinica Neurologica, Università di Tor Vergata, Roma, Italy

Summary. In this review we will briefly examine some physiological and pharmacological aspects of the dopaminergic and non-dopaminergic cells of the midbrain in relationship to pathological conditions such as extrapyramidal disorders, mental illness, drug seeking behaviour and epilepsy.

Introduction

In the last decade the neurons of ventral midbrain have been among the most intensively studied cells of the central nervous system. Of particular interest is their involvement in motor and motivational behaviour and in the control of seizures. Two types of cells have been described in the ventral mesencephalon, the dopaminergic and the non-dopaminergic ones (mainly GABAergic).

The dopaminergic cells of the substantia nigra pars compacta (SNc) and ventral tegmental area (VTA) send projections to various brain areas (e.g. striatum, nucleus accumbens, anterior cingulate nucleus, pyriform and prefrontal cortex) and account for more than 80% of brain dopamine (DA) content. The non-DAergic cells, located in the substantia nigra pars reticulata and in the ventral tegmental area, mainly project to the thalamus, the superior colliculus and pedunculopontine nucleus.

Our knowledge on the physiology and the pathology of DAergic cells has been recently improved by anatomical, biochemical, pharmacological and electrophysiological investigations. The effects of DA in central nervous system were previously thought to be mediated by the activation of two types of receptors, conventionally called D1 and D2. The D2 receptors gained an early interest because they were involved with identifiable effects. It clearly appeared that the blockade of D2 receptors by drugs (e.g. haloperidol or chlorpromazine) produces not only antipsychotic but also extrapyramidal side effects in humans. From these and other findings it appeared that DA is involved in motor, motivational and cognitive processes. The role of the D1 receptor has been instead a Cinderella for neuroscientists. However, pharmacological and electrophysiological studies have recently demonstrated that the

D1 receptors may cooperate with the effects mediated by D2 receptors (Clark and White, 1987; Calabresi et al., 1992; Robertson, 1992). However, this is still a simple view of the complex function of DA in the brain. In fact, recent molecular and biological studies have shown that more than two types of DA receptors exist. They have been finally divided in two subfamily (Seeman, 1992). The D1 subfamily comprehending the classical D1 and the D5 receptors, and the D2 subfamily, including the classical D2, D3 and D4 receptors. A further complication in the comprehension of the whole effect of DA arises from the different localisation of DAergic receptors in different brain areas and on individual cells. For example, it is well known that not only postsynaptic but also pre-synaptic DA receptors exist localised on the nerve terminals and/or the soma and the dendrites of the DA-containing neurons (DA autoreceptors).

Besides the effects mediated by the DAergic cells there are those mediated by the non-DAergic cells of the substantia nigra pars reticulata and the ventral tegmental area. It is well established that these neurons play a key role in the control of movement and are the "common denominator" for the GABAergic mechanisms that limit the tonic and clonic seizures originating in various brain areas (Morimoto and Goddard, 1987; Gale, 1989).

In this brief presentation we will present a small account on the basic research upon themes such as:

— Parkinson's disease and extrapyramidal disorders
— mental illnesses
— drugs of abuse
— epilepsy

which involve DAergic and non-DAergic mechanisms in the ventral mesencephalon.

Parkinson's disease and extrapyramidal disorders

The general notion of "extrapyramidal disorders", as originally formulated, implies a constellation of clinical patterns which are the result of an impaired function of the basal ganglia nuclei.

The term basal ganglia is referred to the striatum (caudate and putamen) and paleostriatum (globus pallidus). Modern conceptions contain also the ventral anterior and lateral nuclei of thalamus and the two divisions of the substantia nigra (pars compacta and pars reticulata) which are functionally connected with the basal ganglia. Since about 70% of total brain DA is localised in the basal ganglia, Carlsson et al. (1959) suggested that this catecholamine might play a key role in the normal "extrapyramidal" motor function. They have found that the catalepsy syndrome in reserpinized animals, was reversed by the exogenous administration of the precursor of DA, L-dopa. Following this early observation subsequent studies have reported a marked diminished DA content in the caudate, putamen and pallidum of brain from patients with both post encephalitic and idiopathic Parkinson's disease. The clinical efficacy of DL-dopa (Birkmayer et al.,

1961; Barbeau et al., 1962) and subsequently the better efficacy of L-dopa (Cotzias et al., 1969) given orally to patients with Parkinson's disease, were confirmed by numerous trials in the late sixties. Accordingly, clinical research quickly become focused upon attempts to augment central DA function. Animal models of Parkinson's disease have been oriented to understand the role of the DAergic neurons in the control of movement. In fact, the unilateral lesion of the substantia nigra in rodents induces a circling behaviour that is reversed by the exogenous administration of DA agonists (Ungerstedt, 1971). More recently it has been discovered that a piperidine derivative, 1-methyl-4-phenyl-1,2,3,6-tetrahydropyridine (MPTP), shows a very selective toxicity for pigmented nigrostriatal DAergic neurons (Snyder and d'Amato, 1986; Di Monte and Smith, 1988) and is capable of inducing a behavioural state, in primate and rodents, that bears striking resemblance to Parkinson's disease. Modern hypothesis on the pathogenesis of Parkinson's disease, suggests an impaired function of the mitochondrial respiratory chain in the substantia nigra that might be linked with abnormal iron metabolism and impaired detoxification of free radicals (Jenner, 1989). In particular several studies have reported a defect of the mitochondrial Complex I (NADH dehydrogenase) in the substantia nigra of Parkinson's disease patients, but the mechanisms responsible for this selective vulnerability is still unclear.

It has been primarily assumed that the striatum is the site of action of DA formed from levodopa. Behavioural, pharmacological and clinical investigations have postulated that the activation of D2 receptors participates to a greater extent than the D1 receptors in reversing parkinsonian symptoms (Seeman, 1980; Clark and White, 1987).

DA is released from the axon terminals of the DA containing neurons in the striatum and from the dendrites of the same cell in the substantia nigra itself (Cubeddu et al., 1979; Cheramy et al., 1981). The activation of the D2 striatal receptors may control the release of glutamate from cortico-striatal fibers and may inhibit the amount of acetylcholine released from striatal interneurons. The stimulation of D1 receptors located on the terminals of the striato-nigral cells increases the release of GABA and may have additional implications for the treatment of Parkinson's disease. The stimulation of DA autoreceptors can inhibit the evoked release of DA into postsynaptic regions. Recently in vitro electrophysiological findings from nigral slices, have delineated the basic mechanisms of DA and DAergic drugs on single neurons (Mercuri et al., 1989a). It is now quite clear that DA D2 receptor activate a GTP-binding protein that opens K+ channels to inhibit substantia nigra pars compacta neurons (Lacey et al., 1987). These findings support the idea that the therapeutic administration of DAergic drugs in parkinsonian patients leads to the inhibition of the remaining mesencephalic DA neurons. Accordingly, electrophysiological studies have demonstrated that L-dopa induces a depression of the substantia nigra zona compacta activity and this depression is due to the activation of D2 autoreceptors (Mercuri et al., 1990). A recent electrophysiological study has shown that the activation of D1 receptors in the substantia nigra enhances the inhibitory potential caused by GABA release on the DAergic cells (Cameron and Williams, 1993).

Thus, there is a synergistic inhibition of the DAergic cells by the stimulation of both D1 and D2 receptors in the substantia nigra. In fact, D2 autoreceptors inhibit DA cells by opening K^+ channels while D1 receptors inhibit the same cells by releasing GABA from striato-nigral boutons. The DAergic mechanisms described above may have implications not only in Parkinson's disease but also in normal and pathological conditions (such as Huntington's chorea).

Additionally, the loss of DAergic neurons in Parkinson's disease is associated with a global disorganisation of basal ganglia activity and, in particular, with an increased activity of the excitatory glutamatergic neurons in the subthalamic nucleus and the substantia nigra. Furthermore, electro-physiological studies have shown that agonists of glutamate receptors, excite DAergic neurons (Mercuri et al., 1992a,b, 1993). More recently other studies have demonstrated that parkinsonian symptoms can be alleviated by selective lesioning of the subthalamic nucleus in monkeys treated with MPTP. These studies support the hypothesis that the subthalamic nucleus and its excitatory projections have an important role in the mechanisms sustaining the expression of the parkinsonian motor changes (Benazzouz et al., 1993).

Mental illnesses

Schizophrenia

The key role of DA in the pathophysiology of schizophrenia was first hypothesised with the induction of paranoid schizophreniform psychosis by DAergic agonists (Randrup and Munkvad, 1965; Snyder et al., 1974) and with the inhibition of the DAergic activity produced by neuroleptics (Seeman et al., 1974, 1976; Carlsson, 1978). The DAergic hypothesis of schizophrenia (Matthysse, 1973) proposes that a hyper-DAergic state is the main responsible for the clinical expression of the disease. Furthermore, receptor binding techniques have demonstrated that the clinical potency of antipsychotic drugs was correlated with their affinity for the D2 receptors (Creese et al., 1975). Since its original conception, this hypothesis was submitted to revisions (Snyder et al., 1974; Seeman, 1987; Carlsson and Carlsson, 1990a; Davis et al., 1991), mainly because of the clear evidence that schizophrenia is a heterogeneous clinical entity. In particular, it was suggested that an increased DA activity and the schizophrenic symptoms may originate from a primary abnormality of serotonin, norepinephrine, glutamate and GABA receptors (Reynolds, 1989; Stein and Wise, 1971; Roberts, 1972), consequently schizophrenia could result from an imbalance between DA and other neurotransmitters. The problem is still unsolved, but the identification of new DA receptors subtypes with different anatomical localizations (Sunahara, 1990; Van Tol et al., 1991; Seeman, 1993) and the demonstration that atypical antipsychotic drugs like clozapine, with a high affinity for D_4 receptors have a great efficacy in reducing the negative symptoms of schizophrenia, have produced new impetus for the DA hypothesis of schizophrenia. The firing of the DAergic cells is certainly important to regulate the DAergic tone in cortical and subcortical regions (Grace, 1991), thus an abnormally intensified DA response due to a disfunction of these neurons may be proposed to underlie part of the symptoms of this disease.

Depression

The hypothesis suggesting DA as implicated in depression was formulated more than 15 years ago. DAergic neurons ascending from the VTA project to the limbic areas (nucleus accumbens, olfactory tubercle, septum) and cortical areas (cingulate, enthorinal, prefrontal and pyriform cortex) and form the mesolimbic and mesocortical pathways. It is well known that these DAergic pathways are involved in the modulation of a behavioural pattern related to motivation and reward. This could be involved in clinical manifestations of depression, since lack of motivation is one of the main symptoms of the disease. Depression is very difficult to be reproduced in animals; a model currently used is the "learned helplessness" (Sherman et al., 1982). The animals are exposed to stressors agents and consequently express a series of behavioural symptoms; a) decreased effort to escape, b) diminished spontaneous activity, c) defects in the reward systems. It has been demonstrated that DA is reduced in the accumbens and striatum of animal in which "learned helplessness" was induced. Moreover, DA antagonists increased the behavioural effects in conditioned animals and prevented the improvement induced by antidepressant drugs (for a rev. see Willner, 1983a,b,c). However, it is problematic to evaluate the connection between the behavioural changes in conditioned rats and the negative fluctuations of the mood in depressed patients. The most consistent finding that supports the hypothesis of a DA involvement in depressed patients is the observation of a decreased turnover of DA in patients affected by depressive disorders (Papeschi and Mc Clure, 1971; Van Praag and Korf, 1971). On the other hand, evaluations of homovanillic acid (HVA), the major metabolite of DA, in cerebrospinal fluid have shown both increase and decrease of it in some depressed patients (Papeschi and Mc Clure, 1971; Van Praag and Korf, 1971; Jimerson, 1987). Apart from that, there is good agreement that the meso-limbic and the nigro-striatal system are underactive in producing the symptomatology of depression. Recent biochemical and electrophysiological findings have also demonstrated that amineptine, a tricyclic antidepressant drug currently used to treat depressed patients, increases the level of DA in the brain by inhibiting the neuronal DA uptake system (Bonnet et al., 1987). Electrophysiological evidence have also shown that this antidepressant is able to inhibit the activity of DA cells in the substantia nigra by elevating the DAergic tone in this structure (Mercuri et al., 1991). This pharmacological result supports the assumption that an increase in the level of DA in the central nervous system exerts an antidepressant action.

F. Stratta et al.

Drugs of abuse

Recent experimental evidences have suggested that the drug-seeking behaviour is the "end-point" common to many drugs such as cocaine, amphetamine, nicotine, ethanol (Stolerman, 1992). The positive reinforcing effects of these drugs are the main responsible for the maintenance of addiction. The increased content of DA in the terminal of the meso-limbic and meso-cortical pathways is known to be essential for self-administration of all drugs of abuse and is considered to be the main cause of reinforcement. Experimental results have suggested that DA transporter, located on the DAergic meso-limbic and meso-cortical neurons, is crucial for the reinforcing properties of drugs (Kuhar et al., 1991). It has been shown by electrophysiological experiments, that cocaine inhibits DA re-uptake and potentiates DAergic transmission (Lacey et al., 1990). In addition, amphetamine has been reported to augment the DAergic tone by increasing the efflux of neuronal DA (Mercuri et al., 1989b). An involvement of midbrain DA neurons in the reinforcing properties of ethanol and nicotine has also been demonstrated by several studies (Calabresi, 1989; Koob, 1992). A good animal model for brain rewarding is also represented by the intracranial self-stimulation of the ventral tegmental area by electrical stimuli in animals. The activation of the DAergic neurons in this area mediates some of the rewarding properties of the electrical stimulation obtained from this brain region (Fibiger et al., 1987).

Epilepsy

Recent studies have shown that the substantia nigra pars reticulata acts as a gating system in the control of motor and limbic seizures (Gale, 1988, 1989; Roberts, 1986). In the early life this structure plays a crucial role in regulating seizures expression. Nigral GABAergic transmission, and particularly $GABA_A$ receptor, seems to be a key factor in controlling seizure suppression (Gale, 1992) with an age-dependent manner (Moshè and Sperber, 1990). The $GABA_A$ receptor is present in two subtypes (low and high affinity binding sites) and is constituted by subunits with several isoforms ($\alpha1$, $\alpha2$, $\beta1$, γ etc). Ontogenetic alterations in the nigral $\alpha1$ isoform may contribute to developmental differences in seizures expression. Intranigral infusion of muscimol, a $GABA_A$ agonist, is proconvulsant in young rats while in adult rats is anticonvulsant (Moshé, 1984). Based on this and other results, it has been suggested that a maturational switch in $GABA_A$ high-affinity receptor gene expression is associated with decreased seizure susceptibility in the mature CNS. With brain age-related maturation the anticonvulsant high-affinity isoform constitutes the majority of the high affinity binding sites (Moshè, 1993). Moreover it is known that GABAergic nigral system expression changes with following seizures. It has been proposed that midbrain GABAergic cells control seizure propagation regardless of the mechanisms responsible for convulsion initiation (Gale, 1989). Thus, an imbalance of the excitation/inhibition of the substantia nigra pars reticulata may determine seizure generalisation.

Acknowledgements

We thank G. Gattoni and M. Tolu for their excellent technical assistance.

References

Barbeau A, Murphy GF, Sourkes TL (1962) Les catecholamines dopamine dans la maladie de Parkinson. In: de Ajuriaguerra J (ed) Monoamines et systeme nerveux central. Georg, Geneva, pp 247–262

Benazzouz A, Gross C, Feger J, Boraud T, Bioulac B (1993) Reversal rigidity and improvement in motor performance by subthalamic high-frequency stimulation in MPTP-treated monkeys. Eur J Neurosci 1: 382–389

Birkmayer W, Hornykiewicz O (1961) Der L-Dioxyphenylalanin-(L-Dopa) Effekt bei der Parkinson — Akinese. Wien Klin Wochenschr 73: 787–788

Bonnet JJ, Chagraoui A, Protais P, Constentin J (1987) Interaction of amineptine with the neuronal dopamine up-take system: neurochemical in vitro and in vivo studies. J Neural Transm 69: 211–220

Calabresi P, Lacey MG, North RA (1989) Nicotinic excitation of rat ventral tegmental neurones in vitro studied by intracellular recording. Br J Pharmacol 98: 135–140

Calabresi P, Maj R, Mercuri NB, Bernardi G (1992) Coactivation of D1 and D2 dopamine receptors is required for long-term depression in neostriatum. Neurosci Lett 142: 95–99

Cameron D, Williams JT (1993) Dopamine D1 receptors facilitate transmitter release. Nature 336: 344–347

Carlsson A (1959) The occurrence, distribution and physiological role of catecholamines in the nervous system. Pharmacol Rev 11: 490–493

Carlsson A (1978) Antipsychotic drugs, neurotransmitter and schizophrenia. Am J Psychiatry 135: 164–173

Carlsson M, Carlsson A (1990) Schizophrenia: a subcortical neurotransmitter imbalance system? Schizophr Bull 16: 425–432

Cheramy A, Leviel V, Glowinski J (1981) Dendritic release of dopamine in the substantia nigra. Nature 269: 537–542

Clark D, White FJ (1987) Review: dopamine receptor — the search for a function: a critical evaluation of the D1/D2 dopamine receptor a classification and its functional implications. Synapse 1: 347–388

Cotzias GC, Papavasiliou PS, Gellene R (1969) Modification of Parkinsonism-chronic treatment with L-dopa. N Engl J Med 280: 337–345

Creese I, Burt DR, Snyder SH (1976) Dopamine receptor binding predicts clinical and pharmacological potencies of antischizophrenics drugs. Science 192: 481–483

Cubeddu LX, Hoffmann IS, Ferrari GB (1979) Metabolism and efflux of [3H]dopamine in rat neostriatum: presynaptic origin of [3,4-3H]dihydroxyphenylacetic acid. J Pharmacol Exp Ther 209: 165–175

Davis KL, Kann RS, Ko G, Davidson M (1991) Dopamine and schizophrenia: a review and a reconceptualization. Am J Psychiatry 148: 1474–1486

Di Monte D, Smith MT (1988) Free radicals, lipid peroxidation and 1-methyl-4-1,2,3,6-tetrahydropyridine (MPTP)-induced parkinsonism. Rev Neurosci 2: 67–81

Fibiger HC, Le Piane FG, Jakubovic A, Philips AG (1987) The role of dopamine in intracranial self-stimulation of the ventral tegmental area. J Neurosci 7: 3888–3896

Filloux FM, Wamsley JK, Dawson TM (1987) Dopamine D2 auto and postsynaptic receptors in the nigrostriatal system of the rat brain: localization by quantitative autoradiography with [3H]sulpiride. Eur J Pharmacol 138: 61–68

Gale K (1985) Mechanisms of seizures control mediated by gaba-aminobutyric acid: role of the substantia nigra. Fed Proc 44: 2414–2424

Gale K (1989) GABA in epilepsy: the pharmacologic basis. Epilepsia 30: S1–S11

Gale K (1992) Subcortical structures and pathways involved in convulsive seizures generalisation. J Clin Neurophysiol 9: 264–277

Grace AA (1991) Phasic versus tonic dopamine release and the modulation of dopamine system responsivity: a hypothesis for the aetiology of schizophrenia. Neuroscience 41: 1–24

Jenner P (1989) Clues to the mechanisms underlying dopamine cell death in Parkinson's disease. J Neurol Neurosurg Psychiatry 52: S22–S28

Jimerson DC (1987) Role of dopamine mechanisms in the affective disorders. In: Meltzer HY (ed) Psychopharmacology: the third generation of progress. Raven Press, New York, pp 505–511

Koob GF (1992) Drugs of abuse: anatomy, pharmacology and function of reward pathways. TIPS 13: 177–184

Kuhar MJ, Ritz MC, Boja JW (1991) The dopamine hypothesis of the reinforcing properties of cocaine. TINS 14(7)

Lacey MG, Mercuri NB, North RA (1987) Dopamine acts on D2 receptors to increase potassium conductance in neurones of the rat substantia nigra zona compacta. J Physiol (Lond) 392: 397–416

Lacey MG, Mercuri NB, North RA (1990) Actions of cocaine on rat dopaminergic neurons in vitro. Br J Pharmacol 99: 731–735

Mercuri NB, Calabresi P, Bernardi G (1989a) Physiology and pharmacology of dopamine D2-receptors: their implications in dopamine-substitute therapy for Parkinson's disease. Neurology 39: 1106–1108

Mercuri NB, Calabresi P, Bernardi G (1989b) The mechanisms of amphetamine induced inhibition of rat substantia nigra compacta neurones investigated with intracellular recordings in vitro. Br J Pharmacol 98: 127–134

Mercuri NB, Calabresi P, Bernardi G (1990) Responses of rat substantia nigra compacta neurones to L-DOPA. Br J Pharmacol 100: 257–260

Mercuri NB, Stratta F, Calabresi P, Bernardi G (1991) Electrophysiological effect of amineptine on neurones of the rat substantia nigra pars compacta: evidence for an inhibition of the dopamine uptake system. Br J Pharmacol 104: 700–704

Mercuri NB, Stratta F, Calabresi P, Bernardi G (1992a) A voltage-clamp analysis of MNDA-induced responses on dopaminergic neurons of the rat substantia nigra zona compacta and ventral tegmental area. Brain Res 593: 51–56

Mercuri NB, Stratta F, Calabresi P, Bernardi G (1992b) Electrophysiological evidence for the presence of ionotropic and metabotropic excitatory amino acid receptors on dopaminergic neurons of the rat mesencephalon: an in vitro study. Funct Neurol 7: 231–234

Mercuri NB, Stratta F, Calabresi P, Bonci A, Bernardi G (1993) Activation of metabotropic glutamate receptors induces an inward current in rat dopamine mesencephalic neurons. Neuroscience 56:2: 399–407

Morimoto K, Goddard GV (1987) The substantia nigra is an important site for the containment of seizure generalisation in the kindling model of epilepsy. Epilepsia 28(1): 1–10

Moshé SL (1993) Seizure in the developing brain. Neurology 43: S3–S7

Moshé SL, Albala BJ (1984) Nigral muscimol infusions facilitate the development of seizures in immature rats. Dev Brain Res 13: 305–308

Moshé SL, Sperber EF (1990) Substantia nigra-mediated control of generalized seizures. In: Gloor G, Koustopulos R, Naquet M, Avoli P (eds) Generalized epilepsy: cellular, molecular and pharmacological approaches. Birkhäuser, Boston, pp 355–367

Papeschi R, Mc Clure DJ (1971) Homovanillic acid and 5-hidroxindoleacetic acid in cerebrospinal fluid of depressed patients. Arch Gen Psychiatry 25: 354–358

Randrup A, Munkvad I (1965) Special antagonism of amphetamine-induced abnormal behaviour. Psychopharmacology 7: 416–422

Reynolds GP (1989) Beyond the dopamine hypothesis. The neurochemical pathology of schizophrenia. Br J Psychiatry 155: 305–316

Roberts E (1972) An hypothesis suggesting that there is a defect in the GABA system in schizophrenia. Neurosci Res Prog Bull 10: 468–481

Roberts E (1986) Failure of GABA-ergic inhibition: a key to local and global seizures. In: Delgado-Escuete AV, Ward AAJ, Woodbury DM, Porter RJ (eds) Advances in neurology. Raven Press, New York, pp 319–341

Robertson HA (1992) Dopamine receptors interactions: some implications for treatment of Parkinson's disease. TINS 15: 201–206

Seeman P (1980) Brain dopamine receptors. Pharmacol Rev 32: 229–313

Seeman, P (1987) Dopamine receptor and the dopamine hypothesis of schizophrenia. Synapse 1: 133–152

Seeman P (1992) Review: dopamine receptor sequences. Therapeutic levels of neuroleptics which occupy D2 receptors, Clozapine occupies D4. Neuropsychopharmacology 7: 261–284

Seeman P, Wong M, Lee T (1974) Dopamine-receptor block and nigral fiber impulse blockade by major tranquillisers. Fed Proc 33: 246

Seeman P, Lee T, Chau Wong M, Wong K (1976) Antipsychotic drugs doses and neuroleptic/dopamine receptors. Nature 261: 717–719

Seeman P, Guan HC, Van Tol UHM, Nizkin H (1993) Low density of dopamine D4 receptor in Parkinson's, schizophrenia, and control brain striata. Synapse 14: 247–253

Sherman AD, Sacquitne JL, Petty F (1982) Specificity of the learned helplessness model of depression. Pharmacol Biochem Behav 16: 449–454

Snyder SH, D'Amato RJ (1986) MPTP: a neurotoxin relevant to the pathophysiology of Parkinson's disease. Neurology 36: 250–258

Snyder S, Banergee S, Yamamura H (1974) Drugs, neurotransmitters and schizophrenia. Science 184: 1243–1253

Stein N, Wise CD (1971) Possible aetiology of schizophrenia: progressive damage to the noradrenergic reward system by 5-hydroxy-dopamine. Science 171: 1032–1036

Stolerman I (1992) Drugs of abuse: behavioural principles, methods and terms. Tips 13: 170–176

Sunahara RK, Guan HC, O'Dowd BF, Seeman P, Laurier LG, Ng G, George S, Torchia J, Van Tol HHM, Nizkin HB (1991) Cloning of the gene for a human dopamine D5 receptor with high affinity for dopamine than D1. Nature 350: 614–619

Ungerstedt U (1971) Striatal dopamine release after amphetamine or nerve degeneration revealed by rotational behaviour. Acta Physiol Scand 367: 49–68

Van Praag HM, Korf J (1971) Retarded depression and the dopamine metabolism. Psychopharmacologia 19: 199–203

Van Tol HHM, Bunzow JR, Guan HC, Sunahara RK, Seeman P, Niznik HB, Civelli O (1991) Cloning of the human dopamine D4 receptor gene with high affinity for the antipsychotic clozapine. Nature 350: 614–619

Willner P (1983a) Dopamine and depression: a review of recent evidence. I Empirical studies. Brain Res Rev 6: 211–224

Willner P (1983b) Dopamine and depression: a review of recent evidence. II. Theoretical approaches. Brain Res Rev 6: 225–236

Willner P (1983c) Dopamine and depression: a review of recent evidence. III. The effects of antidepressant treatments. Brain Res Rev 6: 237–246

Authors' address: Dr. N. B. Mercuri, Clinica Neurologica, Dipartimento di Sanità Pubblica, Università di Roma — Tor Vergata, Via di Tor Vergata 135, I-00133 Roma, Italy.

J Neural Transm (1995) [Suppl] 45: 57–60

Does treatment with dopamine agonists affect utilization of exogenous levodopa in the parkinsonian striatum?

E. Melamed

Department of Neurology, Beilinson Medical Center, and The Felsenstein Research Institute, Petah Tiqva, and The Sackler Faculty of Medicine, Tel Aviv University, Tel Aviv, Israel

Summary. When the nigrostriatal projection is partially destroyed in Parkinson's disease, remaining neurons fire more rapidly and accelerate synthesis and release of dopamine (DA) from endogenous tyrosine and levodopa. It was suggested that such surviving hyperactive nigral neurons can also enhance the utilization of exogenous levodopa and generate adequate amounts of functional dopamine molecules to correct the reduced nigrostriatal neurotransmission. DA agonists stimulate presynaptic DA receptors and suppress nigrostriatal firing rates. Many parkinsonians are treated with a combination of DA agonists and levodopa. This could theoretically suppress both discharge of surviving dopaminergic neurons and their ability to convert exogenous levodopa to dopamine. To test this possibility, rats were injected i.p. with lisuride, bromocriptine or apomorphine alone or one hour after levodopa and decapitated one hour later. The DA agonists suppressed striatal DOPAC and DOPAC/DA ratios indicating attenuation of basic DA turnover. DA agonists given with levodopa did not decrease the levodopa-induced elevations in striatal levodopa, DA and DOPAC. Findings suggest that agonists do not affect entry of levodopa from the circulation into brain and do not alter striatal generation of DA from exogenous levodopa despite inhibition of nigrostriatal firing. Therefore, utilization of levodopa does not seem to depend on the state of discharge rates of nigral neurons and effect of levodopa and DA agonists in Parkinson's disease is additive.

Introduction

Levodopa remains the most potent and widely-used antiparkinsonian medication. Exogenous levodopa is absorbed from the gut into the circulation and traverses the blood brain barrier into brain parenchyma (better with combined administration of peripheral dopa decarboxylase inhibitors). In the striatum (caudate and putamen nuclei), it is converted to dopamine, replenishes the reduced levels of this chemical and corrects the suppressed nigrostriatal dopaminergic neurotransmission. It is not fully established where precisely in the parkinsonian striatum, exogenous levodopa is decarboxylated to dopamine after massive loss of nigrostriatal nerve-terminals and their content of the enzyme dopa decarboxylase (Melamed et al., 1980).

In Parkinson's disease, when the nigrostriatal projection is partially destroyed, the remaining neurons fire more rapidly and accelerate rates of synthesis and release of dopamine from endogenous tyrosine and levodopa (Agid et al., 1973; Bernheimer et al., 1975; Hefti et al., 1980). It was suggested that such surviving hyperactive nigral neurons can also enhance utilization of exogenous levodopa despite their small numbers and generate adequate amounts of functional, receptor accessible dopamine molecules to restore the sluggish nigrostriatal transmission (Hornykiewicz, 1974). This would support the theory that remaining dopaminergic neurons represent the major site for satisfactory conversion of exogenous levodopa to dopamine and the resultant clinical benefit in Parkinson's disease.

Many patients with Parkinson's disease are currently receiving combined treatment with levodopa and dopamine agonists either early or late in their illness to prevent or improve levodopa-associated response fluctuations, respectively. Dopamine agonists including bromocriptine, apomorphine or lisuride, stimulate presynaptic dopaminergic receptors located on the nerve endings in the striatum and thus suppress firing and dopamine turnover (synthesis and release) in nigrostriatal neurons (Bunney et al., 1973; Starke et al., 1978; Hanubrich and Pflueger, 1982). Theoretically, dopamine agonists can also attenuate the firing rates of the surviving hyperactive dopaminergic neurons and thus suppress utilization of exogenous levodopa in the parkinsonian striatum. We, therefore, examined the effects of combined administration of levodopa with dopamine agonists on levodopa-induced elevations of dopamine, its metabolite dihydroxyphenylacetic acid (DOPAC) and levodopa itself in rat striatum.

Materials and methods

Male albino rats (Hebrew University strain, 150 g) were injected i.p. with lisuride (0.5 mg/ kg), bromocriptine (5 mg/kg) or apomorphine (2.5 mg/kg) alone or one hour before levodopa (25 mg/kg, i.p., one hour after carbidopa, 10 mg/kg, i.p.) and decapitated one hour later. Control animals received only saline or levodopa (and carbidopa). The brains were rapidly removed, corpora striata dissected out and frozen on dry ice. Striatal concentrations of dopamine, DOPAC, and levodopa were measured using high performance liquid chromatography with electrochemical detection (HPLC-EC) (Hefti et al., 1980).

Results

Treatment with only each of the dopamine agonists reduced rat striatal levels of DOPAC and the DOPAC/dopamine ratios (data not shown) without affecting dopamine levels (Table 1). This indicates that their systemic administration indeed attenuate basic activity and dopamine turnover in the nigrostriatal neurons. Levodopa given alone, produced (as expected) marked

Table 1. Effect of combined administration of levodopa and dopamine agonists on utilization of levodopa in rat striatum

	DA	DOPAC	Levodopa
		ng/mg protein	
Control	73 ± 3	9.3 ± 0.4	0.6 ± 0.2
Levodopa	$157 \pm 15^*$	$61.3 \pm 5.9^{**}$	$23.0 \pm 4.2^*$
Lisuride	70 ± 5	$6.2 \pm 0.3^*$	0.4 ± 0.1
Lisuride + Levodopa	$152 \pm 8^*$	$62.8 \pm 7.6^{**}$	$24.8 \pm 3.1^*$
Bromocriptine	67 ± 5	$5.3 \pm 0.6^*$	0.4 ± 0.3
Bromocriptine + Levodopa	$149 \pm 10^*$	$59.1 \pm 6.2^{**}$	$21.9 \pm 3.5^*$
Apomorphine	76 ± 9	$4.6 \pm 9.5^*$	0.2 ± 0.2
Apomorphine + Levodopa	$159 \pm 12^*$	$68.1 \pm 6.7^{**}$	$20.1 \pm 2.9^*$

$n = 8$–10 animals in each group; DA (dopamine): * $p < 0.001$ as compared with controls and rats injected with agonists alone; DOPAC (dihydroxyphenylacetic acid): * $p < 0.01$ as compared with controls, ** $p < 0.001$ as compared with controls and with animals injected with agonists alone; levodopa: * $p < 0.001$ as compared with controls and rats injected with agonists only (analysis of variance, followed by Scheffe's test)

increases in striatal concentrations of dopamine, DOPAC and levodopa (Table 1). However, dopamine agonists administered with levodopa did not attenuate the levodopa-induced increases in striatal levels of dopamine, DOPAC and levodopa (Table 1). The latter remained similar to those generated by a challenge with only levodopa.

Discussion

This study shows that coadministration of levodopa with the dopamine receptor agonists lisuride, bromocriptine and apomorphine, does not affect the elevations in dopamine and DOPAC induced by levodopa in rat striatum. Their administration did not interfere also with entry of levodopa from the circulation into the striatum. The generation of dopamine from exogenous levodopa in the striatum remained unchanged despite suppression of nigrostriatal neuronal discharge rates by the dopamine agonists. It is likely that the agonists can inhibit nigrostriatal firing not only when dopaminergic projections are intact but also in conditions of their partial destruction that renders them hyperactive as occurs in Parkinson's disease. We have shown in mice with partial destruction of striatal dopaminergic nerve endings induced by systemic injection of the neurotoxin MPTP that administration of apomorphine can turn off the hyperactivity of surviving neurons (Melamed et al., in preparation). We have also shown that electrical stimulation of the nigra does not affect the metabolism of systemically-administered levodopa in rat striatum (Melamed and Dafni, 1982). All of the above suggest that utilization of exogenous levodopa in the striatum does not depend on the state of firing activity of the dopaminergic neurons. Conversion of levodopa to dopamine goes on in an unchanged manner whether firing of the nigrostriatal neurons is normal, increased or decreased. This indicates that dopamine agonists given to patients with Parkinson's disease do not lower efficacy of levodopa and therefore that their beneficial effects are additive. Our findings do not support the hypothesis that hyperactive nigrostriatal neurons are capable of synthesizing more dopamine from exogenous levodopa. Therefore, there may be a fundamental difference in the manner by which nigrostriatal neurons handle endogenous (tyrosine-derived) and exogenous levodopa (Melamed, 1992). Also, by inference, our study does not lend support to the hypothesis that surviving dopaminergic neurons represent the major or only locus for generation of dopamine from levodopa in the parkinsonian striatum.

Acknowledgement

Supported, in part, by the National Parkinson Foundation, Miami, Florida, U.S.A.

References

Agid Y, Javoy F, Glowinski J (1973) Hyperactivity of remaining dopaminergic neurons after partial destruction of the nigrostriatal dopaminergic system in the rat. Nature (New Biol) 245: 150–151

Bernheimer H, Birkmayer, W, Hornykiewicz O, Jellinger K (1975) Brain dopamine and syndromes of Parkinson and Huntington. J Neurol Sci 30: 415–455

Bunney BS, Aghajanian GK, Roth RH (1973) Comparison of effect of L-dopa, amphetamine and apomorphine or firing rate of rat dopaminergic neurons. Nature (New Biol) 245: 123–125

Haubrich DR, Pflueger AB (1982) The autoreceptor control of dopamine synthesis. An in vitro and in vivo comparison of dopamine agonists. Mol Pharmacol 21: 114–120

Hefti F, Melamed E, Wurtman RJ (1980) Partial lesions of the dopaminergic nigrostriatal system in rat brain: biochemical characterization. Brain Res 195: 123–138

Hornykiewicz O (1974) The mechanisms of action of L-dopa in Parkinson's disease. Life Sci 15: 1249–1259

Melamed E (1992) Biochemical and functional differences between dopamine formed from endogenous tyrosine and exogenous L-dopa in nigrostriatal neurons. Neurochem Int 20 [Suppl]: 1155–1175

Melamed E, Dafni N (1982) Effect of electrical stimulation of nigrostriatal dopaminergic neurons on utilization of exogenous L-dopa in rat striatum. J Pharm Pharmacol 34: 8210–822

Starke K, Reimann W, Zumstein A, Hertting G (1978) Effect of dopamine receptor agonists and antagonists on release of dopamine in the rabbit caudate nucleus in vitro. Naunyn Schmiedebergs Arch Pharmacol 305: 27–36

Authors' address: E. Melamed, M.D., Department of Neurology, Beilinson Medical Center, Petah Tiqva, Israel 49100.

J Neural Transm (1995) [Suppl] 45: 61–66
© Springer-Verlag 1995

The modulation of dopamine receptors in rat striatum

A. Stefani[1], A. Pisani[1], G. Bernardi[1,2], A. Bonci[1], N. B. Mercuri[1], F. Stratta[1], and P. Calabresi[1]

[1] Clinica Neurologica, Università di Roma Tor Vergata, Rome, and
[2] IRCCS Clinica S. Lucia, Rome, Italy

Summary.   In the last decades, the contribution given by basic electrophysiology to the understanding of the nigrostriatal pathway in mammals has been rather important. The main results obtained by our group will be revised in this short review. The most common responses produced by dopamine (DA) on the principal striatal cells (the medium spiny neurons) are the modulation of the corticostriatal synaptic transmission and the decrease of voltage-dependent inward conductances. After blockade of DA transmission, both spontaneous and cortically driven glutamatergic postsynaptic potentials were inhibited by the selective activation of DA D2 receptors. In naive animals, the DA-mediated inhibition of postsynaptic firing activity was mediated by D1 receptor activation. Nevertheless, the two main subclasses of DA receptors seemed to cooperate in the formation of the long-term depression (LTD) of excitatory synaptic transmission in the striatum. The excitotoxic hypothesis of neurodegeneration has further stimulated our interest towards the study of the interactions between DA and other neurotransmitters into the basal ganglia.

Introduction

Almost three decades of electrophysiological studies on mammalian striatal neurons have provided significant contributions in advancing our knowledge of the DAergic pharmacology in the nigrostriatal system. The analysis of the physiological properties of the medium spiny cells and their responses to DA and DAergic agents has opened new therapeutic approaches to the treatment of movement disorders. The actions promoted by DA were initially interpreted as the effects of a fast classical transmitter (Kitai et al., 1976); later on, the activation of DA receptors was considered responsible for a modulatory role on membrane excitability (Bernardi et al., 1978; Mercuri et al., 1985; Calabresi et al., 1987). More recently, DA and DAergic selective agonists were shown to be involved in the synaptic plasticity (Calabresi et al., 1992b). Several pieces of evidence have recently emerged in favour of a excitotoxic pathogenesis of neurodegenerative disorders (Choi, 1988; Lipton and Rosemberg,

1994). It was postulated that Parkinson's disease could possibly benefit from long-term therapies directed to ameliorate an altered energy metabolism (Beal, 1992). Yet, the central core of the therapy of "paralysis agitans" (Parkinson, 1817) is still levodopa (Hornykiewicz, 1966; Cotzias et al., 1969). Bearing in mind those fascinating perspectives, we will briefly outline in this paper the main acquisitions relative to DA actions in mammalian striatum.

Material and methods

Methods concerning the *in vitro* experiments on striatal neurons have been described previously for both slices (Calabresi et al., 1987, 1988) and acutely dissociated neuronal preparations (Stefani et al., 1994a,b).

Adult Wistar rats (1–4 months) were commonly used. Anaesthesia is followed by an heavy blow on the rat neck and rapid decapitation. Brains are quickly removed and 200–350 μm thick coronal slices are prepared from tissue blocks with the use of a vibratome. These slices usually contain the neostriatum, the viciniori corpus callosum and neocortex. A single slice is transferred to the recording chamber and submerged in a continuously flowing Krebs solution (36°C, 2–2.5 ml/min.) gassed with a 95% O_2, 5% CO_2 mixture. Intracellular recording electrodes are filled with 2M KCl or 2M K-acetate (30–60 Mohms); extracellular electrodes are filled with 2M NaCl (5–10 Mohms). Bipolar electrodes are used to promote synaptic stimulation of the corticostriatal pathway. They are located either in cortical areas adjacent to the recording electrode or in the white matter between the cortex and the striatum. When long-term modifications of synaptic transmission are studied, a conditioning tetanus is applied. It is composed by three trains of stimuli of 3 second duration, 100 Hz frequency, at 20 seconds interval. The duration of each individual pulse is 0.01–0.03 ms. In some experiments, the lesioning of the nigrostriatal pathway was obtained by unilateral application of 6-OHDA (see Calabresi et al., 1993a). This lesion caused a loss greater than 95% of DA neurons in the substantia nigra pars compacta (SNc) and the almost complete absence of DA terminals in the striatum. This is detected by an immuno-peroxidase technique, which utilized a monoclonal antibody for tyrosine-hydroxylase (TH).

Results

In vivo

Pioneering intracellular studies *in vivo* showed that DA produced a reduction of striatal firing frequency (Bernardi et al., 1978); such a prevalent inhibitory action was later confirmed by other studies (Herrling and Hull, 1980; Mercuri et al., 1985). Yet, a rather intriguing observation was raised by Bernardi and coauthors (1978): they observed that a slow membrane depolarization could preceed the reduction of the repetitive firing. Since this phenomenon was not observed *In vitro*, its possible mechanism of action was not further investigated. *In vivo* recordings had also shown that DA was able to reduce cortically-evoked excitatory postsynaptic potentials (EPSPs) (Bernardi et al., 1978; Mercuri et al., 1975). *In vivo* studies, however, were hampered by several experimental limitations: the effects of anaesthesia, the alterations caused by surgical preparation, the difficulty to estimate concentration and diffusion of drugs applied either sistemically or iontophoretically. In conclusion, those *in vivo* studies did not allow the pharmacological characterization of the DA receptors involved in the observed electrophysiological effects.

In vitro

The bath application of micromolar concentrations of DA to rat striatal slices usually produced a reduction of the neuronal excitability evoked by depolarizing current pulses. This effect was not coupled to significant modifications of the membrane potential. The D1 agonist SKF 38393, but not the D2 agonist Ly 17555, mimicked this inhibition of action potential discharge (Calabresi et al., 1987). The firing inhibition was associated to a decrease of the tetrodotoxin(TTX)-sensitive membrane rectification present in the depolarized voltage-range of the membrane potential. In other words, DA, by acting on the voltage-dependent sodium current, reduced the probability of action potential discharge. The observed D1-mediated modulation was dependent upon the direct, postsynaptic activation of DA receptors on striatal neurons. In fact, it persisted in low calcium-cadmium containing media. In naive animals, the action on the evoked firing was coupled with analogous modulation of intrastriatally evoked excitatory postsynaptic potentials (EPSPs) (Calabresi et al., 1987). The EPSP reduction by exogenous DA was antagonized by SCH 23390. Moreover, low micromolar doses of amphetamine, known to release endogenous DA from striatal slices, mimicked the effects of exogenous D1 receptor agonists on intrastriatal EPSP (Calabresi et al., 1988). Again, SCH 23390, but not sulpiride, antagonized or prevented the d-amphetamine induced reduction of intrastriatal excitation. These results suggested that coactivation of both subclasses of DA receptors was required to induce and maintain LTD. In fact, selective antagonists of either D1 or D2 receptor could block LTD. Moreover, in denervated rats, we failed to reproduce LTD. We hypothesized that the integrity of nigrostriatal pathway and the release of endogenous striatal DA are crucial conditions to produce LTD. In fact, when DA-denervated striata were incubated in both D1 and D2 agonists, LTD could be restored (Calabresi et al., 1992b). Striatal LTD could be blocked by chronic lithium treatment or by antagonists of glutamate metabotropic receptors (Calabresi et al., 1993b). These findings suggest that a modulation of phosphoinositides (PI) turnover is involved in this form of synaptic plasticity.

Discussion

Taken together, these results describe a quite coherent picture in which DA, by a concomitant activation of D1 and D2 receptors, causes both a short-term and a long-term reduction of cellular excitability. This result is a consequence of both a direct effect on intrinsic properties (in particular the modulation of the sodium conductance) and a presynaptic action on glutamate release.

However, some interesting unanswered questions are to be addressed by future experimental studies. Among these, we would like to indicate the following:

1. D2 DA responses in control condition. What is the role of D2 striatal receptors under control conditions? In fact, we are able to observe a D2-mediated decrease of corticostriatal transmission only in DA-denervated striatum. Nevertheless, we have suggested the participation of D2 DA receptors in striatal synaptic plasticity (Calabresi et al., 1992b).

2. D3/D4 receptors. What is the functional role of the new subclasses of receptors, namely D3 and D4, in striatal pharmacology? Although the endogenous DA, released by nigrostriatal terminals, plays a direct inhibitory role in the control of striatal neuronal activity through interaction with D1 receptors. In contrast, in naive animals, D2 receptor activation did significantly affect neither the intrinsic membrane properties nor the synaptic potentials measured from the recorded neurons (Calabresi et al., 1992a).

In order to examine the DA pharmacology in experimental conditions which may mimic Parkinson's disease, we evaluated the effects of DA agonists in DA-depleted animals (Ungerstedt et al., 1971, see methods). In this condition, Ly 17555 produced a significant reduction of excitatory synaptic transmission. In particular, both the frequency and the amplitude of glutamate-mediated spontaneous postsynaptic potentials were reversibly decreased by 1–$10\,\mu M$ of LY 17555. Also cortically driven striatal EPSPs, which are mediated by AMPA-like glutamate receptors (Calabresi et al., 1992a), were inhibited by the D2 agonist at low micromolar doses. This presynaptic effect of LY 17555 was antagonised by sulpiride, but not by SCH 23390 (Calabresi et al., 1993a).

Recently, we have studied whether, similarly to the cerebellum and the hippocampus, also the striatum can express long-term modifications of synaptic transmission. Induction of both long-term potentiation (LTP) and long-term depression (LTD) could be obtained depending on the ionic composition of the media. In control conditions (physiological magnesium concentration: $1.2\,mM$), LTD is commonly generated by a conditioning tetanic stimulation (see methods). LTD of the corticostriatal EPSP is also associated with the long-term reduction of extracellularly recorded field potentials. In contrast, when magnesium was omitted from the external medium (to remove voltage-dependent magnesium block of NMDA receptor) the same tetanic stimulation produced LTP.

3. Possible synergism between D1 and D2 receptors. The prevalent synergism of action between D1 and D2 receptors, as shown by our studies on synaptic plasticity (Calabresi et al., 1992b) is in accordance with previous biochemical findings (Bertorello et al., 1990). Surprisingly, the vast majority of postsynaptic DA receptors were suggested to be segregated in striatonigral (D1) and striatopallidal (D2) neurons (Gerfen, 1992). It would not be easy to reconcile the observed effects with such a receptor segregation. Patch-clamp studies, however, performed on acutely isolated striatal cells previously identified as projection neurons to SN, revealed that D1 and D2 receptors colocalize on the same cells (Surmeier et al., 1992). Moreover, activation of both receptors produced a prevalent inhibitory modulation of sodium current, in agreement with our results in slices (Surmeier et al., 1992).

4. Ach/DA balance. The balance between DA and acetylcholine (Ach) within the striatum is still an important target for the therapy of extrapyramidal disorders. The complex interactions among cholinergic interneurons, subpopulations of striatal projecting cells and DA have received a great attention from anatomical and biochemical studies (Gerfen, 1992). Much has still to be done at the pharmacological and physiological level.

5. DA and cellular metabolism. Excitotoxicity and the energy metabolism failure have recently been indicated as playing an important role in the pathogenesis of neurodegenerative disorders. In this regard, the analysis of the interaction between excitatory amino acids, cellular metabolism and DA will probably represent a main goal for many laboratories in the next future. Recent observations by Cepeda and coworkers (1993), who claimed that D1 agonists could potentiate the NMDA responses, were not confirmed by our group (Calabresi et al., 1995). In conclusion, interactions between these two classes of transmitters remain a main matter of future investigation.

Acknowledgements

We are greatly thankful to G. Gattoni and M. Tolu for their excellent technical assistance.

References

Beal FM (1992) Does impediment of energy metabolism result in excitotoxic neuronal death in neurodefenerative illnesses? Ann Neurol 31: 119–130

Bernardi G, Marciani MG, Morocutti C, Pavone F, Stanzione P (1978) The action of dopamine on rat caudate neurons intracellularly recorded. Neurosci Lett 8: 35–240

Bertorello AM, Hopfield JF, Aperia A, Greengard P (1990) Inhibition by dopamine of (Na+/K+)ATPase activity in neostriatal neurones through D1 and D2 dopamine receptor synergism. Nature 347: 386–388

Calabresi P, Mercuri NB, Stanzione P, Stefani A, Bernardi G (1987) Intracellular studies on the dopamine-induced firing inhibition of neostriatal neurons. Neuroscience 20: 757–771

Calabresi P, Benedetti M, Mercuri NB, Bernardi G (1988) Endogenous dopamine and dopaminergic agonists modulate synaptic excitation in neostriatum: intracellular studies from naive and catecholamine-depleted rats. Neuroscience 27: 145–157

Calabresi P, De Murtas M, Mercuri NB, Bernardi G (1992a) Chronic neuroleptic treatment: D2 receptor supersensitity and striatal glutamatergic transmission. Ann Neurol 31: 366–373

Calabresi P, Maj R, Pisani A, Mercuri NB, Bernardi G (1992b) Long-term synaptic depression in the striatum: physiological and pharmacological characterization. J Neurosci 12: 4224–4233

Calabresi P, Mercuri NB, Sancesario G, Bernardi G (1993a) Electrophysiology of dopamine-denervated striatal neurons. Brain 116: 433–452

Calabresi P, Pisani A, Mercuri NB, Bernardi G (1993b) Lithium treatment blocks LTD in the striatum. Neuron 10: 955–962

Calabresi P, DeMurtas M, Pisani A, Sancesario G, Mercuri NB, Bernardi G (1995) Vulnerability of medium spiny striatal neurons to glutamate; role of Na+/K+ AT-Pase. Eur J Neurosci (in press)

Cepeda C, Buchwald NA, Levine MS (1993) Neuromodulatory actions of dopamine in the neostriatum are dependent upon the excitatory amino acid receptor subtypes activated. Proc Natl Acad Sci USA 90: 9576–9580

Choi DW (1988) Glutamate neurotoxicity and disease of the nervous system. Neuron 1: 623–634

Cotzias GC, Papavasiliou PS, Gellene R (1969) Modifications of parkinsonism: chronic treatment with 1-DOPA. N Engl J Med 280: 337–345

Gerfen C (1992) The neostriatal mosaic: multiple levels of compartmental organization in the basal ganglia. Ann Rev Neurosci 15: 285–320

Herrling PL, Hull CD (1980) Iontophoretically applied dopamine depolarizes and hyperpolarizes the membrane of cat caudate neuron. Brain Res 192: 441–452

Hornykiewicz O (1966) Dopamine and brain function. Pharmacol Rev 18: 925–964

Kitai ST, Sugimori M, Kocsis JD (1976) Excitatory nature of dopamine in the nigrocaudate pathway. Exp Brain Res 24: 351–363

Lipton SA, Rosenberg PA (1994) Excitatory amino acids as a final common pathway for neurologic disorders. N Engl J Med 330: 613–622

Mercuri NB, Bernardi G, Calabresi P, Cotugno A, Levi G, Stanzione P (1985) Dopamine decreases cell excitability in rat striatal neurons by pre- and postsynaptic mechanisms. Brain Res 358: 110–121

Parkinson J (1817) An essay on the shaking palsy. Neely and Jones, Sherwood, p 66

Stefani A, Surmeier DJ, Bernardi G (1994a) The μ-agonist DAGO decreases HVA calcium currents in acutely dissociated neostriatal neurons. Brain Res 642: 339–343

Stefani A, Pisani, Mercuri NB, Bernardi G, Calabresi P (1994b) Activation of metabotropic glutamate receptors inhibits calcium currents and GABA-mediated synaptic potentials in rat striatal neurons. J Neurosci 14: 6734–6743

Surmeier DJ, Eberwine J, Wilson CJ, Cao Y, Stefani A, Kitai ST (1992) Dopamine receptor subtypes colocalize in rat striatonigral neurons. Proc Natl Acad Sci USA 89: 10178–10182

Ungerstedt U (1971) Striatal dopamine release after amphetamine or nerve degeneration revealed by rotational behaviour. Acta Physiol Scand [Suppl] 367: 69–93

Authors' address: Dr. A. Stefani, Clinica Neurologica, Università di Roma Tor Vergata, Via di Tor Vergata 135, I-00135 Rome, Italy.

J Neural Transm (1995) [Suppl] 45: 67–74

On the functional significance of primate retinal dopamine receptors

I. Bodis-Wollner[1] and **A. Antal**[2]

[1] Department of Neurology, State University of New York — Health Science Center at Brooklyn, Brooklyn, New York, U.S.A.
[2] Department of Physiology, Szent-Gyorgyi Albert Medical University, Szeged, Hungary

Summary.   Diverse dopamine receptors have been identified in the primate retina. Evidence summarized from human and monkey retinal electrophysiological studies (ERG) suggests that separate D1 and D2 receptor activation results in stimulus dependent antagonistic effects. Studies were performed using Haloperidol, l-sulpiride, CY 208-243 and dopamine. It is inferred that the antagonistic functions of D1 and D2 receptors synergistically determine the inverted U-shaped spatial contrast response function of the primate retina. An understanding of the logic performed by retinal D1 and D2 receptors may be useful to discern properties of the role of diverse dopamine receptors in basal ganglia DA circuits.

Introduction

Over the last decade and a half our understanding of the morphology and pharmacological diversity of electrical and chemical coupling between neurons has increased at a dramatic rate. Information concerning the *dynamics* of neural organization corresponding to this diversity is lacking. Dopaminergic circuits of the primate retina offer the opportunity to study input-output and feedback relations and — as a model system — to explore the diversity of function and timing of neural events tied to different receptors within the same neurotransmitter system. In addition, studies of dopaminergic retinal mechanisms provide in vivo methods (Marx et al., 1986; Gottlob et al., 1987; Ellis et al., 1988; Harnois and di Paolo, 1990; Gelmi et al., 1992; Stanzione et al., 1992; Nguyen-Legros et al., 1993; Ikeda et al., 1994) to evaluate for Parkinson's disease putative therapeutic agents with selective affinity for diverse receptors.

From a therapeutic point of view, one of the most challenging pharmacological discoveries has been the demonstration of the diversity of pre-and post-synaptic dopamine receptors of the CNS including the retina (Schorderet and Nowak, 1990). While since the original studies of Makman et al. (1980) it has become apparent that beyond D1 and D2 receptors subtypes D3, D4, D5 also exist, at present our knowledge of the functional role of these subtypes is limited (Cohen et al., 1992).

In this chapter current understanding of the functional and logic role of D1 and D2 retinal receptors in the primate will be reviewed. We report results obtained in the monkey, contrasting results obtained with DA cell destruction and postsynaptic receptor blockade. Finally we shall relate these conclusions to those reached in humans with retinal dopaminergic deficiency, as it occurs in Parkinson's disease (Ellis and Ikeda, 1988; Harnois and di Paolo, 1990; Nguyen-Legros et al., 1993; Ikeda et al., 1994).

Method

Electrophysiological retinal responses (ERG) were registered both in man and monkey. Human studies performed in Parkinson's disease patients and controls will be compared with results obtained in monkeys (Rhesus and Cynomolgous) with various manipulations of their dopaminergic systems. In man the ERG was recorded using either C-glide corneal electrodes or DTL fiber electrodes while in monkey the active electrode was a pediatric EEG needle electrode inserted into the fold of the lower lid (Marx et al., 1988). The reference electrode was placed on the ipsilateral temple. Recordings were monocular. Monkeys were under light ketamine anesthesia (5 mgm. kg., on the average). Animals were restrained and comfortably seated in a special monkey chair. One experimenter watched the monkey's eyes and halted the recording whenever the reflexion of the screen was not centered on the pupil. The animal studies conformed to the ARVO guidelines and resolutions concerning the use of primates. All human studies were approved by institutional review boards and confirmed to guidelines for the protection of human subjects.

Stimuli were sinusoidal gratings produced under software control on a high resolution, high luminance, large monitor. The stimuli were variable in spatial frequency, and contrast. Other parameters were not varied in this study.

A homogeneous field (0 spatial frequency) was used for studying flicker responses (temporal modulation) or without modulation for studying as a control condition "blank" responses of the eye.

Results

— The effect of retinal DA deficiency on visual processing of the monkey.
  - 6-OHDA
  - MPTP
— The effect of Haloperidol on the flash ERG in the monkey.
— The effect of l-Sulpiride on the pattern ERG in the monkey: the importance of the PERG tuning ratio.
— The effect of Parkinson's disease on the spatial properties of the PERG in man.

The effect of retinal DA deficiency on visual processing in the monkey

a) The effect of intravitreally administered 6-hydroxydopamine (6-OHDA) on the pattern electroretinogram and pattern visual evoked potential of 3 aphakic monkeys was studied (Ghilardi et al., 1989). Because of the aphake condition, several complexities of intravitreal injection of 6-OH-DA could be avoided. Nevertheless, following monocular 6-OHDA treatment, both the phase and the amplitude of pattern electroretinogram and pattern visual evoked potential became abnormal. This abnormality was most pronounced for the peak spatial frequencies (2.5 and 3.5 cycles per degree), whereas responses to lower spatial frequencies (0.5 and 1.2 cycles per degree) were less impaired. The non-injected eye was not affected. The effects of systemically administered MPTP (see below) on pattern electroretinogram and pattern visual evoked potential are similar to the effects of intravitreal injections of 6-OHDA.

b) Systemically administered N-methyl, 4-phenyl, 1-2-3-6 tetrahydropyridine (MPTP) was used to produce a chronic parkinsonian syndrome in monkeys. The pattern visual evoked potential (PVEP) and pattern electroretinogram (PERG) were studied in 5 cynomolgus monkeys before and during the development of the parkinsonian syndrome induced by MPTP (Ghilardi et al., 1988). Besides motor impairment spatial frequency-dependent visual abnormalities developed both in the pattern electroretinogram and visual evoked potential following MPTP. The stimuli were vertical gratings of four spatial frequencies (0.5, 1.2, 2.5 and 3.5 cycles/degree (cpd) modulated at temporal rates of 1, 4, 6, and 8 Hz. Following MPTP administration, the monkeys developed typical motor signs of Parkinsonism accompanied by changes in the amplitude and latency of the PVEP and PERG. Sinemet (L-dopa/carbidopa) administration produced temporary recovery of both PVEP and PERG. Two of the monkeys were followed for a prolonged period (30–40 days) after MPTP and the parkinsonian signs showed partial recovery; the PVEP latency and amplitude to 2.5 and 3.5 cpd stimuli and the latency to 1.2 cpd showed improvement but remained abnormal. The latencies of PERGS were normal, but the amplitudes were significantly reduced when stimuli of 2.5 and 3.5 cpd were used. Both PVEP and PERG to 0.5 cpd stimuli returned to normal, but not to peak spatial frequency stimuli even when recordings were performed 6 months 1 year later. These studies demonstrate that spatial frequency-dependent electrophysiological abnormalities characterize both the MPTP and the intravitreal 6-OHDA treated monkey, a result found in human Parkinson's disease which shows an attenuation of peak spatial frequency responses.

The effect of Haloperidol on the flash ERG in the monkey

We examined the effect of dopaminergic blockade on signal processing in the primate retina (Bodis-Wollner et al., 1989). Both light and dark adapted flash electroretinograms (flash ERGS) were measured in 5 normal Cynomolgus monkeys prior to and following the systemic administration of Haloperidol, a mixed blocker of dopamine receptors. Flash ERG amplitude was measured from the trough of the a-wave to the peak of the b-wave. The flash stimulus is broad band in respect to spatial frequency. Haloperidol 0.1 mg/kg i.m. caused a statistically significant increase in the amplitude of both light-and dark-

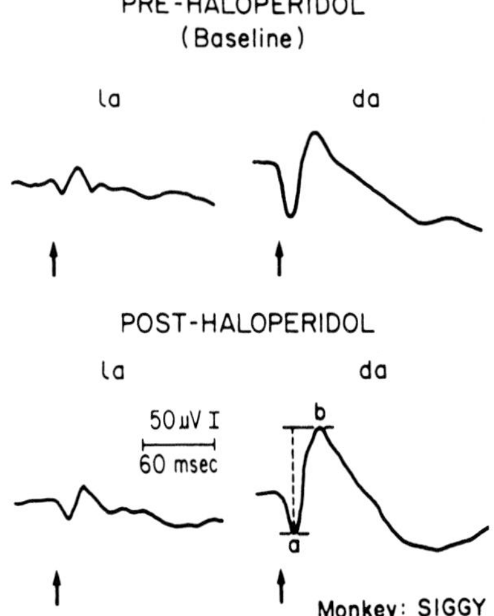

Fig. 1. Both light-adapted (la) and dark-adapted (da) flash ERG (FERG) waveforms are shown for one monkey: Siggy. Positivity of the waveforms is upward. In this figure, the la FERGs were recorded after 5 min of light adaptation and the da FERGs were recorded following 25 min of dark adaptation. The FERGs recorded pre-haloperidol (i.e. baseline) are presented on the top row; FERGs recorded post-haloperidol are presented on the bottom row. The vertical arrows at the beginning of each waveform indicate when the flash stimulus was presented. Amplitude was measured from the peak of the a-wave to the peak of the b-wave, represented by the vertical dashed line on the FERG in the lower right corner. Amplitude and latency calibrations are indicated (from Bodis-Wollner et al., 1989)

adapted flash ERGs in all monkeys (Fig. 1) We concluded that mixed (predominantly D1) receptor blockade in the primate retina enhances both light and dark adapted flash ERGs a result which suggests that dopamine is active in both the light and the dark in response to flash stimulation. Secondly this result suggests that D1 receptors are involved in luminance (or low spatial frequency) responses possibly in an inhibitory manner.

The effect of L-sulpiride on the pattern ERG in the monkey:
the importance of the PERG tuning ratio

The effect of systemic D2 receptor blockade was studied on retinal responses in the monkey (Tagliati et al., 1994). We studied one cynomolgous and two rhesus monkeys. The ERG was recorded to pattern stimulation before and 20′ following the I. M. administration of L-sulpiride, a selective D2 blocker (Spano et al., 1979). The ERG was recorded to four different spatial frequencies of stimulation in each monkey in repeated sessions. Two different doses of L-sulpiride (0.07 and 0.35 mgm/kg) were used. The results showed that prior to the administration of L-sulpiride the ERG response amplitude was lower to the lowest spatial frequency of stimulation (0.5 cpd), than to either 2.3 or 4.6 cpd. Hence the PERG shows tuning in respect to spatial frequency.

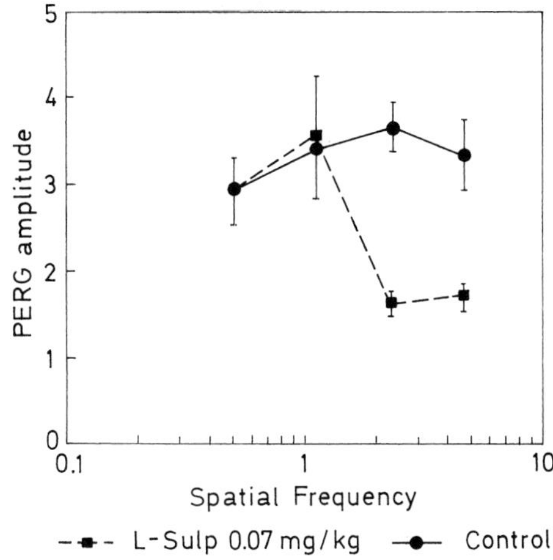

Fig. 2. The effect of low dose of l-sulpiride on the PERG spatial transfer function in one monkey: Marci. A clear attenuation at the peak of the function is evident while response amplitude is unaffected for low spatial frequencies (after Tagliati et al., 1994)

This result is consistent with the results of other normative studies performed in our laboratory, using moderate (less than 16 degree) visual field size. L-sulpiride had no effect on pupil size. Following l-sulpiride the response to the peak spatial frequencies decreased while ERG amplitude did not change to the 0.5 cpd spatial frequency (course pattern) (Fig. 2). As a result the amplitude ratio of *peak* versus *low* spatial frequency response, we called tuning ratio, normally above one, became less than unity. This result is consistent with the ERG results we obtained for presynaptic DA neuron destruction by either 6-OHDA or MPTP (see above): i.e. either by DA deficiency or by D2 receptor blockade the spatial tuning ratio inverted. Since D2 receptor blockade and DA deficiency cause similar effects all three results taken together suggest that systemic D2 receptor blockade primarily affects postsynaptic D2 receptors.

The effect of Parkinson's disease on the spatial properties
of the pattern ERG in man

We used essentially similar methods to the monkey studies to quantify the pattern electroretinogram in normal controls and in Parkinson's disease patients. Most of these patients were undergoing chronic treatment with dopaminergic agents with mixed affinities to D1 and D2 receptors. As described for the monkeys, we studied the response to diverse spatial frequencies of stimulation. The results, compared to age matched controls, were across the whole population not very impressive. When, however, patients with advanced Parkinson's disease, or those without treatment were separately evaluated, an *inversion* of the normally larger than unity PERG tuning ratio became evident. This result is qualitatively similar to the results obtained by Stanzione and his colleagues (1993) using L-sulpiride in normal human volunteers. Our studies in Parkinson's disease also suggested that a correlation exists between the decrease in the ERG tuning ratio and the severity of Parkinson's disease.

Discussion

Several of the reviewed studies suggest that although details of retinal dopaminergic mechanisms are not well known in primates, one can conclude that D2 receptor mediated actions do relate to elementary aspects of pattern vision. The property of the normal primate retinal ganglion cells to be selective for pattern size is understood as the result of antagonistic center-surround interaction of the pre-ganglionic receptive field organization. The pattern ERG predominantly reflects retinal ganglion cell activity (Maffei and Fiorentini, 1986). The lack of spatial frequency tuning of the PERG as a result of various manipulations of the dopaminergic system, as we summarized above, suggests that a normal spatially selective bandpass behaviour is linked to D2 receptor function. Our Haloperidol results (see above and Bodis-Wollner et al., 1989) and some new data obtained with a direct D1 receptor agonist (CY208-243) suggests that conversely, low spatial frequency responses are linked to D1 receptors, which may attenuate the response. However, D1 receptors may also play a smaller role in peak spatial frequency responses. Indeed an interaction of Cy 208-243 a D1 receptor agonist with D2 receptors have been reported (Robertson et al., 1992).

Studies of the primate retina suggest that while DA neurons are located in the inner retina, D2 receptors (and recently discovered subclasses of D4 and D5) are located both in inner and outer retinal layers (Mariani et al., 1984; McGonigle et al., 1988; Storman et al., 1990; Van Tol et al., 1991; Djamgoz and Wagner, 1992). Receptors in the inner layers may be in the near proximity of DA cells and possibly respond to conventional synaptic release and dynamics of DA neurons, while modulating amacrine cell gap functions (Hampson et al., 1992). The timing of these processes would be in the milliseconds range. On the other hand, if DA is released proximally and affects distal D2 receptors (Piccolino et al., 1987) in a paracrine mode of operation, a longer time constant needs to be considered as can be inferred from the results of studies using steady-state stimulation in primates (Bodis-Wollner et al., 1983; Marx et al., 1986; Stanzione et al., 1991). At present studies concerning the dynamics of DA retinal circuits in lower vertebrates yield conflicting data (Umino et al., 1991; Doug and McReynolds, 1992).

Studies reviewed here have not revealed precise timing data for the retinal domaminergic circuits. However, we found in both Parkinson's disease patients (Marx et al., 1986) and in the monkey using l-sulpiride (unpublished data) that the most pronounced ERG amplitude attenuation occurred when the stimulus was modulated between 4 and 8 Hz. This result is also consistent with human psychophysical (Bodis-Wollner et al., 1986) and electrophysiological (Marx et al., 1986) studies in Parkinson's disease. This type of temporal frequency dependent effect suggests that if DA is involved in a modulatory feedback circuit, the time constant of this circuit is relatively slow, compared to conventional electrical transmission. It remains to be seen however whether or not the suggested paracrine retinal DA circuit modulating the gain of a slow feedback loop (Bodis-Wollner, 1990) could serve as a generalizable concept in the logic of brain DA circuits.

Additionally future studies need to address experimental questions concerning the role of DA and dopamine receptors role in promoting or blocking (Yazulla and Kleinschmidt, 1982; Kamisaki et al., 1991) the release of other retinal neurotransmitters (Imperato et al., 1993), which may act in parallel or sequentially (Wu, 1994).

References

Bodis-Wollner I (1990) Visual deficits related to dopamine deficiency in experimental animals and Parkinson's disease. TINS 13: 296–301

Bodis-Wollner I, Harnois C, Bobak P, Mylin LH (1983) On the possible role of temporal delays of afferent processing in Parkinson's disease. J Neural Transm [Suppl] 19: 243–252

Bodis-Wollner I, Mark M, Ghilardi MD (1989) Systemic haloperidol administration increases the amplitude of the light-and-dark-adapted flash ERG in the monkey. Clin Vis Sci 4: 19–26

Bodis-Wollner I, Marx MS, Mitra S, Bobak P, Mylin L, Yahr M (1987) Visual dysfunction in Parkinson's disease-loss in spatiotemporal contrast sensitivity. Brain 110: 1675–1698

Cohen AI, Todd RD, Harmon S, O'Malley KL (1992) Photoreceptors of mouse retinas posses D4 receptors coupled to adenylate cyclase. Proc Natl Acad Sci USA 89: 12093–12097

Dong CJ, McReynolds JS (1992) Comparison of the effects of flickering and steady light on dopamine release and horizontal cell coupling in the mudpuppy retina. J Neurophys 67: 364–372

Djamgoz MBA, Wagner HJ (1992) Localization and function of dopamine in the adult vertebrate retina. Neurochem Int 20: 139–191

Ellis CJK, Ikeda H (1988) Evidence for retinal dopamine deficiency in Parkinson's disease. In: Bodis-Wollner I, Piccolino M (eds) Dopaminergic mechanisms in vision. Alan R Liss, New York, pp 239–251

Gelmi C, Sandrini G, Martignoni E, Bruno A, Nappi G, Trimarchi F (1992) Electroretinograms and visual evoked potentials in Parkinsonian patients with or without L-Dopa treatment. Neuroophthalmol 12: 125–132

Ghilardi MF, Bodis-Wollner I, Onofrj M, Marx MS, Glover A (1988) Spatial frequency-dependent abnormalities of the pattern electroretinogram and visual evoked potentials in a parkinsonian monkey model. Brain lll: 131–149

Ghilardi MF, Marx MS, Bodis-Wollner I, Camras CB, Glover AA (1989) The effect of intraocular 6-hydroxidopamine on retinal processing of primates. Ann Neurol 25: 357–364

Gottlob I, Schneider E, Heider W, Skrandies W (1987) Alteration of visual evoked potentials and electroretinograms in Parkinson's disease. Electroencephalogr Clin Neurophysiol 66: 349–357

Hampson ECGM, Vahey DI, Weiler Z (1992) Dopaminergic modulation of gap junction permeability between amacine cells in mammalian retina. J Neurosci 12: 4911–4922

Harnois C, Di Paolo T (1990) Decreased dopamine in the retinas of patients with Parkinson's disease. Invest Ophthalmol Vis Sci 31: 2473–2475

Ikeda H, Head GM, Ellis GM (1994) Electrophysiological signs of retinal dopamine deficiency in recently diagnosed Parkinson's disease and a follow up study. Vision Res 34: 2629–2638

Imperato A, Obinu MC, Gessa GL (1993) Stimulation of both dopamine D1 and D2 receptors facilitates in vivo acetylcholine release in the hippocampus. Brain Res 618: 341–345

Kamisaki Y, Hamahashi T, Mita E, Ipoh T (1991) D2 dopamine receptors inhibit release of aspartate and glutamate in rat retina. J Pharmacol Exp Ther 256: 634–638

Maffei L, Fiorentini A (1986) Generator sources of the pattern ERG in man and animals. In: Bodis-Wollner I, Cracco R (eds) Evoked potentials. Alan R Liss, New York, pp 101–116

Makman MJ, Dvorkin B, Horowitz SG, Thal LJ (1980) Properties of dopamine agonist and antagonist binding sites in mammalian retina. Brain Res 194: 403–418

Mariani AP, Kolb H, Nelson R (1984) Dopamine-containing amacrine cells of the rhesus monkey retina parallel rods in spatial distribution. Brain Res 322: 1–7

Marx MS, Bodis-Wollner I, Bobak P, Harnois C, Mylin L (1986) Temporal frequency-dependent VEP changes in Parkinson's disease. Vision Res 26: 185–193

Marx MS, Podos SM, Bodis-Wollner I, Lee PY, Wang RF, Severine C (1988) Signs of early damage in glaucomatous monkey eyes: low spatial frequency losses in the pattern ERG and VEP. Exp Eye Res 46: 173–184

McGonigle P, Wax MB, Molinoff PB (1988) Characterization of binding sites for 3H-spiroperidol in human retina. Invest Ophtalmol Vis Sci 29: 687–694

Nguyen-Legros J, Harnois C, Di Paolo T, Simon A (1993) The retinal dopamine system in Parkinson's disease. Clin Vis Sci 1: 1–12

Piccolino M, De Montis G, Witkovsky P, Bodis-Wollner I, Mirolli M (1987) D1 and D2 dopamine receptors involved in the control of electrical transmission between retinal horizontal cells. In: Biggio G, Spano PF, Toffano G, Gessa GL (eds) Symposium in neuroscience. Springer, Berlin Heidelberg New York, pp 1–12

Robertson HA, Peterson MR, Worth GG (1992) Synergistic and persistent interaction between the D2 agonist bromocriptine and the D1 selective agonist CY 208-243. Brain Res 593: 332–334

Schorderet M, Nowak JZ (1990) Retinal dopamine D1 and D2 receptors: characterization by binding or pharmacological studies and physiological functions. Cell Mol Neurobiol 10: 303–325

Spano PF, Stefanini E, Trabucchi M, Fresia P (1979) Stereospecific interaction of sulpiride with striatal and nonstriatal dopamine receptors. In: Spano PF, Trabucchi M, Corsini GU, Gessa GL (eds) Sulpiride and other benzamides. Italian Brain Research Foundation Press, Milan, pp 11–31

Stanzione P, Tagliati M, Pierantozzi M, Bodis-Wollner I (1991) The role of D2 receptors in retinal processing in humans. Ann Neurol 30: 293

Stanzione P, Traversa R, Pierantozzi M, Semprini R, Marciani MG, Bernardi G (1992) An electrophysiological study of D2 dopaminergic actions in human retina: a tool in Parkinson's disease. Neurosci Lett 136: 125–128

Stormann T, Gdula D, Weiner D, Brann M (1990) Molecular cloning and expression of a dopamine D2 receptor from human retina. Mol Pharmacol 37: 1–6

Tagliati M, Bodis-Wollner I, Kovanecz I, Stanzione P (1994) Spatial frequency tuning of the monkey pattern ERG depends on D2 receptor-linked action of dopamine. Vision Res 34: 2051–2057

Umino Q, Lee YL, Dowling JE (1991) Effects of light stimuli on the release of dopamine from interplexiform cells in the white perch retina. Neurosci Lett 87: 205–209

Van Tol HMH, Bunzow JR, Guan HC, Sunahara RK, Seeman P, Niznik HP, Civelli O (1991) Cloning of the gene for the human dopamine D4 receptor with high affinity for the antipsychotic clozapine. Nature 350: 610–611

Wu SM (1994) Synaptic transmission in the outer retina. Annu Rev Physiol 56: 141–168

Yazulla SK, Kleinschmidt J (1982) Dopamine blocks carrier-mediated release of GABA from retinal horizontal cells. Brain Res 233: 211–215

Authors' address: Dr. I. Bodis-Wollner, Department of Neurology, Box 1213, State University of New York — Health Science Center at Brooklyn, 450 Clarkson Avenue, Brooklyn, NY 11203, U.S.A.

J Neural Transm (1995) [Suppl] 45: 75–81

Intranigral injections of glutamate antagonists modulate dopamine D₁-mediated turning behavior and striatal c-fos expression

S. Fenu, A. Carta, and **M. Morelli**

Department of Toxicology, University of Cagliari, Cagliari, Italy

Summary. The contribution of the substantia nigra (SN) in the positive interaction between dopamine D_1 receptor agonists and glutamate antagonists was studied in rats with a unilateral 6-hydroxydopamine (6-OHDA) lesion of dopaminergic nigro-striatal pathway. Local infusion into the SN of the 6-OHDA lesioned side of NMDA glutamate antagonists MK 801 and CPP or the AMPA antagonist NBQX at doses inducing none or minimal behavioral effects, significantly increased the turning behavior and the expression of c-fos induced, in the lesioned caudate-putamen (CPu), by a parenteral administration of SKF 38393. High doses of MK 801 or CPP infused into the SN produced intense contralateral turning per-se but induced only sparse c-fos expression in the lesioned CPu. The results show that a depression of SN pars reticulata efferent neurons, potentiates D_1-mediated responses and suggest that this area may play a role in the positive interaction between glutamate antagonists and D_1 receptor agonists.

Introduction

Blockade of the N-methyl-D-aspartate (NMDA) or α-amino-3-hydroxy-5-methyl-4-isoxazolepropionate (AMPA) type of glutamate receptor, modulates in a positive manner the motor responses induced by dopamine (DA) agonists in 6-hydroxydopamine (6-OHDA) and MPTP models of Parkinson's disease (Morelli et al., 1990; Löschman et al., 1991; Wachtel et al., 1992) or in reserpine treated rodents (Carlsson and Carlsson, 1989; Klockgether et al., 1990, 1991; Goodwin et al., 1992; Svensson et al., 1992). Thus, parenteral administration of MK 801 potentiated the turning behavior induced by the D_1 agonist SKF 38393 in rats with a unilateral 6-OHDA lesion of the DA nigro-striatal pathway (Morelli et al., 1990; Boldry et al., 1993) and increased the number of Fos-positive nuclei induced by SKF 38393 in the lesioned caudate-putamen (CPu) (Morelli et al., 1992).

The substantia nigra pars-reticulata (SNr), is an area rich of glutamate receptors (Albin et al., 1991; Burns et al., 1993) which plays an important role in the mediation of motor responses originated in the CPu (Olianas et al., 1978; Di Chiara et al., 1979a; Morelli et al., 1980). Therefore, to evaluate its possible contribution in the positive interaction between DA D_1 agonists and NMDA or AMPA receptor antagonists, we have performed local infusions of NMDA (MK 801 or CPP) or AMPA antagonists (NBQX) into the SN of rats with a unilateral 6-OHDA lesion of the DA nigro-striatal pathway in combination with a parenteral administration of the D_1 agonist SKF 38393. In these rats we have then correlated the turning behavior contralateral to the 6-OHDA lesioned side, with the expression of the early gene c-fos as an index of neuronal activation (Morgan and Curran, 1989) in the lesioned CPu.

Materials and methods

Male Sprague-Dawley rats (275–300 g) anesthetized with chloral hydrate (400 mg/kg) were injected in the left medial forebrain bundle with 6-OHDA-HCl (8 μg in 4 μl) in order to lesion the DA nigrostriatal pathways. Eleven days after 6-OHDA lesions, rats were implanted in the SN of the 6-OHDA lesioned side of the brain, with chronic stainless steel guide cannulae for acute injection of drugs. Three days after implant of cannulae, rats were screened on the basis of their contralateral rotation in response to benserazide (30 mg/kg i.p.) + L-dopa (50 mg/kg i.p.) and treated three days later with the various drugs. Turning behavior was counted by automated rotameters.

Two hours after drug administration, rats were anesthetized and perfused with paraformaldehyde and their brains were cut coronally on a vibratome (40 μm) two days later. Sections were incubated with a Fos primary antibody (C.R.B., England) and the reaction was visualized using biotinylated secondary antisera and by standard avidin-biotin-horseradish peroxidase technique as described previously (Morelli et al., 1992). Neurons showing Fos-like-immunoreactivity were quantified with an image analyzer (IBAS) by counting the number of Fos-positive nuclei.

Statistics

Mean and S.E.M. were calculated. Significance between groups was evaluated by analysis of variance.

Results

Turning behavior

Intranigral infusion of MK 801 (1.5, 5.9, 14.8 nmol) or CPP (1.2, 4 nmol) dose-dependently induced contralateral turning hehavior as shown in Table 1. Parenteral administration of SKF 38393 (1.5 mg/kg s.c.) at a dose which induced only a few contralateral turns per-se caused intense contralateral turning when combined with intranigral MK 801 (1.5 nmol), CPP (1.2 nmol), or NBQX (0.6 nmol) at doses which induced none or a few contralateral turns by themselves (Fig. 1).

Fos immunohistochemistry

Infusion of MK 801 (1.5 nmol), CPP (1.2 nmol) or NBQX (0.6 nmol) into the 6-OHDA lesioned SN did not induce any significant increase in fos-like-

Table 1. Number of Fos-positive nuclei in the CPu of 6-OHDA lesioned rats and total turning behavior

Drug in SN	Fos positive nuclei (1 mm² grid)		Total turns (2 h)
	medial	dorso-lateral	
MK 801 (1.5)	6 ± 2	4 ± 3	8 ± 3
MK 801 (5.9)	10 ± 4	11 ± 2	68 ± 13
MK 801 (14.8)	23.7 ± 9	19.7 ± 4	988 ± 168
CPP (1.2)	12 ± 2	10 ± 3	6 ± 2
CPP (4)	32.4 ± 8	27.1 ± 4	898 ± 162

The doses of drugs injected into the SN were expressed in nmol. Total number of turns were measured in two hours

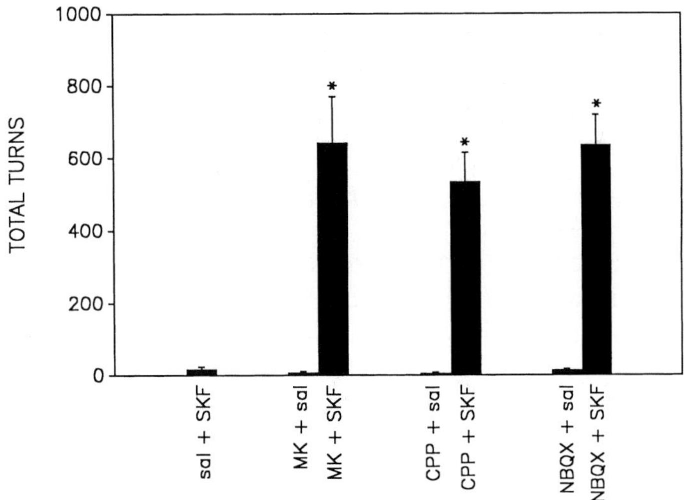

Fig. 1. Contralateral turning in response to MK 801 (1.5 nmol), CPP (1.2 nmol) and NBQX (0.6 nmol) injected into the 6-OHDA lesioned SN + saline s.c. and contralateral turning in response to the same drugs or saline into the SN plus SKF 38393 (1.5 mg/kg s.c.). MK 801, CPP or NBQX and SKF 38393 were injected at the same time. The data are the mean ± SEM of the total number of contralateral turns. Each group consisted of 6–11 rats. *p < 0.05 versus saline + SKF 38393

immunoreactivity in the lesioned CPu (Fig. 2). SKF 38393 (1.5 mg/kg s.c.), which induced sparse Fos-positive nuclei, when combined with intra-nigral infusions of MK 801, CPP or NBQX, caused strong activation of Fos-like-immunoreactivity in the lesioned CPu (Fig. 2). The distribution of Fos-positive neurons after combined administration of the two drugs followed a nedio-lateral gradient with a significant difference between the medial and the dorso-lateral part of the CPu in all the experimental groups (Fig. 2).

Intra-nigral infusion of higher doses of MK 801 (14.8 nmol) or CPP (4 nmol) although producing intense contralateral turning with a total number of turns similar to that obtained after lower doses plus parenteral SKF 38393, induced only few Fos-positive nuclei in the lesioned CPu (Table 1).

                                    S. Fenu et al.

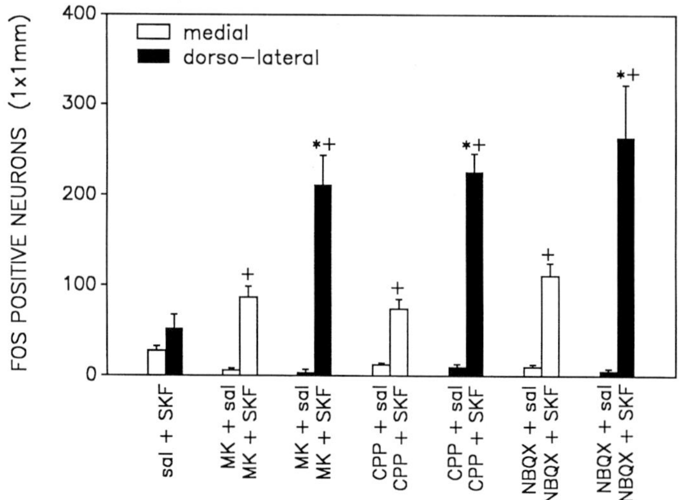

Fig. 2. Number of Fos-positive-nuclei in the medial and dorso-lateral part of the CPu after intranigral saline + SKF 38393 (1.5 mg/kg s.c.) or intranigral MK 801 (1.5 nmol), CPP (1.2 nmol), NBQX (0.6 nmol) + saline or SKF 38393 (1.5 mg/kg s.c.). p < 0.05 *versus saline in SN + SKF 38393; + dorso-lateral CPu versus medial CPu

Specificity of the injection sites

To check the specificity of the injection sites MK 801, CPP and NBQX were injected 2 or 3 mm above the SN. MK 801 (1.5 nmol), CPP (1.2 nmol) and NBQX (0.6 nmol) infused above the SN failed to induce contralateral turning behavior or to potentiate the c-fos expression induced in the CPu by SKF 38393 (1.5 mg/kg s.c.). In all rats the injection sites were checked after perfusion of the brains. Besides rats used for the site specificity studies, only rats in which the cannula tip was located in the SN were used for the immunohistochemical studies and included in the final results.

Discussion

The present results show that in unilaterally 6-OHDA lesioned rats, blockade of nigral NMDA or AMPA receptors by local infusion of MK 801, CPP or NBQX, potentiated DA D_1-mediated turning behavior and striatal c-fos expression indicating that blockade of the excitatory input to the SNr induces potentiation of D_1-mediated responses.

In 6-OHDA lesioned rats, stimulation of D_1 receptors results in an increased activity of striato-nigral GABA neurons (Trugman and Wooten, 1987; Gerfen et al., 1990) therefore, the results of this study suggest that a blockade of the excitatory input to the SNr might facilitate the inhibitory effect of a subthreshold stimulation of D_1 receptors, thus potentiating D_1-mediated responses.

Previous studies have suggested that the motor impairments caused by the loss of DA in the CPu are due to an increased activity of the GABAergic output from the SNr, leading to an excessive inhibition of talamo-cortical neurons (Albin et al., 1989; DeLong, 1990); moreover, local cerebral infusions of drugs have shown that the SN and the thalamic motor nuclei control neurotransmitter release in the CPu (Barbeito et al., 1989; De Boer and Abercrombie, 1993).

All together these results suggest that NMDA and AMPA antagonists when infused into the SN in combination with parenteral SKF 38393 might, by a disfacilitation or inhibition of GABA neurons projecting to the talamus, increase the activity of cortico-striatal glutamate neurons, thus potentiating c-fos expression in the CPu (Beretta et al., 1992).

Quantification of Fos-positive nuclei showed that SKF 38393 alone induced c-fos expression in a uniform manner in the CPu, while when SKF 38393 is administered in combination with intranigral NMDA and AMPA antagonists, c-fos expression is particularly stimulated in the dorso-lateral part of the CPu. This pattern of Fos distribution can be related to the fact that the cortico-striatal projections, which are organized in a general topographic manner (Alexander et al., 1986; Gerfen, 1992), innervate the dorso-lateral part of the CPu through their glutamatergic projections originating from the motor cortex (Walaas, 1981; Kelly et al., 1982).

High doses of MK 801 or CPP applied into the SN caused contralateral turning of a similar degree to that obtained after combined intra SN administration of lower doses of MK 801 or CPP plus parenteral SKF 38393. This treatment however, induces sparse fos-like-immunoreactivity in the 6-OHDA lesioned CPu. An explanation of this difference is that the SNr project through two different GABAergic pathways, to the ventromedial thalamus and to the superior colliculus/mesencephalic reticular formation (Di Chiara et al., 1979b; Morelli et al., 1981), therefore turning behavior may be mediated by two separate SNr efferent pathways, one ascending to the thalamus and innervating the CPu which in the presence of a subtreshold stimulation of D-1 receptors activates c-fos, the other projecting to the superior colliculus/ mesencephalic reticular formation which does not influence c-fos expression in the CPu.

C-fos induction in the CPu therefore, would not always reflect turning behavior. Evidence from studies on D$_1$-mediated contralateral turning and Fos are in line with this observation (Robertson et al., 1989).

In conclusion the results reported in this study suggest that although the mechanism of the synergism between D$_1$ agonists and glutamate antagonists may be complex and involve several sites in the basal ganglia circuits, a depression of SNr efferent neurons by glutamate antagonists, modulates in a positive manner the responses obtained by stimulation of D$_1$ receptors.

                    S. Fenu et al.

References

Albin RL, Young AB, Penney JB (1989) The functional anatomy of basal ganglia disorders. TINS 12: 366–375

Albin RL, Makowiec RL, Hollingsworth SR, Dure LS, Penney JB, Young AB (1991) Excitatory amino acid binding sites in the basalganglia of the rat: a quantitative autoradiographic study. Neuroscience 46: 35–48

Alexander GE, DeLong MR, Strick P (1986) Parallel organization of functionally segregated circuits linking basal ganglia and cortex. Annu Rev Neurosci 9: 357–381

Barbeito L, Girault JA, Godeheu G, Pittaluga A, Glowinski J, Cheramy A (1989) Activation of the bilateral corticostriatal glutamatergic projection by infusion of GABA into thalamic motor nuclei in the cat: an in vivo release study. Neuroscience 28: 365–374

Beretta S, Robertson HA, Graybiel AM (1992) Dopamine and glutamate agonists stimulate neuron specific expression of fos-like protein in the striatum. J Neurophysiol 68: 767–777

Boldry RC, Chase TN, Engber TM (1993) Influence of previous exposure to L-dopa on the interaction between dizocilpine and dopamine D1 and D2 agonists in 6-hydroxydopamine lesioned rats. J Pharmacol Exp Ther 267: 1454–1459

Burns LH, Sato K, Wullner U, Isacson O (1993) Intra-nigra infusion of AMPA attenuates dopamine-dependent rotation in the rat. Neuroreport 4: 1075–1078

Carlsson M, Carlsson A (1989) Dramatic synergism between MK-801 and clonidine with respect to locomotor stimulatory effect in monoamine-depleted mice. J Neural Transm 77: 65–71

De Boer P, Abercrombie ED (1993) Amphetamine-induced modulation of striatal acetylcholine efflux: mechanisms of action. Soc Neurosci Abstr 19: 304.5

DeLong R (1990) Primate models of movement disorders of basal ganglia origin. Trends Neurosci 13: 281–285

Di Chiara G, Porceddu ML, Morelli M, Mulas ML, Gessa GL (1979a) Substantia nigra as an out-put station for striatal dopaminergic responses: role of a GABA-mediated inhibition of pars reticulata neurons. Naunyn Schmiedebergs Arch Pharmacol 306: 153–159

Di Chiara G, Porceddu ML, Morelli M, Mulas ML, Gessa GL (1979b) Evidence for a gabaergic projection from the substantia nigra to the ventromedial thalamus and to the superior colliculus of the rat. Brain Res 176: 273–284

Gerfen CR (1992) The neostriatal mosaic: multiple levels of compartmental organization. Trends Neurosci 15: 133–139

Gerfen CR, Engber TM, Mahan LC, Susel Z, Chase TN, Monsma FJ, Sibley DR (1990) D_1 and D_2 dopamine receptor-regulated gene expression of striatonigral and striatopallidal neurons. Science 250: 1429–1432

Goddwin P, Starr BS, Starr MS (1992) Motor responses to dopamine D_1 and D_2 agonists in the reserpine-treated mouse are affected differentially by the NMDA receptor antagonist MK 801. J Neural Transm [PD-Sect] 4: 15–26

Kelly AE, Domesick VB, Nauta WJH (1982) The amygdalostriatal projection in the rat an anatomical study by anterograde tracing methods. Neuroscience 7: 615–630

Klockgether T, Turski L (1990) NMDA antagonists potentiate antiparkinsonian actions of L-Dopa in monoamine-depleted rats. Ann Neurol 28: 539–546

Klockgether T, Turski L, Honoré T, Zhang Z, Gash DM, Kurlan R, Greenamyre JT (1991) The AMPA receptor antagonist NBQX has antiparkinsonian effects in monoamine-depleted rats and MPTP-treated monkeys. Ann Neurol 30: 717–723

Löschmann P-A, Lange KW, Kunow M, Rettig K-J, Jähnig P, Honoré T, Turski L, Wachtel H, Jenner P, Marsden CD (1991) Synergism of the AMPA-antagonist NBQX and the NMDA-antagonist CPP with L-DOPA in models of Parkinson's disease. J Neural Transm [PD Sect] 3: 203–213

Morelli M, Porceddu ML, Di Chiara G (1980) Lesions of substantia nigra by kainic acid: effects on apomorphine-induced stereotyped behaviour. Brain Res 191: 67–78

Morelli M, Imperato A, Porceddu ML, Di Chiara G (1981) Role of dorsal mesencephalic reticular formation and deep layers of superior colliculus in turning behaviour elicited from the striatum. Brain Res 215: 337–341

Morelli M, Di Chiara G (1990) MK-801 potentiates dopaminergic D_1 but reduces D_2 responses in the 6-hydroxydopamine model of Parkinson's disease. Eur J Pharmacol 182: 611–612

Morelli M, Fenu S, Pinna A, Di Chiara G (1992) Opposite effects of NMDA receptor blockade on dopaminergic D_1- and D_2-mediated behavior in the 6-hydroxydopamine model of turning: relationship with c-fos expression. J Pharmacol Exp Ther 260: 402–406

Morgan JI, Curran T (1989) Stimulus-transcription coupling in neurons: role of cellular immediate-early genes. TINS 12: 459–462

Olianas MC, De Montis GM, Mulas G, Tagliamonte A (1978) The striatal dopaminergic function is mediated by the inhibition of a nigral, non-dopaminergic neuronal system via a strionigral GABAergic pathway. Eur J Pharmacol 49: 233–241

Robertson HA, Peterson MR, Murphy K, Robertson GS (1989) D_1-dopamine receptor agonists selectively activate striatal c-fos independent of rotational behaviour. Brain Res 503: 346–349

Svensson A, Carlsson A, Carlsson ML (1992) Differential locomotor interactions between dopamine D1/D2 receptor agonists and the NMDA antagonist dizocilpine in monoamine-depleted mice. J Neural Transm [Gen Sect] 90: 199–217

Trugman JM, Wooten GF (1987) Selective D_1 and D_2 dopamine agonists differentially alter basal ganglia glucose utilization in rats with unilateral 6-hydroxydopamine substantia nigra lesions. J Neurosci 7: 2927–2935

Wachtel H, Kunow M, Löschmann PA (1992) NBQX (6-nitro-sulfamoyl-benzo-quinoxaline-dione) and CPP (3-carboxy-piperazin-propyl phosphonic acid) potentiate dopamine agonist induced rotations in substantia nigra lesioned rats. Neurosci Lett 142: 179–182

Walaas I (1981) Biochemical evidence for overlapping neocortical and allocortical glutamate projections to the nucleus accumbens and rostral caudatoputamen in the rat brain. Neuroscience 6: 399–405

Authors' address: Dr. M. Morelli, Department of Toxicology, Viale A. Diaz 182, I-09100 Cagliari, Italy.

J Neural Transm (1995) [Suppl] 45: 83–90

Dopamine mediated responses in 6-hydroxydopamine lesioned rats involve changes of the signal transduction

P. Barone[1], **M. Popoli**[1], **M. Morelli**[3], **G. Cicarelli**[1,2], **G. Campanella**[1], and **G. Di Chiara**[3]

[1] Department of Neurology, University of Napoli, Federico II, [2] IRCCS Sanatrix, Pozzilli, and [3] Department of Toxicology, University of Cagliari, Italy

Summary. A single dose of the D_1 agonist SKF 38393 (3 mg/kg) produces contralateral turning in unilaterally 6-hydroxydopamine lesioned rats only after a previous exposure of the animals to a dopamine agonist. This priming phenomenon is here investigated by studying the phosphorylation of DARPP-32, a dopamine- and cyclic AMP-regulated phosphoprotein functionally linked to D_1 receptors in striatum. Dephospho-form of DARPP-32 in striatal tissue was measured by a back-phosphorylation assay. While the levels of DARPP-32 protein, as measured by quantitative immunoblotting, remained unchanged, a significant decrease of dephospho-DARPP-32 was observed in the denervated striatum of primed rats, indicating an increased phosphorylation in vivo of DARPP-32 in response to the D_1 agonist. This study shows that an alteration of the dopamine-dependent signal transduction is related to the behavioral response to dopamine agents, suggesting a possible mechanism involved in the effects of these drugs in parkinsonian patients.

Introduction

The unilateral lesion of the nigro-striatal pathway induced by 6-hydroxydopamine (6-OHDA) in rat provides an experimental model of Parkinson's disease generally used to test anti-parkinsonian effects of dopaminergic drugs (Ungerstedt, 1971). In these animals, a single administration of either selective D_2 receptor agonists or mixed D_1/D_2 receptor agonists, but not D_1 agonists, induces contralateral turning behavior (Herrera-Marschitz and Ungerstedt, 1984; Morelli and Di Chiara, 1987). Consistently in parkinsonian patients, unlike all D_2 agonists, D_1 agonists have not shown a clear anti-parkinsonian action (Barone et al., 1987; Braun et al., 1987; Kebabian et al., 1992).

Recently, it has been shown that in animals previously primed with either a DA agonist or the DA precursor L-Dopa a low dose of the dopamine D_1 receptor agonist SKF 38393 is able to induce contralateral turning (Morelli and DiChiara, 1987). This sensitization phenomenon cannot be related to the alterations in DA receptors. In fact, striatal D_1 receptors are modified neither by denervation of the dopamine pathway nor by DA agonist exposure following the lesion (Morelli et al., 1990). As an alternative hypothesis, D1 agonist efficacy after priming might be related to the modification of the transduction pathway as a consequence of intracellular adaptative changes to both DA denervation and DA-ergic stimulation.

The role of signal transduction in the development of DA-mediated sensitization might be studied by evaluating the phosphorylation state of DARPP-32, a neuron-specific phosphoprotein which is regulated by DA and cyclic AMP (cAMP) (Hemmings et al., 1987). DARPP-32 is phosphorylated by the cAMP-dependent protein kinase (PKA) which is activated by the increased cAMP levels following D_1 receptor stimulation. Therefore, the phosphorylation state of DARPP-32 appears to be an excellent index of the activity of transduction mechanisms regulated by D_1 receptors and can be determined by a back-phosphorylation assay "in vitro" (Hemmings et al., 1987; Walaas et al., 1983). According to this technique, a decrease of $[^{32}P]$-phosphate tissue incorporation following "in vitro" incubation reflects an increase of phosphorylation state of DARPP-32 "in vivo". Conversely, an increase of $[^{32}P]$-phosphate incorporation indicates a reduction of DARPP-32 phosphorylation "in vivo".

In the present study, we evaluated the effect of D_1 agonist administration on DARPP-32 phosphorylation in striata of both primed and drug-naive rats with unilateral 6-OHDA induced nigral lesion. Characterization of alterations in signal transduction in response to both DA denervation and DA stimulation might be relevant to better understand the effects of DA-ergic drugs in parkinsonian patients.

Materials and methods

Animals

Male, Sprague-Dawley rats, weighing 250–300 g were anaesthetized with chloral hydrate (400 mg/kg i.p.), positioned in a David Kopf stereotaxic apparatus and injected into the left medial forebrain bundle (coordinates A: −2.2, L: 1.5, V: 7.4, according to the atlas of Pellegrino et al., 1979) with 8 μl of a 6-OHDA solution (1 mg/ml) containing 0.05% ascorbic acid. In order to avoid damage of noradrenergic neurons all rats were injected subcutaneously with desipramine (25 mg/kg) prior to the lesion. Fourteen days after lesioning, rats randomly received either saline (drug-naive rats) or L-Dopa, 50 mg/kg i.p., plus the Dopa decarboxylase inhibitor benserazide, 30 mg/kg i.p. (primed rats). Three days later, animals from both groups were injected with the test drug, either saline or the D_1 agonist SKF 38393 (3 mg/kg, s.c.), and placed in plastic hemispheric individual cages. Turning behavior was recorded for 30 min after the test drug. The last 5 min recording was considered for the analysis. Immediately after the behavioral recording all rats were sacrificed by decapitation and the striata of both sides were dissected out on ice and frozen in liquid nitrogen.

Backphosphorylation of the striatal protein extracts

Frozen striata were immersed in ice-cold homogenization buffer, 10 mM TRIS HCl (pH 7.4) containing 2 mM EDTA and 0.1 mM PMSF (Sigma) and homogenized with 10 strokes in a teflon-glass Potter homogenizer. Proteins were precipitated by adding 350 μl of homogenate to 5 ml of ice-cold 5 mM zinc acetate and pelleted by centrifugation at 2,000 × g for 15 min. The pellet was resuspended in 1 ml of 10 mM citric acid (pH 2.8) containing 0.1% Triton × 100 (Baker) and the suspension was centrifuged at 27,000 × g for 15 min. The supernatant was collected, adjusted to pH 6.5 by adding 0.5 M Na_2HPO_4 and left on ice 10 min. After centrifugation at 16,000 × g for 15 min, the final supernatant was collected and kept on ice. Protein concentration was measured according to Lowry et al. (1951) using bovine serum albumin as a standard.

The state of phosphorylation of DARPP-32 was evaluated by back-phosphorylation of acid-extracted tissues according to Walaas et al. (1983). Briefly, phosphorlation reactions were carried out for 60 min at 30°C in a final volume of 100 μl containing 50 mM HEPES (pH 7.4), 10 mM $MgCl_2$, 1 mM EGTA, 1 mM EDTA, 10 nM catalytic subunit of protein kinase A (Sigma), 10 μM $[\gamma\text{-}^{32}P]$ ATP (Dupont, 20 Ci/mmol) and 40 μg of striatal proteins. The reaction was stopped by adding 50 μl of SDS sample buffer (3X concentrated). Following one dimensional SDS-polyacrylamide gel electrophoresis (10% acrylamide, 0.3% bis-acrylamide) gels were stained with Coomassie Brilliant Blue, destained, dried and autoradiographed on Kodak XAR 5 films. The amount of $[^{32}P]$-phosphate incorporated in the DARPP-32 band was determined by excision of the band from the gel followed by solubilization and liquid scintillation counting.

Quantitative immunoblotting of DARPP-32

Both identification of the DARPP-32 band on polyacrylamide gels and quantification of the phosphoprotein were performed by an immunoblotting technique according to Hemmings and Greengard (1986). The band was detected using a chemiluminiscent method (ECL, Amersham).

Protein bands were analyzed with regard to density and area using a Macintosh image analysis system (IMAGE 1.47). Band densities were within the linear range of the camera sensitivity (not shown).

Data analysis

Both differences in $[^{32}P]$-phosphate incorporation in DARPP-32 bands and differences in band densities of immunoblot experiments were analyzed by 2-way analysis of variance (ANOVA).

Drugs and antibodies

6-OHDA and L-Dopa were purchased from Sigma Chem. (St. Louis, USA). SKF 38393, benserazide and desipramine were respectively donated by Smith Kline and French (Welwyn Garden City, UK), Hoffman La Roche (Switzerland) and Ciba-Geigy (Basel, Switzerland). DARPP-32 monoclonal antibodies were kindly provided by Dr. G. Snyder and Dr. P. Greengard.

  P. Barone et al.

Results

Both primed and unprimed rats did not exhibit turning behavior following the injection of saline (control groups). Similarly, no turning behavior was observed in lesioned rats never exposed to L-Dopa and tested with 3 mg/kg of SKF 38393 (unprimed group). On the other hand, the same dose of the D_1 agonist was able to induce contralateral turning behavior in the primed group. The circling behavior occurred approximately 10 min after the injection of SKF 38393 (Fig. 1).

DARPP-32 phosphorylation was not modified by saline administration in both primed and not primed animals. No difference was found in [^{32}P]-phosphate incorporation between the intact and the denervated striatum following saline injection (Fig. 2). On the other hand, the injection of SKF 38393 significantly diminished the incorporation of [^{32}P]-phosphate in DARPP-32 only in the denervated striatum of primed rats (Fig. 2). Such a reduction reflects the decrease of dephospho-DARPP-32 available "in vitro" for the back-phosphorylation and conversely indicates the increase of phospho-DARPP-32 "in vivo".

No variation in the levels of DARPP-32 was revealed by quantitative immunoblotting in either intact or denervated striatum of both primed and unprimed animals (Fig. 3). These data indicate that the reduced amount of dephospho-DARPP-32 occurring in the denervated striatum of primed rats is due to the change in protein phosphorylation rather than to the variation of the phosphoprotein levels.

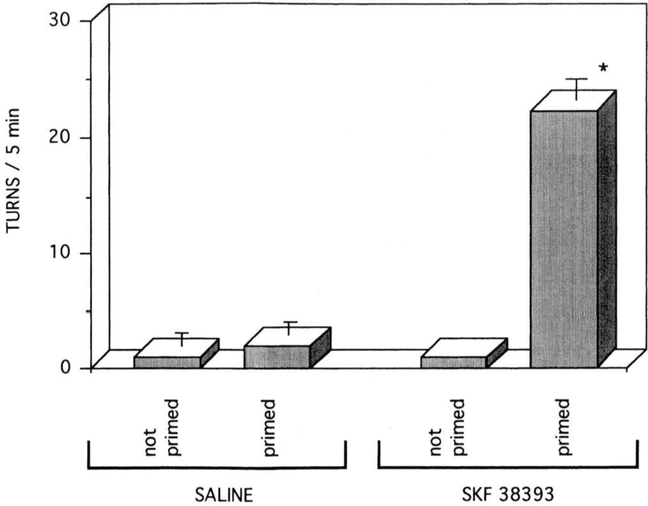

Fig. 1. Effects of a single administration of either saline or SKF 38393 (3 mg/kg) on turning behavior of both unprimed and primed 6-OHDA lesioned rats. Values represent mean ± SD of four experiments using six animals for each treatment. Circling behavior was recorded during 5 min prior to the sacrifice. *p < 0.01

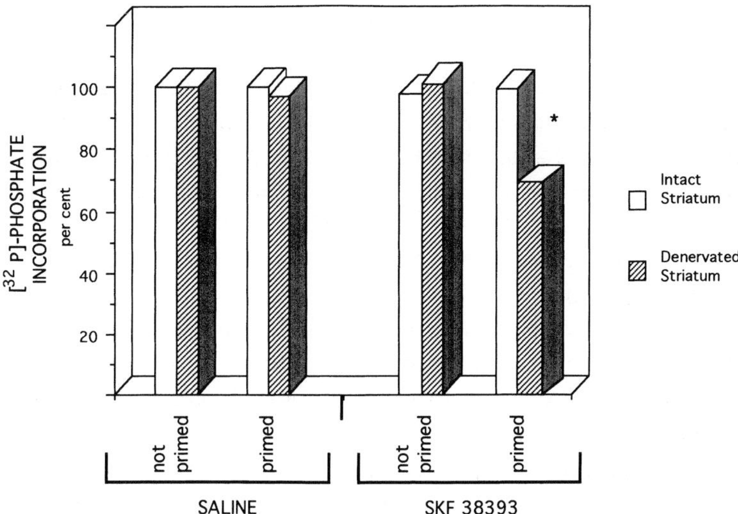

Fig. 2. Effects of a single administration of either saline or SKF 38393 (3 mg/kg) on DARPP-32 phosphorylation in striata of both unprimed and primed 6-OHDA lesioned rats. The reduced incorporation of [³²P]-phosphate in DARPP-32 of primed denervated striatum reflects an increase of phosphorylation state of DARPP-32 "in vivo". *p < 0.01 (n = 6 animals for each treatment group)

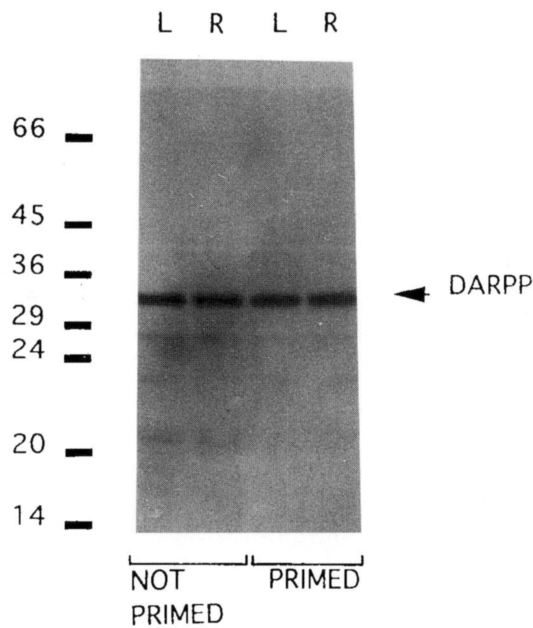

Fig. 3. Immunoblot with DARPP-32 monoclonal antibody of striatal proteins from two representative rats, respectively unprimed and primed, following treatment with SKF 38393. No difference in optical density was found, indicating no alteration of the levels of the protein between denervated (L) and intact (R) striata of primed and unprimed animals. Bars and numbers indicate molecular weight × 10³

Discussion

The present results show that the $[^{32}P]$-phosphate incorporation in DARPP-32, as revealed by back-phosphorylation assay, is significantly decreased in striata of the denervated side, in primed as compared to drug-naive rats. Since the $[^{32}P]$-phosphate incorporation in vitro reflects the opposite situation in vivo (Forn and Greengard, 1978), it is possible that, following priming, the D_1 receptor stimulation results in an increased phosphorylation of DARPP-32 in the denervated striatum.

This observation closely correlates with behavioral studies showing that low doses of SKF 38393 induce contralateral turning in 6-OHDA lesioned rats only after exposure to a dopamine agonist (this paper and Morelli and Di Chiara, 1987). Analysis of D_1 receptor binding in the striatum of both primed and unprimed rats showed no change in the number and affinity of the receptors (Morelli and Di Chiara, 1990). In contrast, dopamine-stimulated adenylate cyclase showed an increase in the affinity of the enzyme for DA in the lesioned side of primed rats as compared with drug-naive rats (Morelli and Di Chiara, 1990). Taken together these results strongly support the hypothesis that changes in signal transduction mechanisms, rather than in recognition sites, are involved in the development of D_1 mediated behavioral sensitization. Conceivably, priming might alter the cAMP cascade in striatal neurons in the sense of an increased sensitivity to D_1 receptor stimulation. All components of this cAMP cascade may be potentially involved, namely the GTP-binding proteins and the PKA (Birnbaumer, 1990). The latter, catalyzing the phosphorylation of DARPP-32, might be involved in the functional changes induced by priming (Walaas and Greengard, 1991).

Further evidence for a PKA involvement in the priming development is provided by the fact that priming seems to act preferentially through a modification of the phosphorylation state rather than neo-synthesis of DARPP-32. In fact, in the present study neither the 6-OHDA induced lesion nor the priming nor the combination of both modified the total amount of phosphoprotein as revealed by quantitative immunoblotting. These results are in line with previous studies showing no change in the level of DARPP-32 protein or mRNA in the striata of parkinsonian patients and of 6-OHDA lesioned rats (Girault et al., 1989; Raisman-Vozari et al., 1990).

The consistency among behavioral studies and the finding of an alteration of DARPP-32 phosphorylation only in the denervated striatum of primed rats supports the view of an involvement of post-synaptic signal transduction in the mechanism of expression of priming. Well established relationships between sensitization phenomena and alteration of the signal transduction are provided by studies on the effect of antidepressants and drugs of abuse chronically administered (Nestler et al., 1989; Guitart and Nestler, 1992; Beitner-Johnson et al., 1992). Also in these studies supersensitivity is not related to modification of receptors density but to the increased activity of adenylate cyclase and PKA suggesting that a common biochemical mechanism involving signal transduction might be relevant to the development of behavioral sensitization.

The adaptative changes of striatal neurons to DA denervation and DA-ergic stimulation might explain the wide range of responses to dopaminergic agents in parkinsonism. Unlike all D_2 agonists, D_1 agonists have not generally shown antiparkinsonian effects in both MPTP-lesioned monkeys and parkinsonian patients (Barone et al., 1987; Braun et al., 1987; Kebabian et al., 1992). We suggest that D_1 agonist efficacy might be related to the development of intracellular adaptative changes similar to those induced by the priming in 6-OHDA lesioned rats. Conceivably, early or late exposure of humans to drugs acting on DA system might result in different therapeutic effects. Similarly, the effects of long term exposure to L-Dopa, such as on-off phenomena occurring in parkinsonians, might be explained by adaptative changes of signal transduction as a consequence of the chronic treatment.

References

Barone P, Bankiewicz KS, Corsini GU, Kopin IJ, Chase TN (1987) Dopaminergic mechanisms in hemiparkinsonian monkeys. Neurology 37: 1592–1595

Beitner-Johnson D, Guitart X, Nestler EJ (1992) Common intracellular actions of chronic morphine and cocaine in dopaminergic brain reward regions. Ann NY Acad Sci: 71–87

Birnbaumer L (1990) G proteins in signal transduction. Annu Rev Pharmacol Toxicol 30: 675–705

Braun AR, Fabbrini G, Mouradian MM, Serrati C, Barone P, Chase TN (1987) Selective D1 dopamine receptor agonist treatment of Parkinson's disease. J Neural Transm 68: 41–50

Forn J, Greengard P (1978) Depolarizing agents and cyclic nucleotides regulate the phosphorylation of specific neuronal proteins in rat cerebral cortex slices. Proc Natl Acad Sci USA 75: 5195–5199

Girault JA, Raisman-Vozari R, Agid Y, Greengard P (1989) Striatal phosphoproteins in Parkinson disease and progressive supranuclear palsy. Proc Natl Acad Sci 86: 2493–2497

Guitart X, Nestler J (1992) Chronic administration of lithium or other antidepressants increases levels of DARPP-32 in rat frontal cortex. J Neurochem 59: 1164–1167

Hemmings HC, Greengard P (1986) DARPP-32, a dopamine and 3′-5′-monophosphate-regulated phosphoprotein: regional, tissue and phylogenetic distribution. J Neurosci 6: 1469–1481

Hemmings HC, Walaas SI, Ouimet CC, Greengard P (1987) Dopaminergic regulation of protein phosphorylation in the striatum: DARPP-32. Trends Neurosci 10: 377–383

Herrera-Marschitz M, Ungerstedt U (1984) Evidence that apomorphine and pergolide induce rotation in rats by different action on D1 and D2 receptor sites. Eur J Pharmacol 98: 165–171

Kebabian JW, Britton DR, DeNinno MP, Perner R, Smith L, Jenner P, Schoenleber R, Williams M (1992) A-77636: a potent and selective dopamine D1 receptor agonist with antiparkinsonian activity in marmosets. Eur J Pharmacol 229: 203–209

Lowry OH, Rosenbrough NJ, Farr AR, Randall RJ (1951) Protein measurement with the Folin phenol reagent. J Biol Chem 193: 265–275

Morelli M, Di Chiara G (1987) Agonist-induced homologus and heterologous sensitization to D1 and D2 dependent contraversive turning. Eur J Pharmacol 141: 101–107

Morelli M, De Montis G, Di Chiara G (1990) Changes in the D1 receptoradenylate cyclase complex after priming. Eur J Pharmacol 180: 365–367

Nestler EJ, Terwilliger RZ, Duman RS (1989) Chronic antidepressant administration alters the subcellular distribution of cyclic AMP-dependent protein kinase in rat frontal cortex. J Neurochem 53: 1644–1647

Pellegrino LJ, Pellegrino AS, Cushman AJ (1979) A stereotaxic atlas of the rat brain. Plenum Press, New York

Raisman-Vozari R, Girault JA, Moussaoui S, Fererstein C, Jenner P, Marsden CD, Agid Y (1990) Lack of change in striatal DARPP-32 levels following nigrostriatal dopaminergic lesions in animals and in parkinsonian syndromes in man. Brain Res 507: 45–50

Ungerstedt U (1971) Postsynaptic supersensitivity after 6-hydroxydopamine induced degeneration of the nigro-striatal dopamine system. Acta Physiol Scand [Suppl] 367: 69–93

Walaas SI, Greengard P (1991) Protein phosphorylation and neuronal function. Pharmacol Rev 43: 229–349

Walaas SI, Aswad DW, Greengard P (1983) A dopamine and cyclic AMP-regulated phosphoprotein enriched in dopamine-innervated brain regions. Nature 301: 69–71

Authors' address: P. Barone, MD, PhD, Clinica Neurologica, Università di Napoli Federico II, Via S. Pansini 5, I-80131 Napoli, Italy.

J Neural Transm (1995) [Suppl] 45: 91–102

Is in vivo striatal acetylcholine output under a tonic inhibitory control by dopamine?

A. Imperato, M. C. Obinu, and **G. L. Gessa**

"G. M. Everett" Laboratory of Neuropsychopharmacology, Department of
Neuroscience "Bernard B. Brodie", University of Cagliari, Italy

Summary.   The role of dopamine transmission on striatal acetylcholine release was investigated by using brain microdialysis. Blockade of dopamine D_2 receptors with $(-)$-sulpiride or haloperidol increased acetylcholine release to a maximum of 80% (after 50 and 0.5 mg/kg, respectively). This effect was prevented by blockade of dopamine D_1 receptors with 0.5 mg/kg SCH 39166 or by depletion of dopamine stores after 5 mg/kg reserpine + 150 mg/kg α-methyltyrosine.

Treatment with SCH 39166 or reserpine + α-methyltyrosine reduced acetylcholine release by about a maximum of 30%. Stimulation of dopamine D_2 receptors with LY 171555 (quinpirole) at a low, sedative dose (0.05 mg/kg), reduced acetylcholine release by about 30% with no further reduction at higher doses up to 1 mg/kg. Moreover, LY 171555 (0.1 mg/kg) given to SCH 39166 (0.5 mg/kg) or SKF 38393 (20 mg/kg)-pretreated rats did not decrease acetylcholine release, suggesting that its effect is through a dopamine D_1 receptor-mediated mechanism.

In contrast, in dopamine depleted rats, LY 171555 0.1 mg/kg became more effective in decreasing acetylcholine release (about 70%) also after SCH 39166 (0.5 mg/kg) pretreatment (about 80%), thus acting independently of dopamine D_1 receptor mechanisms.

These results indicate that, in normal circumstances, endogenous dopamine facilitates striatal acetylcholine release through dopamine D_1 receptors. The results argue against the commonly accepted view that dopamine D_2 receptors exert a tonic inhibitory control on acetylcholine release. Moreover, they suggest that dopamine D_2 receptors, in circumstances of dopamine depletion, may exert an inhibitory control on acetylcholine release independent of dopamine D_1 receptor mechanisms.

Introduction

Many studies in the last two decades have led to the concept that nigrostriatal dopaminergic neurons exert an inhibitory influence on striatal acetylcholine release by an action of dopamine on D_2 receptors located on cholinergic interneurons (Stoof et al., 1992). Accordingly, in vitro and in vivo studies have shown that blockade of D_2 receptors by neuroleptics results in increased striatal acetylcholine release (Bertorelli and Consolo, 1990; Damsma et al., 1990a; Marien and Richard, 1990; Stoof et al., 1979) whereas selective stimulation of D_2 receptors causes inhibition of striatal acetylcholine output (Damsma et al., 1990a; Stoof et al., 1979).

These results support the contention that endogenous dopamine exerts a tonic inhibitory control on acetylcholine release under normal conditions (De Boer et al., 1992; Stoof et al., 1992).

However, in contrast to the in vitro studies, where no consistent evidence has been obtained for a role of D_1 receptors in the regulation of acetylcholine release (Stoof and Kebabian, 1982; Plantjè et al., 1984; Gorell and Czarnecki, 1986; Gorell et al., 1986), microdialysis studies have indicated that D_1 receptor agonists increase, and antagonists decrease, acetylcholine release in the striatum, suggesting that D_1 receptors play a facilitatory control on acetylcholine release in vivo (Consolo et al., 1987; Damsma et al., 1990b; Imperato et al., 1992b).

Therefore the question arises whether acetylcholine release is tonically inhibited by endogenous dopamine acting upon D_2 receptors or is tonically activated by dopamine acting on D_1 receptors. In order to answer this question, the microdialysis technique in freely moving rats was used to investigate the modification of acetylcholine release following blockade or stimulation of D_2 receptors in combination with D_1 receptor blockade. Moreover, the role of D_2 receptors in the regulation of striatal acetylcholine release was studied in rats with prolonged dopamine depletion.

Materials and methods

Animals

Male Sprague-Dawley (Charles River, Italy) (225–250 g) were housed in groups of 3 per cage for at least 10 days before use. Food and water were freely available and animals were maintained under an artificial 12/12 light/dark cycle (lights were on from 7 a.m. to 7 p.m.). Experiments were carried out between 8.30 a.m. and 5 p.m.

Microdialysis implantation and experimental procedure

Rats were anesthetized with chloralhydrate (0.4 g/kg i.p.) and implanted with dialysis tubes (AN 69-HF, wet tube o.d. is 320 µm; Hospal-Dasco, Bologna, Italy) at the level of dorsal striata according to the König and Klippel atlas (König and Klippel, 1963) (A + 1.5 from bregma, V-5.0 from the skull). Surgery was carried out by using the transversal microdialysis technique recently revised in order to induce less tissue damage and to reduce glia reaction around the dialysis tube (Imperato et al., 1992a).

Ringer solution containing (mM) KCl 3, NaCl 125, $CaCl_2$ 1.3, $MgCl_2$ 1.0, $NaHCO_3$ 23, potassium phosphate buffer 1.5, pH 7.3 and neostigmine 0.1 µM, was pumped through the dialysis probe at a constant rate of 2 µl/min. The extracellular concentration of acetylcholine was measured by high performance liquid chromatography (HPLC) with electrochemical detection according to the technique described by Damsma and Westerink (1991). Samples were collected every 20 min (40 µl) and the average concentration of acetylcholine in the last 3 pre-drug samples, obtained after 1 h of perfusion, was taken as 100% and all subsequent post-treatment values were expressed as mean ($\pm$ S.E.M. percent variation of basal values. The baseline acetylcholine concentration in 20 min samples from the striatum was 4.5 ± 0.38 pmol (mean $\pm$ S.E.M. of 9 rats). The datection limit for acetylcholine was 0.05 pmol/injection. Experiments started 24 h after the implantation of the dialysis tube.

Drugs

Haloperidol (Janssen, Belgium), ($-$)-sulpiride (Ravizza, Italy) and reserpine (Sigma, Italy) were dissolved by adding a minimum amount of glacial acetic acid and then adjusting to pH 6 with NaOH. SCH 39166 HCl (Schering Research Laboratories), SKF 38393 HCl (Research Biochemicals Incorporated), LY 171555 HCl (Research Biochemicals Incorporated) and α-methyltyrosine methyl ester hydrochloride (Sigma, Italy) were dissolved in distilled water. All drugs were administered intraperitoneally in a volume of 0.3 ml/100 g.

For data presented in Fig. 5, the treatment with reserpine (5 mg/kg i.p.) and α-methyltyrosine (150 mg/kg i.p.) was performed 6 h before vehicle, ($-$)-sulpiride or haloperidol injection. The control group received the injection of vehicle 6 h before the experiment.

For data presented in Figs. 6 and 7, the treatment with reserpine (5 mg/kg i.p.) + α-methyltyrosine (100 mg/kg i.p.) was performed 24 h before, and the injection of α-methyltyrosine was repeated 8 h before the administration of LY 171555 or SCH 39166. The control groups received the injection of saline or vehicle 24 and 8 h before the experiment.

Statistics

Between-groups comparisons were performed using a two-way ANOVA for repeated measures, the factors being treatment (2 levels = two doses for drug as in Fig. 2, or saline pretreatment compared to drug pretreatment as in Fig. 3; or 3 levels = 3 doses for each drug as in Fig. 1) and time points (10 levels =0 to 180 min as in Figs. 1 and 3, or 7 levels =0 to 120 min as in Figs. 2 and 7). Data presented in Fig. 4 were analyzed by two-way ANOVA, the factors being pretreatment (2 levels =saline, SKF 38393) and treatment (2 levels =saline, LY 171555). Data presented in Fig. 5 were analyzed by one-way ANOVA.

The results presented in Fig. 6 were analyzed by two-way ANOVA, the factors being pretreatment (2 levels =vehicle and reserpine/α-methyltyrosine) and treatment (6 levels = saline, LY 1711555 0.025 mg/kg, LY 171555 0.05 mg/kg, LY 171555 0.1 mg/kg, LY 171555 0.5 mg/kg, LY 171555 1 mg/kg). For data presented in Fig. 7, the factors being: treatment (4 levels = reserpine/α-methyltyrosine)+ saline, reserpine/α-methyltyrosine + LY 171555, vehicle + saline, vehicle + LY 171555).

Post hoc analysis was performed by Student's t-test for paired and unpaired data.

Results

Dopamine D_2 receptor blockade

The administration of D_2 receptor antagonists ($-$)-sulpiride (20 up 100 mg/kg i.p.) or haloperidol (0.25 up to 1 mg/kg i.p.) produced a dose-related increase

                                    A. Imperato et al.

in acetylcholine release. Maximal increase of about 70–80% was observed within 20 min after treatment with 50 mg/kg of (−)-sulpiride and 0.5 mg/kg of haloperidol (Fig. 1A,B). Higher doses of (−)-sulpiride and haloperidol (100 and 1 mg/kg, respectively) no further increased but prolonged the effect (Fig. 1A,B).

Dopamine D_1 receptor blockade

The administration of the D_1 receptor antagonist SCH 39166 (Chipkin et al., 1988) (0.25 mg/kg and 0.5 mg/kg i.p.) produced a dose-related decrease in acetylcholine release (Fig. 2). Maximal reduction of about 30% was produced by 0.5 mg/kg SCH 39166. Higher doses of compound did not further reduce the release of acetylcholine (not shown).

Pretreatment with SCH 39166 (0.5 mg/kg i.p., 40 min beforehand completely prevented the enhancement in acetylcholine release produced by either (−)-sulpiride (50 mg/kg i.p.) or haloperidol (0.5 mg/kg i.p.) (Fig. 3A,B).

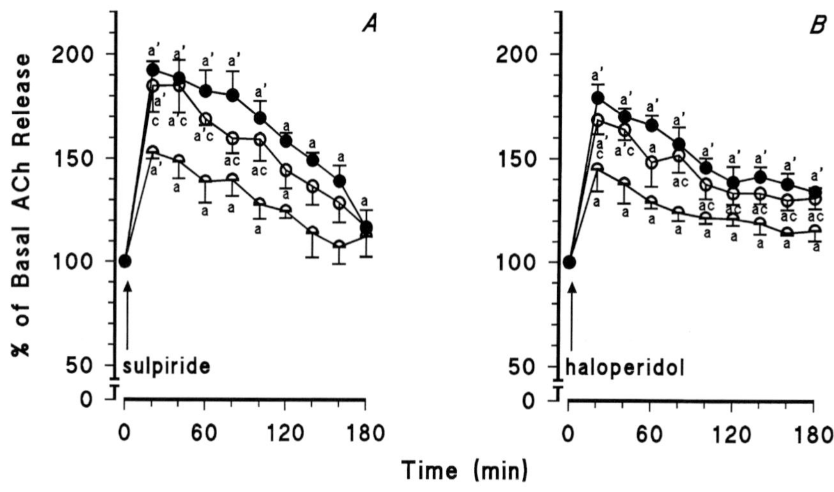

Fig. 1. Effect of (−)-sulpiride 20 (○); 50 (○) and 100 (●) mg/kg i.p. (panel A), and haloperidol 0.25 (○); 0.5 (○) and 1 (●) mg/kg i.p. (panel B) on the extracellular concentration of striatal acetylcholine (ACh). Data are expressed as mean (± S.E.M.) percent variation of basal values. For (−)-sulpiride (panel A): ANOVA revealed a significant main effect of treatment (F(2,119) = 26.763; P < 0.001) and a significant main effect of repeated measures (F(9,119) = 33.478; P < 0.001)). n = 4 for each group. For haloperidol (panel B): ANOVA revealed a significant main effect of treat-ment (F(2,119) = 254.963; P < 0.001), a significant main effect of repeated measures (F(9,119) = 41.056; P < 0.001) and a significant interaction between factors (F(18,119) = 2.144; P < 0.01). n = 4 for each group. ᵃP < 0.05 and ᵃ′P < 0.01 in comparison to baseline values; ᶜP < 0.05 in comparison with the effect of the lower dose at the same time-point. For more details see text (Materials and methods)

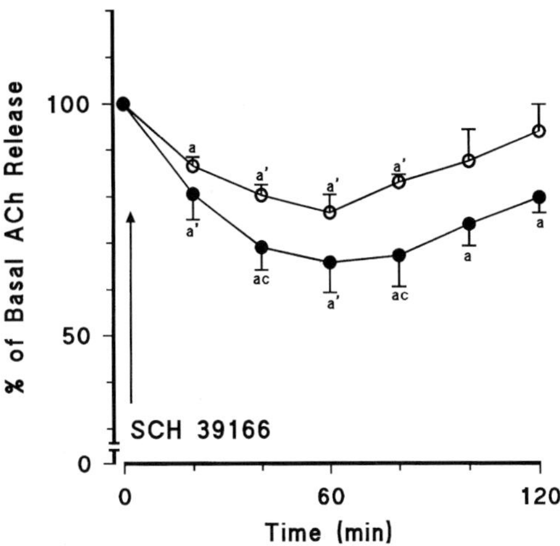

Fig. 2. Effect of SCH 39166 0.25 (○) and 0.5 (●) mg/kg i.p. on the extracellular concentration of striatal acetylcholine (ACh). Data are expressed as mean (± S.E.M.) percent variation of basal values. ANOVA revealed a significant main effect of treatment ($F_{(1,55)}$ = 67.105; $P < 0.001$). and a significant main effect of repeated measures ($F_{(6,55)}$ = 18.819; $P < 0.001$). n = 4 for each dose. [a]$P < 0.005$ and [a']$P < 0.0005$ in comparison with baseline values. [c]$P < 0.05$ in comparison with the effect of the lower dose at the same time-point. For more details see text (Materials and methods)

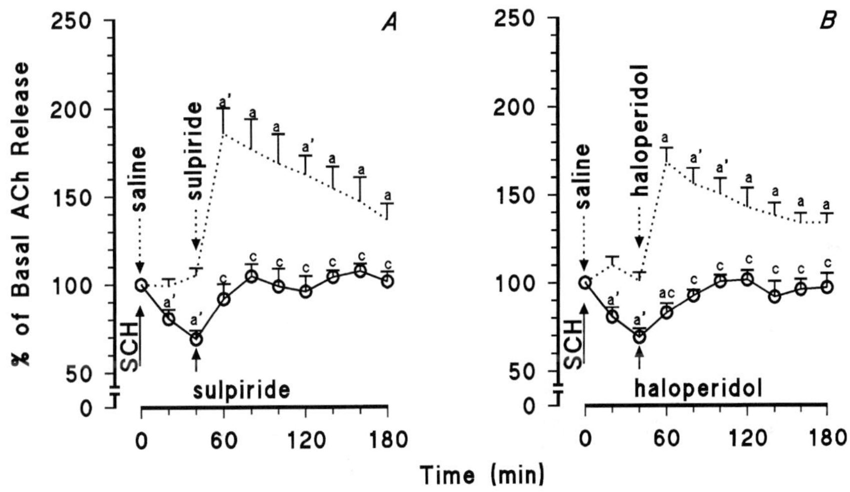

Fig. 3. SCH 39166 0.5 mg/kg i.p. (administered 40 min before neuroleptic drugs) is able to prevent the enhancement of acetylcholine (ACh) release induced by (−)-sulpiride 50 mg/kg i.p. (panel A) and by haloperidol 0.5 mg/kg i.p. (panel B). Data are expressed as mean (± S.E.M.) percent variation of basal values. For the interaction SCH 39166-sulpiride compared to saline-sulpiride (panel A) ANOVA revealed a significant main effect of pretreatments ($F_{(1,79)}$ = 224.825; $P < 0.001$), a sgnificant main effect of repeated measures ($F_{(9,79)}$ = 19.644; $P < 0.001$)) and a significant interaction between factors ($F_{(9,79)}$ = 9.79) = 9.342; $P < 0.001$). n = 4 for each curve. For the interaction SCH 39166-haloperidol compared to saline-haloperidol (panel B) ANOVA revealed a significant main effect of pretreatments ($F_{(1,79)}$ = 554.719; $P < 0.001$), a significant main effect of repeated measures ($F_{(9,79)}$ = 20.126; $P < 0.001$)) and a significant interaction between factors ($F_{(9,79)}$ = 12.502; $P < 0.001$). n = 4 for each each surve. [a]$P < 0.01$ and [a']$P < 0.001$ in comparison with baseline values; [c]$P < 0.05$ in comparison with the effects of saline-sulpiride or saline-haloperidol respectively, at the same time-point. For more details see text (Materials and methods)

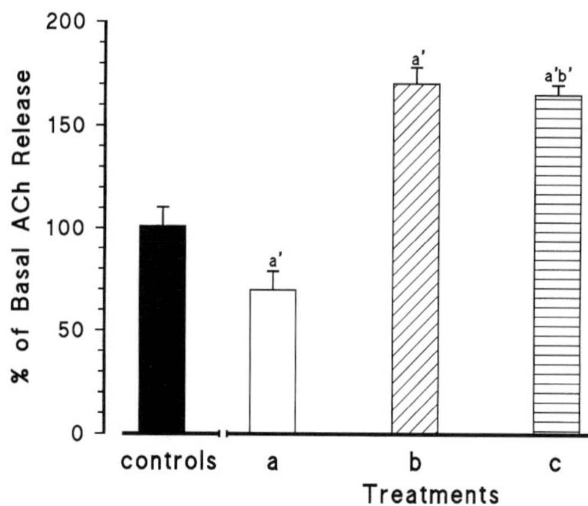

Fig. 4. SKF 38393 (20 mg/kg i.p.) increases the output of acetylcholine (column b) and prevents (column c) the reduction of acetylcholine release induced by LY 171555 (0.1 mg/kg i.p.) (column a). Treatments: controls = saline + saline; column a = saline + LY 171555; column b = SKF 38393 + saline; column c = SKF 38393 + LY 171555. Saline or SKF 38393 were administered 40 min before saline or LY 171555. Data are expressed as mean ($\pm$ S.E.M.) percent variation of basal values. ANOVA revealed a significant main effect of pretreatments ($F(1,15) = 294.040$; $P < 0.001$), a significant main effect of treatments ($F(1,15) = 13.888$; $P < 0.005$)) and a significant interaction between factors ($F(1,15) = 6.652$; $P < 0.05$. n = 4 for each group. [a']$P < 0.001$ in comparison with controls; [b']$P < 0.001$ in comparison with the effect of the group pre treated with saline. For more details see text (Materials and methods)

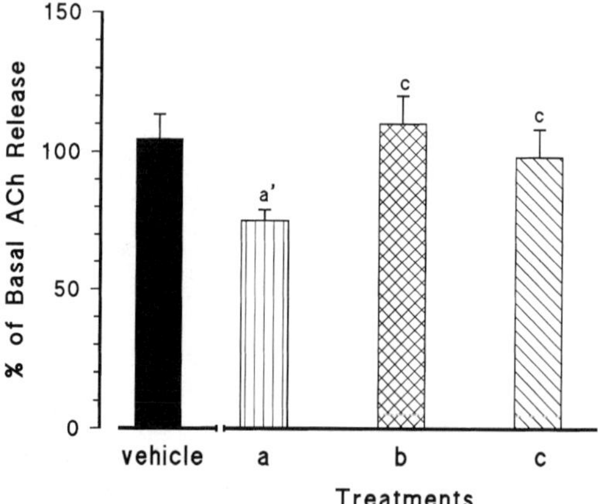

Fig. 5. Treatment with reserpine (5 mg/kg i.p.) and α-methyltyrosine (150 mg/kg i.p.), 6 h beforehand, reduces the output of acetylcholine (ACH) (column a) and prevents the enhancement of acetylcholine release induced by ($-$)-sulpiride (50 mg/kg i.p.) (column b) and by haloperidol (0.5 mg/kg i.p.) (column c). For more details see text: Materials and methods. Data are expressed as mean ($\pm$ S.E.M.) percent variation of basal values. n = 5 or more for each group. [a']$P < 0.001$ in comparison with controls (vehicle injected rats) at the same time-point. [c]$P < 0.05$ in comparison with the reserpine + α-methyltyrosine pretreated group

Dopamine D₁ receptor stimulation

The stimulation of D_1 receptors with the selective agonist, SKF 38393 (Damsma et al., 1990b; Imperato et al., 1993a), increased acetylcholine release (Fig. 4, column b).

Figure 4 (column c) also shows that SKF 38393 (20 mg/kg i.p.) prevents the reduction of acetylcholine release induced by LY 171555 (0.1 mg/kg i.p.) (column a).

Depletion of dopamine stores and inhibition of dopamine synthesis

As previously shown (Imperato et al., 1992b) the combined administration of reserpine (5 mg/kg i.p.) and α-methyltyrosine (150 mg/kg i.p.), aimed at simultaneously depleting dopamine stores and inhibiting dopamine synthesis, reduced acetylcholine release with a maximal reduction of about 30% (Fig. 5, column a) which is present from 4 up to at least 24 h after treatment. Moreover, this combined treatment blocked the increase in acetylcholine release induced by either (−)-sulpiride (50 mg/kg i.p.) or haloperidol (0.5 mg/kg i.p.). (Fig. 5, columns b and c, respectively), administered 6 h afterwards.

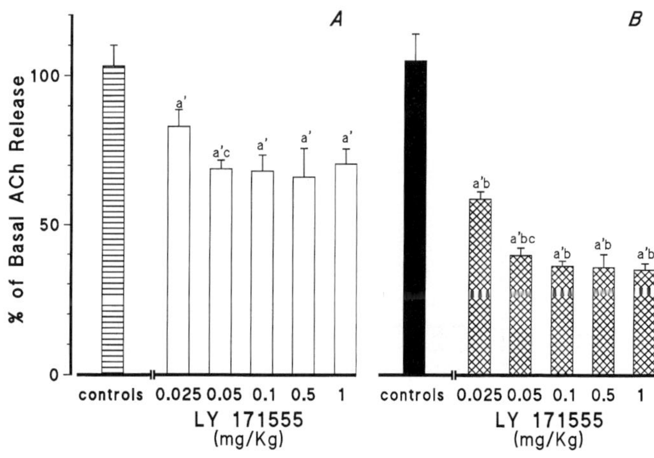

Fig. 6. Effects of various doses of LY 171555 (0.025 up to 1 mg/kg) on the output of acetylcholine (ACh) in the striatum in normal (vehicle-injected, 24 beforehand) rats (panel A) and in dopamine depleted rats (treated with 5 mg/kg reserpine and 100 mg/kg α-methyltyrosine, 24 h beforehand; for more details see text: Results) (panel B). The values reported represent the effect of LY 171555 at 40 min after the injection (time point of the peak effect). Control rats include: vehicle + saline-injected rats (panel A) and reserpine/α-methyltyrosine + saline-injected rats (panel B). Acetylcholine values are expressed as mean (± S.E.M.) percent variation of basal values. ANOVA revealed a significant main effect of pretreatment ($F_{(1,59)}$ = 200.838; $P < 0.001$), a significant effect of treatment ($F_{(5,59)}$ = 92.153; $P < 0.001$) and a significant interaction between factors ($F_{(5,59)}$ = 12.090; $P < 0.001$). n = 5 or more for each group. [a]$P < 0.001$ in comparison with respective controls; [b] < 0.05 versus the same dose in normal rats; [c] $< P < 0.05$ in comparison with previous dose

                            A. Imperato et al.

Stimulation of dopamine D_2 receptors in normal and dopamine depleted rats

In agreement with previous results (Bertorelli and Consolo, 1990; Robertson et al., 1992; Imperato et al., 1993b), the administration of the D_2 receptor agonist LY 171555 reduced acetylcholine release (Fig. 6A). However, we found that the maximum reduction (about 30%) was already produced by a minute dose of 0.05 mg/kg i.p. which induces hypomotility (Koller et al., 1987; Eilam and Szechtman, 1989). While no further reduction was obtained with higher doses up to 1 mg/kg i.p. inducing behavioral stimulation (Eilam and Szechtman, 1989) (Fig. 6A).

Figure 6B shows that, instead, depletion of dopamine stores (with 5 mg/kg i.p. reserpine and 100 mg/kg α-methyltyrosine 24 h beforehand, with the α-methyltyrosine injection repeated 8 h before the experiment) enhanced the ability of LY 171555 to decrease striatal acetylcholine release. In such animals, the maximal reduction was about 70% at the dose of 0.1 mg/kg i.p.

Finally, as shown in Fig. 7, the injection of LY 171555 (0.1 mg/kg i.p.), 20 min after SCH 39166 (0.5 mg/kg i.p.), failed to further decrease the

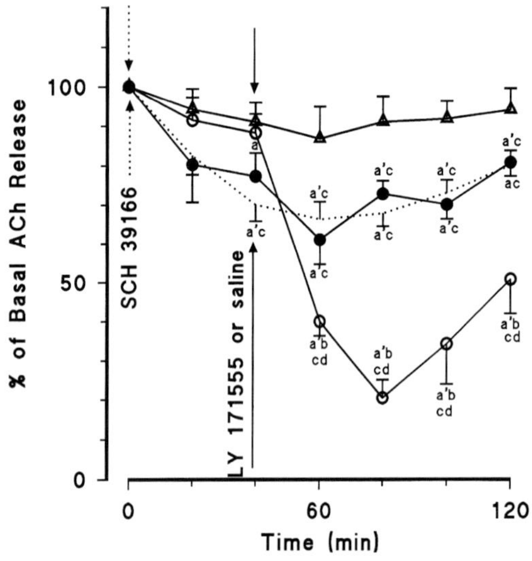

Fig. 7. Effect of SCH 39166 alone and in presence of LY 171555 on the output of acetylcholine (ACh) in normal rats (vehicle injected, 24 h beforehand) and in dopamine depleted rats (pretreated with 5 mg/kg reserpine + 100 mg/kg α-methyltyrosine, 24 h beforehand; for more details see text: Results). SCH 39166 (0.5 mg/kg i.p.) was administered 40 min before saline in normal rats (dotted line) and in dopamine depleted rats (empty triangles), or before LY 171555 (0.1 mg/kg i.p.) in normal rats (full line, filled circles) and dopamine depleted rats (full line, empty circles). For details see text (Materials and methods). Data are expressed as mean (± S.E.M.) percent variation of basal values. ANOVA revealed a significant main effect of treatments ($F_{(3,111)}$ = 87.733; P < 0.001), a significant main effect of repeated measures ($F_{(6,111)}$ = 60.012; P < 0.001)) and a significant interaction between factors ($F_{(18,111)}$ = 14.104; P < 0.001). n = 4 for each curve. [a]P < 0.001 in comparison with basal values; [b]P < 0.05 in comparison with the effect of SCH 39166 + saline in normal rats at the same time-point; [c]P < 0.05 in comparison with the effect of SCH 39166 + saline in depleted rats at the same time-point; [d]P < 0.05 in comparison with the effect of SCH 39166 + LY 171555 in normal rats at the same time-point

release of acetylcholine in normal (vehicle-injected) rats while it strongly reduced acetylcholine output in rats with prolonged dopamine depletion (about 80%).

Discussion

The concept that endogenous dopamine, under normal conditions, exerts a tonic inhibitory control on the release of acetylcholine by an action on D_2 receptors is mainly based on the finding that acetylcholine release is enhanced by drugs that block and reduced by drugs which stimulate D_2 receptors.

However, our results have shown that the stimulant effect of $(-)$-sulpiride and haloperidol, on acetylcholine release is suppressed by blockade of D_1 receptors with SCH 39166. Thus, the enhancement in acetylcholine release following D_2 receptor blockade is not due to the loss of the inhibitory dopaminergic control on cholinergic neurons, but to the stimulant action of endogenously released dopamine on D_1 receptors. Indeed, it is known that blockade of D_2 receptors results in the compensatory activation of dopaminergic neuronal firing (Bunney et al., 1973; Mereu et al., 1983) and enhanced dopamine release (Zetterstrom et al., 1984; Imperato and Di Chiara, 1985). The latter event should, consequently, lead to stimulation of the unblocked D_1 receptors. Consistent with this concept is our finding that the effects of haloperidol and $(-)$-sulpiride can be prevented by the depletion of dopamine stores with reserpine and α-methyltyrosine, suggesting that this effect is mediated by endogenous dopamine. If endogenous dopamine tonically inhibits the release of acetylcholine in the striatum, one would expect an increase in acetylcholine output after depletion of dopamine stores combined with inhibition of dopamine synthesis. In contrast, this treatment produced a reduction in acetylcholine release by about 30%, which is similar to that observed after blockade of D_1 receptors pointing to the existence of a stimulatory action of dopamine, through D_1 receptors, on the output of acetylcholine.

As mentioned before, another argument in favor of the concept that D_2 receptors play an inhibitory control on acetylcholine release in vivo is that the systemic administration of D_2 receptor agonists reduces acetylcholine release in the striatum. Indeed, we have confirmed that LY 171555 reduces acetylcholine output, but we have also observed that this compound was maximally effective at small doses inducing hypomotility within the dose-range that is considered to stimulate presynaptic D_2 receptors (Brown et al., 1985; Clark et al., 1985; Koller et al., 1987; Eilam and Szechtman, 1989). Moreover, no additional effect was produced by higher, postsynaptic doses of the drug which induce behavioral stimulation (Koller et al., 1987; Eilam and Szechtman, 1989).

Therefore, the inhibition of acetylcholine output produced by quinpirole appears to be the result of the inhibition of dopaminergic firing (White, 1987) and dopamine release (Imperato et al., 1988) and, consequently, of reduced stimulation of D_1 receptors by endogenous dopamine.

This possibility is supported by the finding that, in normal rats, LY 171555 was not able to reduce acetylcholine release further after blockade of D_1 receptors, suggesting that LY 171555 may reduce acetylcholine release through a D_1 receptor mechanism. In agreement with previous findings (Robertson et al., 1992), we found that LY 171555 is more potent in decreasing the output of acetylcholine in dopamine depleted rats in a situation where D_2 receptor function, due to functional denervation, has changed. This is in line with behavioral studies demonstrating the development of supersensitivity of D_2 receptors to agonists after depletion of catecholamine-containing neurons 16 h after reserpine pretreatment (Morelli et al., 1986). We have also shown that in dopamine depleted rats LY 171555 is able to reduce the output of acetylcholine after blockade of D_1 receptors with SCH 39166. This finding suggests that, in case of denervation, stimulation of D_2 receptor may become independent of D_1 receptor mechanisms. In line with these results, it has been shown that D_1 and D_2 receptors are coupled in a normally innervated system and may be uncoupled as a result of denervation supersensitivity (Arnt, 1985a, b) or even after denervation itself without development of receptor supersensitivity) (Longoni et al., 1987; Breese and Mueller, 1985).

In conclusion, our results and previous data support the view that in vivo striatal acetylcholine release is under a tonic facilitatory control by dopamine acting on D_1 receptors while they seriously challenge the widely accepted view that endogenous dopamine, through activation of D_2 receptors, plays a tonic inhibitory control on the release of striatal acetylcholine in normal circumstances.

Moreover, we have also shown that D_2 receptor-mediated inhibition of acetylcholine release becomes relevant in case of dopamine depletion and dopamine receptor supersensitivity, suggesting that this can occur in pathological and/or pharmacological conditions such as Parkinson's Disease or extrapyramidal syndromes during prolonged treatment with neuroleptics. Therefore, our results also suggest that differences may exist in the dopaminergic regulation of striatal acetylcholine release in normal conditions and in states of altered dopamine D_2 receptor sensitivity.

Acknowledgements

We wish to thank SANDOZ Prodotti Farmaceutici S.p.A. Italy for having generously supported this research with a grant "Project in Neuroscience" dedicated to A. R. Lurija.

References

Arnt J (1985a) Behavioral stimulation is induced by separate dopamine D-1 and D-2 receptor sites in reserpine-pretreated but not in normal rats. Eur J Pharmacol 113: 79–88

Arnt J (1985b) Hyperactivity induced by stimulation of separate dopamine D-1 and D-2 receptors in rats with bilateral 6-OHDA lesions. Life Sci 37: 717–723

Bertorelli R, Consolo S (1990) D_1 and D_2 dopaminergic regulation of acetylcholine release from striata of freely-moving rats. J Neurochem 54: 2145–2148

Breese GR, Mueller RA (1985) SCH 23390 antagonism of a D-2 dopamine agonist depends upon catecholaminergic neurons. Eur J Pharmacol 113: 109–144

Brown F, Campbell W, Mitchell PJ, Randall K (1985) Dopamine autoreceptors and the effects of drugs on locomotion and dopamine synthesis. Br J Pharmacol 84: 853

Bunney BS, Walters JR, Roth RH, Aghajanian GK (1973) Dopaminergic neurons: effect of antipsychotic drugs and amphetamine on single cell activity. J Pharmacol Exp Ther 195: 560–564

Chipkin RE, Iorio LC, Coffin VF, Mcquade RD, Berger JG, Barnett B (1988) Pharmacological profile of SCH 39166: a dopamine D1 selective benzonaphthazepine with potent antipsychotic activity. J Pharmacol Exp Ther 247: 1093–1102

Clark D Hjorth S, Carlsson A (1985) Dopamine-receptor agonists: mechanisms underlying autoreceptor selectivity. J Neural Transm 62: 1–52

Consolo S, Wu CF, Fusi R (1987) D-1 receptor-linked mechanism modulates cholinergic neurotransmission in the rat striatum. J Pharmacol Exp Ther 242: 300–305

Damsma G Westerink BHC (1991) A microdialysis and automated on-line analysis approach to study central cholinergic transmission in vivo. In: Robinson TE, Justice JB (eds) Microdialysis in neurosciences. Elsevier, Amsterdam, pp 237–252

Damsma G, De Boer P, Westerink BHC, Fibiger HC (1990a) Dopaminergic regulation of striatal cholinergic interneurons: an in vivo microdialysis study. Naunyn Schmiedebergs Arch Pharmacol 342: 523–527

Damsma G, Tham C, Robertson GS, Fibiger HC (1990b) Dopamine D1 receptor stimulation increases striatal acetylcholine release in the rat. Eur J Pharmacol 186: 335–338

De Boer P, Damsma G, Schram Q, Stoof JC, Zaagsma J, Westerink BHC (1992) The effect of intrastriatal application of directly and indirectly acting dopamine agonists and antagonists on the in vivo release of acetylcholine measured by brain microdialysis. Naunyn Schmiedebergs Arch Pharmacol 345: 144–152

Eilam D, Szechtam H (1989) Biphasic effect of quinpirole on locomotion and movements. Eur J Pharmacol 161: 151–157

Gorell JM, Czarnecki B (1986) Pharmacologial evidence for direct dopaminergic regulation of striatal acetylcholine release. Life Sci 38: 2239–2246

Gorell JM Czarnecki B, Hubbel S (1986) Fuctional antagonism of D-1 and D-2 dopaminergic mechanisms affecting striatal acetylcholine release. Life Sci 38: 2247–2254

Imperato A, Di Chiara G (1985) Dopamine release and metabolism in awake rats after systemic neuroleptics as studied by trans-striatal dialysis. J Neurosci 5: 297–306

Imperato A, Tanda GL, Frau R, Di Chiara G (1988) Pharmacological profile of dopamine receptor agonists as studied by brain dialysis in behaving rats. J Pharmacol Exp Ther 245: 257–264

Imperato A, Angelucci L, Zocchi A, Casolini P, Puglisi-Allegra S (1992a) Repeated stressful experiences differently affect limbic dopamine release during and following stress. Brain Res 577: 194–199

Imperato A, Obinu MC, Demontis MV, Gessa GL (1992b) Cocaine releases limbic acetylcholine by action of endogenous dopamine onto D_1 receptors. Eur J Pharmacol 229: 265–267

Imperato A, Obinu MC, Gessa GL (1993a) Stimulation of both dopamine D_1 and D_2 receptors facilitates in vivo acetylcholine release in the hippocampus. Brain Res 618: 341–345

Imperato A, Obinu MC, Casu MA, Mascia MS, Dazzi L, Gessa GL (1993b) Evidence that neuroleptics increase striatal acetylcholine release through stimulation of dopamine D_1 receptors. J Pharmacol Exp Ther 266: 577–562

Koller W, Herbster G, Anderson D, Wack R, Gordon J (1987) Quinpirole hydroghloride a potential antiparkinson drug. Neuropharmacology 26(8): 1031–1036

König JFR, Klippel RA (1963) The rat brain. Williams and Wilkins, Baltimore

Longoni R, Spina L, Di Chiara G (1987) Permissive role of D-1 receptor stimulation by endogenous dopamine for the expression of postsynaptic D-2 mediated behavioral responses. Yawning in rats. Eur J Pharmacol 134: 163–173

Marien MR, Richard JW (1990) Drug effects on the release of endogenous acetylcholine in vivo: measurement by intracerebral dialysis and gas chromatography-mass spectrometry. J Neurochem 54: 2016–2023

Mereu GP, Casu M, Gessa GL (1983) (−)Sulpiride activates the firing activity and tyrosine hydroxylase activity of dopaminergic neurons in unanesthetized rats. Brain Res 264: 105–107

Morelli M, Longoni R, Spina L, Di Chiara G (1986) Antagonism of apomorphine-induced yawning by SCH 23390: Evidence against the autoreceptor hypothesis. Psychopharmacology 89: 259–260

Plantjé JF, Hansen HA, Daus FJ, Stoof JC (1984) SCH 23390, TM 09151-2, (+)−3-ppp and some classical neuroleptics on D1 and D2 receptors in rat neostriatum in vivo. Naunyn Schmiedebergs Arch Pharmacol 105: 73–83

Robertson GS, Hubert GW, Tham CS, Fibiger HC (1992) Lesions of the mesotelencephalic dopamine system enhance the effects of selective dopamine D1 and D2 receptor agonists on striatal acetylcholine release. Eur J Pharmacol 219: 323–325

Stoof JC, Kebabian JW (1982) Independent in vitro regulation by D2 dopamine receptors of dopamine-stimulated efflux of cyclic AMP and K$^+$ stimulated release of acetylcholine from rat neostriatum. Brain Res 250: 263–270

Stoof JC, Thieme RE, Vrijmoed-de Vries MC, Mulder AH (1979) In vitro acetylcholine release from the rat caudate nucleus as a model for testing drugs with dopamine-receptor activity. Naunyn Schmiedebergs Arch Pharmacol 309: 119–124

Stoof JC, Drukarch B, De Boer P, Westerink BHC, Groenewegen HJ (1992) Regulation of the activity of striatal cholinergic neurons by dopamine. Neuroscience 47: 755–770

White FJ (1987) D-1 dopamine receptor stimulation enables the inhibition of nucleus accumbens neurons by a D-2 receptor agonist. Eur J Pharmacol 135: 101–105

Zetterstrom T, Sharp T, Ungerstedt U (1984) Effect of neuroleptic drugs on striatal dopamine release and metabolism in awake rats studied by intracerebral dialysis. Eur J Pharmacol 106: 27–31

Authors' address: A. Imperato, Ph.D., "Bernard B. Brodie" Department of Neuroscience, Via Porcell 4, I-09124 Cagliari, Italy.

J Neural Transm (1995) [Suppl] 45: 103–112

DOPA-induced "peak dose" dyskinesia: clues implicating D2 receptor-mediated mechanisms using dopaminergic agonists in MPTP monkeys

P. J. Blanchet[1], **B. Gomez-Mancilla**[1], and **P. J. Bédard**[1,2]

[1] Neurobiology Research Centre, Enfant-Jésus Hospital, Québec City, and
[2] Pharmacology Department, Laval University, Québec City, Québec, Canada

Summary. Dopa-induced "peak dose" dyskinesia (DID) observed during the treatment of Parkinson's disease patients has traditionally been linked primarily to dopamine D_1 receptor-mediated mechanisms. However, in MPTP-induced parkinsonian monkeys with DID, the administration of selective dopamine D_1 or D_2 agonists will, in the case of D_1 agonists result in similar antiparkinsonian effect but with much less dyskinesia. Thus, once primed, enhanced D_1 neural transmission might in fact benefit DID. In drug-naive MPTP monkeys, the high dyskinetic potential of several selective D_2 agonists and the more favorable outcome on dyskinesia resulting from the continuous stimulation of D_2 receptors (leading to D_2 receptor down regulation) are important clues suggesting the primary role played by D_2 receptor-mediated mechanisms in the dyskinesia priming process. Further clinical studies using drugs selective for the various dopamine receptor subtypes and of different efficacy half-lives are needed to validate our primate data.

Introduction

Dyskinesia frequently complicates long-term levodopa treatment in patients with Parkinson's disease and often interferes with optimization of therapy. It most commonly occurs when parkinsonian symptoms are corrected (conventionally refered to as "peak dose" or "on" dyskinesia) and manifests as choreoathetoid or dystonic movements of variable intensity, Severe nigrostriatal system denervation in the presence of an intact striatal outflow, and chronic levodopa treatment usually for several months to years are necessary conditions for its development (Mones et al., 1971; Schneider, 1989; Boyce et al., 1990a; Horstink et al., 1990; Nutt, 1990). The duration of levodopa treatment before induction of dyskinesia varies remarkably between patients and young-onset patients (those developing symptoms before age 40) develop dyskinesia more frequently and sooner after levodopa initiation (Quinn et al., 1987; Golbe et al., 1991) for unknown reasons (Gibb and Lees, 1988).

Thus far, the intimate mechanisms conducive to the development of dyskinesia following levodopa initiation and the respective contribution of the two main neostriatal dopamine receptors (namely the D_1 and D_2 subtypes) continue to elude us. Current hypotheses on the pathophysiology of dopa-induced dyskinesia (DID) have been undoubtedly biased by the lack of selective, full dopamine D_1 agonists to generate comparative clinical data. However, over the past decade, the 1-methyl-4-phenyl-1,2,3,6-tetrahydropyridine (MPTP)-induced primate model of parkinsonism has greatly contributed to our understanding of DID since monkeys with moderately severe, stable parkinsonism develop dyskinesia similar to the human counterpart following exposure to levodopa for 4–8 weeks (Bédard et al., 1986; Clarke et al., 1987). We herein review the experimental data looking at the involvement of D_1 or D_2 receptor-mediated mechanisms using selective agonists in levodopa "primed" (dyskinetic) and "de novo" (drug-naive) MPTP monkeys. We propose that no single receptor or pathway is exclusively linked to dyskinesia production but that D_2 mechanisms are most important and sufficient in the induction process.

D_1 receptor-mediated mechanisms and dyskinesia

The concept that D_1 mechanisms are potentially responsible for dyskinesia induction stems mainly from behavioral observations obtained with bromocriptine, an ergot derivative with dopamine D_2 receptor agonistic properties also displaying an antagonistic profile at D_1 receptors in vitro (Trabucchi et al., 1976; Markstein et al., 1978). Unlike levodopa (D_1/D_2 proagonists), bromocriptine shows a much lower dyskinetic potential when administered alone (Rascol et al., 1979; Lees and Stern, 1981) or in combination with levodopa (Rinne, 1987) to parkinsonian patients, or in monotherapy to "de novo" MPTP primates, even when large doses producing antiparkinsonian activity comparable to levodopa are used (Bédard et al., 1986). The low incidence of dyskinesia seen with bromocriptine has been assumed to be related to its D_1 antagonism. Other preclinical data like the demonstration that the D_1 receptor-linked adenylate cyclase system is more sensitive following prolonged levodopa treatment in dopamine-denervated rats (Parenti et al., 1986) or the fact that a D_1 receptor antagonist (SCH 23390) can effectively block levodopa-induced chorea in MPTP primates (Boyce et al., 199b) have given credit to the relation between D_1 receptor stimulation and dyskinesia. The effective suppression of DID with clozapine in 6 parkinsonian subjects has also been linked primarily to D_1 receptor blockade (Bennett et al., 1993). Evidence for long-lasting sensitization following repeated D_1 receptor stimulation in dopamine-denervated rat neonates exposed to 6-hydroxydopamine (6-OHDA) (Criswell et al., 1989) has been used in support of the idea that an imbalance in striatal output favoring D_1 receptor-mediated mechanisms underlies the development of DID (Trugman and Wooten, 1993). Other arguments in support of this idea are listed in Table 1.

Table 1. Summary of arguments favoring D_1 receptor-mediated mechanisms in dopa-induced dyskinesia (DID)

- Lower dyskinetic potential of bromocriptine (D_2 agonists/D_1 antagonists
- Enhanced adenylate cyclase activity after levodopa treatment in 6-OHDA rats
- Antichoreic activity of SCH 23390 (D_1 antagonist) in MPTP parkinsonism primates with DID
- Antidyskinetic activity of clozapine (atypical neuroleptic) in parkinsonian patients
- Sensitization of D_1 receptors after repeated D_1 agonist exposure in 6-OHDA rat neonates
- Further upregulation of striatal D_1 receptors after chronic levodopa treatment in MPTP parkinsonism primates with DID (few studies)

The D_1 hypothesis was recently fueled by the demonstration of an increase in regional striatal D_1 receptor binding in MPTP primates rendered dyskinetic following chronic exposure to levodopa or apomorphine (Graham et al., 1993), supporting similar earlier findings in levodopa-treated parkinsonian patients in whom striatal D_1 receptor binding was also increased, particularly in those subjects with dyskinesia (Rinne et al., 1985). However, these latter results could not be reproduced subsequently by the same group using a more selective D_1 antagonist as radioligand (Rinne et al., 1991). In another primate study (Alexander et al., 1993), D_1 receptors remained essentially unchanged after MPTP or levodopa treatment, even in dyskinetic animals. Our own primate data have pointed toward a decreased sensitivity (-28%) of striatal D_1 receptors following chronic levodopa treatment compared to untreated MPTP animals (Gagnon et al., 1990), although a more recent experiment has allowed us to observe a trend toward further upregulation ($+20\%$) of putaminal D_1 receptors in MPTP monkeys with DID (Blanchet et al., 1995). The functional significance of these receptor findings in the scheme of the dyskinesia induction process remains unclear.

Nonetheless, other data obtained in 6-OHDA adult rats contradict the D_1 hypothesis and favor the opposite idea that the D_1 receptor-linked, striatal efferent pathway is not functionally supersensitive but rather subsensitive following daily intermittent exposure to levodopa, as suggested by the reduced responsiveness of these animals to D_1 agonists (Engber et al., 1989; Weick et al., 1990; Britton et al., 1991). In vitro (Barton and Sibley, 1990; Balmforth et al., 1990) and in vivo (Winkler and Weiss, 1989; Britton et al., 1991) studies have shown the unique susceptibility of D_1 receptors to agonist-induced desensitization, an intrinsic regulatory process that may be physiologically relevant to DID and could potentially tilt the balance of neural stimulation in certain conditions toward the D_2 subsystem. The D_1 hypothesis was further challenged by experiments conducted in our laboratory in 5 cynomolgous (Macaca fascicularis) monkeys bearing a stable parkinsonian syndrome following MPTP exposure and studied whilst consistently exhibiting DID after each dose of oral levodopa (Gomez-Mancilla and Bédard, 1991). At that stage, the substitution of CY-208243 [$(-)$-(6aR)(12bR)-4,6,6a,7,8,12b-hexahydro-7-methylindolo[4,3-ab]-phenanthridine] (0.1 and

0.5 mg/kg s.c.), a partial, functional D_1 agonist for levodopa produced good antiparkinsonian activity but no dyskinesia at the lower dose. Dyskinesia of lesser intensity to that seen with levodopa was reproduced with a dose 5 times higher. This more favorable therapeutic window dissociating dyskinesia and antiparkinsonian relief was not observed after substitution with the D_2-like receptor agonist quinpirole (0.001, 0.01 and 0.1 mg/kg s.c.) or single dosing with D_2 agonists like (+)-PHNO [(+)-4-propyl-9-hydroxynaphthoxazine], bromocriptine, terguride and (−)-3PPP [(−)-3-(3-hydroxyphenyl)-N-n-propylpiperidine], which always reproduced dyskinesia in association with antiparkinsonian efficacy. In another study using 4 dyskinetic monkeys "primed" with various dopamine agonists, the effective full D_1 agonists SKF 82958 [(±)6-chloro-7,8-dihydroxy-3-allyl-1-phenyl-2,3,4,5-tetrahydro-1H-3-benzazepine hydrobromide] (0.25, 0.5 and 1 mg/kg s.c.) and A-77636 [(1R,3S)3-(1'adamantyl)-1-aminomethyl-3,4-dihydro-5,6-dihydroxy-1H-2-benzopyran hydrochloride] (0.5 and 2 mg/kg s.c.) also produced far less dyskinesia for a similar antiparkinsonian potency than levodopa and D_2 agonists (Fig. 1), for a comparable peak antiparkinsonian response (Blanchet et al., 1993). Thus, once DID is primed, avoiding excessive stimulation of the D_2

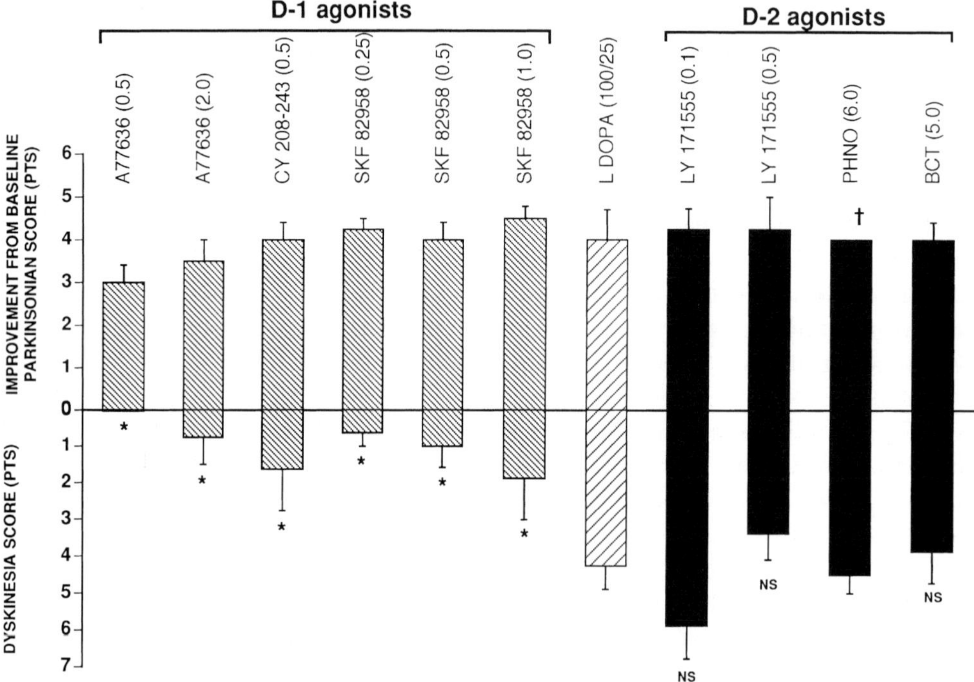

Fig. 1. Peak response profile of various D_1 and D_2 agonists compared to levodopa in 4 dyskinesia-primed monkeys with MPTP-induced parkinsonism. Improvement in parkinsonian scores (on a 10-point scale) and dyskinesia scores are provided. The agonists used were administered s.c. (bromocriptine was given orally) at the dose indicated (in mg/kg), whilst levodopa/benserazide was given orally as one standard 100 mg/25 mg capsule. Each bar represents the mean score ± SEM. Values were compared using the nonparametric Friedman's test and a posteriori multiple comparison t tests. *p < 0.01 compared to levodopa. *NS* not significantly different from levodopa. ††Results for 2 monkeys only

receptors by the administration of an optimal dose of a D_1 agonists could well offer an interesting alternative strategy, at odds with the D_1 hypothesis of dyskinesia induction. We have hypothesized that if the striatal dopamine D_1 and D_2 receptors are largely segregated on separate striatonigral and striatopallidal efferent neurons, respectively (Gerfen et al., 1990; Gerfen and Keefe, 1994; Bloch and Le Moine, 1994; not supported by Surmeier et al., 1993), selective D_1 agonism could then leave untouched the inhibitory pallido-subthalamic neurons that receive striatopallidal efferents and are thought to be overactive in DID (Crossman, 1990). A more balanced effect could then result downstream from the striatum at the level of the internal segment of the globus pallidus, one of the main output stations in the basal ganglia circuitry (see Fig. 3 in Blanchet et al., 1993).

D_2 receptor-mediated mechanisms and dyskinesia

The D_1 hypothesis of dyskinesia induction and the encouraging results obtained with bromocriptine have spawned the study of various dopamine D_2 agonists thought to represent the optimal treatment approach for Parkinson's disease. Evidence emerged showing that the development of behavioral sensitization following dopaminergic agonist treatment is not a phenomenon restricted to the D_1 subsystem since the rat D_2 subsystem is also prone to sensitization following repeated daily exposure to levodopa (Engber et al., 1989) or single dosing with a selective D_2 agonist (Morelli and Di Chiara, 1987). Furthermore, the administration of the potent and selective D_2 agonist (+)-PHNO to parkinsonian patients with DID (Grandas et al., 1987) and MPTP-treated cynomolgous monkeys (Clarke et al., 1988) reproduced the choreoathetoid movements seen with levodopa. Although one subsequent report in MPTP-treated squirrel monkeys failed to reproduce chorea after challenge with (+)-PHNO (Boyce et al., 1990b), the same drug administered at a dose of 6 µg/kg s.c. to 4 drug-naive, MPTP cynomolgous monkeys rapidly induced a combination of choreic and dystonic movements in all animals (Gomez-Mancilla and Bédard, 1992). Similar results have been obtained with (+)-PHNO in drug-naive parkinsonian monkeys by Clarke et al. (1988) and Luquin et al. (1992a, 1994), suggesting a link between dyskinesia induction and the D_2 receptor in non primed conditions. The pharmacological imbalance of neural stimulation created by selective D_2 agonism in a dopamine-denervated striatum is detrimental, perhaps because it ultimately leads to excessive inhibition of the subthalamic nucleus (Crossman, 1990). This can be counteracted by the administration of D_2 receptor blocking agents (Klawans and Weiner, 1974; Tarsy et al., 1975; Luquin et al., 1992b) (impractical due to a return in parkinsonian disability) or partial dopamine D_2 agonists (which may also act as functional antagonists) in parkinsonian primates (Goldstein et al., 1990) and patients (Baronti et al., 1992) that provide antidyskinetic activity and additional support to the role played by D_2 receptors in DID. Other clues favoring the latter hypothesis are summarized in Table 2.

Table 2. Summary of arguments favoring D_2 agonists receptor-mediated mechanisms in dopa-induced dyskinesia (DID)

- High dyskinetic potential of most D_2 in de novo MPTP parkinsonian primates
- Dyskinesia of higher intensity after administration of selective D_2 agonists compared to D_1 agonists in "dyskinesia-primed" MPTP primates
- Antidyskinetic activity of conventional D_2 receptor blocking agents
- Antidyskinetic activity of partial D_2 agonists
- Supersensitive D_2 receptors/subsensitive D_1 receptors following chronic levodopa treatment in 6-OHDA rats
- Lower susceptibility to dyskinesia with striatal D_2 receptor desensitization following continuous D_2 receptor stimulation in MPTP primates and perhaps parkinsonian patients (Cedarbaum et al., 1990)

In our experience, bromocriptine stands out as the only D_2 agonists with such a low dyskinetic potential in drug-naive subjects. In addition to its D_1 receptor antagonism, bromocriptine is also a longer-acting drug than (+)-PHNO and levodopa, and acts as an alpha-adrenergic receptor antagonists (Jackson et al., 1988). Furthermore, in primate experiments where chronic treatment of MPTP cynomolgous monkeys with levodopa and bromocriptine were compared, bromocriptine therapy affected denervated striatal dopamine receptors differently, with [^{3}H]spiperone binding density values 10–67% lower than following chronic levodopa treatment (Bédard et al., 1986; Falardeau et al., 1988; Gagnon et al., 1990). This difference may underlie the progressive lack of clinical efficacy seen with chronic bromocriptine therapy and raises once more the possible pathophysiological link between D_2 receptors and dyskinesia. Recently, we investigated further the dyskinetic potential of D_2 agonists by administering the novel and highly selective D_2 agonist U-91356A [(R)-5-(propylamino)-5,6-dihydro-4H-imidazo[4,5,1-ij]-quinolin 2(1H)-one hydrochloride] to 6 MPTP parkinsonian monkeys for 4 weeks (Blanchet et al., 1995). Three monkeys received the drug in a pulsatile fashion twice daily at 600 µg/kg/dose s.c. whilst 3 others were treated with the same drug but in a continuous fashion using Alzet osmotic minipumps implanted s.c. in the back of each animal, for an infusion rate of approximately 50–60 µg/kg/h. These animals were compared to 3 MPTP subjects treated with oral levodopa/benserazide for a similar length of time. After a good initial antiparkinsonian response, 2/3 animals treated continuously with U-91356A unequivocally displayed reduced responsiveness and a partial return of their parkinsonian symptoms within the first 10 days despite plasma drug levels that were still well above threshold. Only one animal treated in a continuous fashion developed transient choreic dyskinesia (Fig. 2). In contrast, all animals treated with levodopa or given pulsatile U-91356A showed a good antiparkinsonian response for 3 hours (levodopa) to 4–5 hours (U-91356A) as well as evidence for behavioral sensitization with locomotor hyperactivity and choreic dyskinesia developing within the first 2 weeks of therapy and increasing thereafter (Fig. 2). All treatments desensitized putaminal D_2 receptors compared to untreated MPTP controls, but the behavioral desensitization observed with continuous drug administration was correlated with a more significant downregulation of these receptors with a density 10% lower than

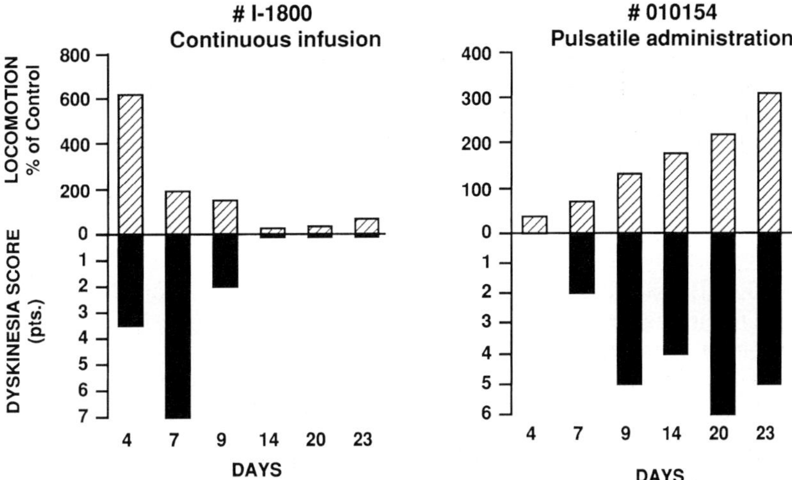

Fig. 2. One illustrative example of the response of 2 different MPTP-induced parkinsonian monkeys treated either continuously through an Alzet osmotic pump (left) or in a pulsatile fashion twice daily (right) with the D_2 agonist U-91356A over 23 days. Absolute dyskinesia score values and 24-hour locomotor counts (provided by a computer-assisted program linked to photocells mounted on each cage) expressed as the percentage increase over a control initial day are shown for 6 different days. A robust response was observed during the first week of continuous therapy but desensitization then supervened; with pulsatile administration however, behavioral sensitization is apparent

the animals given pulsatile U-91356A. Animals with or without U-91356A-induced dyskinesia did not differ in striatal D_1 receptor density and affinity. Therefore, D_2 receptor downregulation with bromocriptine or continuous U-91356A seems to benefit dyskinesia, an indication that D_2 receptor stimulation is not necessarily bound to dyskinesia and that the mode of stimulation of D_2 receptors is physiologically important. Similar results have been reported following continuous forms of administration of (+)-PHNO to parkinsoni an patients (Cedarbaum et al., 1990) or MPTP monkeys (Alexander et al., 1991).

Admittedly, the data generated with selective D_2 agonists may not entirely apply to the context of chronic levodopa therapy. Agonists-induced and levodopa-induced dyskinesia may emerge from different mechanisms and complex interactions with other dopamine receptor subtypes or other neurotransmitter systems may also contribute more strongly in one case than the other. Nonetheless, selective short-acting D_2 agonism does not appear to hold promise in the treatment of Parkinson's disease. Further clinical studies with selective D_1 agonists of different efficacy half-lives in dyskinetic and non dyskinetic subjects appears warranted.

Acknowledgements

The authors wish to express their gratitude to M .F. Piercey (the Upjohn Co.) and D. R. Britton (Abbott Laboratories) for their generous gift of compounds without which these studies would not have been possible. C. Gagnon, F. Calon, J.-C. Martel and T. Di Paolo

110 P. J. Blanchet et al.

are greatly acknowledged for performing the in vitro dopamine receptor binding assays. The authors also thank R. Boucher, L. Grégoire and G. Côté for skillful assistance.

P. Blanchet held a grant from the FRSQ. This work has been supported by the MRC of Canada and the Parkinson Foundation of Canada.

References

Alexander GM, Brainard DL, Gordon SW, Hichens M, Grothusen JR, Schwartzman RJ (1991) Dopamine receptor changes in untreated and (+)-PHNO-treated MPTP parkinsonian primates. Brain Res 547: 181–189

Alexander GM, Schwartzman RJ, Grothusen JR, Brainard L, Gordon SW (1993) Changes in brain dopamine receptors in MPTP parkinsonian monkeys following L-dopa treatment. Brain Res 625: 276–282

Balmforth AJ, Warburton P, Ball SG (1990) Homologous desensitization of the D_1 dopamine receptor. J Neurochem 55: 2111–2116

Baronti F, Mouradian MM, Conant KE, Giuffra M, Brughitta G, Chase TN (1992) Partial dopamine agonist therapy of levodopa-induced dyskinesias. Neurology 42: 1241–1243

Barton AC, Sibley DR (1990) Agonist-induced desensitization of D_1-dopamine receptors linked to adenylyl-cyclase activity in cultured NS20Y neuroblastoma cells. Mol Pharmacol 38: 531–541

Bédard PJ, Di Paolo T, Falardeau P, Boucher R (1986) Chronic treatment with L-Dopa, but not bromocriptine induces dyskinesia in MPTP-parkinsonian monkeys. Correlation with [³H]spiperone binding. Brain Res 379: 294–299

Bennett JP Jr, Landow ER, Schuh LA (1993) Suppression of dyskinesias in advanced Parkinson's disease. II. Increasing daily clozapine doses suppress dyskinesias and improve parkinsonism symptoms. Neurology 43: 1551–1555

Blanchet P, Bédard PJ, Britton DR, Kebabian JW (1993) Differential effect of selective D-land D-2 dopamine receptor agonists on levodopa-induced dyskinesia in 1-methyl-4-phenyl-1,2,3,6-tetrahydropyridine-exposed monkeys. J Pharmacol Exp Ther 267: 275–279

Blanchet PJ, Calon F, Martel JC, Bédard PJ, Di Paolo T, Walters RR, Piercey MF (1995) Continuous administration decreases and pulsatile administration increases behavioral sensitivity to a novel dopamine D-2 agonist (U-91356A) in MPTP monkeys. Pharmacol Exp Ther 272: 854–859

Bloch B, Le Moine C (1994) Letter to the editor. TINS 17: 3–4

Boyce S, Rupniak NMJ, Steventon MJ, Iversen SD (1990a) Nigrostriatal damage is required for induction of dyskinesias by L-DOPA in squirrel monkeys. Clin Neuropharmacol 13: 448–458

Boyce S, Rupniak NMJ, Steventon MJ, Iversen SD (1990b) Differential effects of D_1 and D_2 agonists in MPTP-treated primates: functional implications for Parkinson's disease. Neurology 40: 927–933

Britton DR, Kebabian JW, Curzon P (1991) Rapid reversal of denervation supersensitivity of dopamine D_1 receptors by L-Dopa or a novel dopamine D_1 receptor agonists, A68390. Eur J Pharmacol 200: 89–93

Cedarbaum JM, Clark M, Toy LH, Green-Parsons A (1990) Sustained-release (+)-PHNO [MK-458 (HPMC)] in the treatment of Parkinson's disease: evidence for tolerance to a selective D_2-receptor agonist administered as a long-acting formulation. Mov Disord 5: 298–303

Clarke CE, Boyce S, Sambrook MA, Stahl SM, Crossman AR (1988) Behavioral effects of (+)-4-propyl-9-hydroxynaphthoxazine in primates rendered parkinsonian with 1-methyl-4-phenyl-1,2,36-tetrahydropyridine. Naunyn Schmiedebergs Arch Pharmacol 338: 35–38

Clarke CE, Sambrook MA, Mitchell IJ, Crossamn AR (1987) Levodopa-induced dyskinesia and response fluctuations in primates rendered parkinsonian with 1-methyl-4-phenyl-1,2,3, 6-tetrahydropyridine (MPTP). J Neurol Sci 78: 273–280

Criswell H, Mueller RA, Breese GA (1989) Priming of D_1-dopamine receptor responses: long-lasting behavioral supersensitivity to a D_1-dopamine agonist following repeated administration to neonatal 6-OHDA-lesioned rats. J Neurosci 9: 125–133

Crossman AR (1990) A hypothesis on the pathophysiological mechanisms that underlie levodopa or dopamine agonists-induced dyskinesia in Parkinson's disease: implications for future strategies in treatment. Mov Disord 5: 100–108

Engber TM, Susel Z, Juncos JL, Chase TN (1989) Continuous and intermittent levodopa differentially affect rotation induced by D-1 and D-2 dopamine agonists. Eur J Pharmacol 168: 291–298

Falardeau P, Bouchard S, Bédard PJ, Boucher R, Di Paolo T (1988) Behavioral and biochemical effect of chronic treatment with D-1 and/or D-2 dopamine agonists in MPTP monkeys. Eur J Pharmacol 150: 59–66

Gagnon C, Bédard PJ, Di Paolo T (1990) Effect of chronic treatment of MPTP monkeys with dopamine D-1 and/or D-2 receptor agonists. Eur J Pharmacol 178: 115–120

Gerfen CR, Keefe KA (1994) Letter to the editor. TINS 17: 2–3

Gerfen CR, Engber TM, Mahan LC, Susel Z, Chase TN, Monsma Jr FJ, Sibley DR (1990) D_1 and D_2 dopamine receptor-regulated gene expression of striatonigral and striatopallidal neurons. Science 250: 1429–1432

Gibb WRG, Lees AJ (1988) A comparison of clinical and pathological features of young- and old-onset Parkinson's disease. Neurology 38: 1402–1406

Golbe LI (1991) Young-onset Parkinson's disease: a clinical review. Neurology 41: 168–173

Goldstein M, Lieberman AN, Takasugi N, Shimizu Y, Kuga S (1990) The antiparkinsonian activity of dopamine agonists and their interaction with central dopamine receptor subtypes. In: Streifler MB, Korczyn AD, Melamed E, Youdim MBH (eds) Advances in neurology, vol 53. Parkinson's disease: anatomy, pathology, and therapy. Raven Press, New York, pp 101–106

Gomez-Mancilla B, Bédard PJ (1991) Effect of D_1 and D_2 agonists and antagonists on dyskinesia produced by L-DOPA in 1-methyl-4-phenyl-1,2,3,6-tetrahydropyridine-treated monkeys. J Pharmacol Exp Ther 259: 409–413

Gomez-Mancilla B, Bédard PJ (1992) Effect of chronic treatment with (+)-PHNO, a D_2 agonists in MPTP-treated monkeys. Exp Neurol 117: 185–188

Graham WC, Sambrook MA, Crossman AR (1993) Differential effect of chronic dopaminergic treatment on dopamine D_1 and D_2 receptors in the monkey brain in MPTP-induced parkinsonism. Brain Res 602: 290–303

Grandas F, Quinn N, Critchley P, Rohan A, Marsden CD, Stahl SM (1987) Antiparkinsonian activity of a single oral dose of PHN O. Mov Dis 2: 47–51

Horstink MWIM, Zijlmans JCM, Pasman JW, Berger HJC, van't Hof MA (1990) Severity of Parkinson's disease is a risk factory for peak-dose dyskinesia. J Neurol Neurosurg Psychiatry 53: 224–226

Jackson DM, Jenkins OF, Ross SB (1988) The motor effects of bromocriptinea review. Psychopharmacology 95: 433–446

Klawans Jr HL, Weiner WJ (1974) Attempted use of haloperidol in the treatment of L-Dopa induced dyskinesias. J Neurol Neurosurg Psychiatry 37: 427–430

Lees AJ, Stern GM (1981) Sustained bromocriptine therapy in previously untreated patients with Parkinson's disease. J Neurol Neurosurg Psychiatry 44: 1020–1023

Luquin MR, Laguna J, Obeso JA (1992a) Selective D2 receptor stimulation induces dyskinesia in parkinsonian monkeys. Ann Neurol 31: 551–554

Luquin MR Guillén J, Martinez-Vila E, Laguna J, Martinez-Lage JM (1994) Functional interaction between dopamine D_1 and D_2 receptors in "MPTP" monkeys. Eur J Pharmacol 253: 215–224

Markstein R, Herrling PL, Bürki HR, Asper H , Ruch W (1978) The effect of bromocriptine on rat striatal adenylate cyclase and rat brain monoamine metabolism. J Neurochem 31: 1163–1172

Mones RJ, Elizan TS, Siegel GJ (1971) Analysis of L-dopa induced dyskinesias in 51 patients with parkinsonism. J Neurol Neurosurg Psychiatry 34: 668–673

Morelli M, Di Chiara G (1987) Agonist-induced homologous and heterologous sensitization to D-1- and D-2-dependent contraversive turning. Eur J Pharmacol 141: 101–107

Nutt JG (1990) Levodopa-induced dyskinesia: review, observations, and speculations. Neurology 40: 340–345

Parenti, M, Flauto C, Parati E, Vescovi A, Groppetti A (1986) Differential effect of repeated treatment with L-DOPA on dopamine-D1 or-D2 receptors. Neuropharmacology 25: 331–334

Quinn N, Critchley P, Marsden CD (1987) Young onset Parkinson's disease. Mov Dis 2: 73–91

Rascol A, Guiraud B, Montastruc JL, David J, Clanet M (1979) Long-term treatment of Parkinson's disease with bromocriptine. J Neurol Neurosurg Psychiatry 42: 143–150

Rinne JO, Rinne JK, Laakso K, Lönnberg P, Rinne UK (1985) Dopamine D-1 receptors in the parkinsonian brain. Brain Res 359: 306–310

Rinne JO, Laihinen A, Lönnberg P, Marjamäki P, Rinne UK (1991) A post-mortem study on striatal dopamine receptors in Parkinson's disease. Brian Res 556: 117–122

Rinne UK (1987) Early combination of bromocriptine and levodopa in the treatment of Parkinson's disease: a 5-year follow-up. Neurology 37: 826–828

Schneider JS (1989) Levodopa-induced dyskinesias in parkinsonian monkeys: relationship to extent of nigrostriatal damage. Pharmacol Biochem Behav 34: 193–196

Surmeier DJ, Reiner A, Levine MS, Ariano MA (1993) Are neostriatal dopamine receptors co-localized? TINS 16: 299–305

Tarsy D, Parkes JD, Marsden CD (1975) Metoclopramide and pimozide in Parkinson's disease and levodopa-induced dyskinesias. J Neurol Neurosurg Psychiatry 38: 331–335

Trabucchi M, Spano PF, Tonon GC, Frattola L (1976) Effects of bromocriptine of central dopaminergic receptors. Life Sci 19: 225–232

Trugman JM, Wooten GF (1993) A common pathophsiological mechanism for levodopa-induced and tardive dyskinesia (abstract). Mov Dis 8: 415

Weick BG, Engber TM, Susel Z, Chase TN, Walters JR (1990) Responses of substantia nigra pars reticulata neurons to GABA and SKF 38393 in 6-hydroxydopamine-lesioned rats are differentially affected by continuous and intermittent levodopa administration. Brain Res 523: 16–22

Winkler JD, Weiss B (1989) Effect of continuous exposure to selective D_1 and D_2 dopaminergic agonists on rotational behavior in supersensitive mice. J Pharmacol Exp Ther 249: 507–516

Authors' address: Dr. P. J. Bédard, Neurobiology Research Center, Hôpital de l'Enfant-Jésus, 1401, 18e Rue, Québec, Québec, Canada G1J 1Z4.

J Neural Transm (1995) [Suppl] 45: 113–122
© Springer-Verlag 1995

Alterations of striatal dopamine D2 receptors contribute to deteriorated response to l-dopa in Parkinson's disease: a [123I]-IBZM SPET study

G. Pizzolato[1], F. Chierichetti[2], A. Rossato[1], A. Cagnin[1], M. Fabbri[1], M. Dam[1], G. Ferlin[2], and L. Battistin[1]

[1] Department of Neurology, University of Padova School of Medicine, Padova, and
[2] Division of Nuclear Medicine, Hospital of Castelfranco Veneto (TV), Italy

Summary. Single photon emission tomography with the ligand [123I]-IBZM was used to image central dopamine D2 receptors in Parkinson's disease patients. The aim was to assess striatal receptor densities in relation to response to L-Dopa therapy. In the parkinsonian patients group who were untreated until SPET study and in the group of patients with a sustained response to chronic L-Dopa, striatal [123I]-IBZM uptake did not differ significantly from mean values of the control group. On the contrary, significantly diminished uptake of [123I]-IBZM was found in the basal ganglia regions of the group of patients who developed a complicated/fluctuating response to chronic L-Dopa treatment. Our results indicate that striatal D2 receptor alterations in Parkinson's disease may contribute to the altered response to L-Dopa.

Introduction

Approximately 50% of the Parkinson's disease (PD) patients experience an altered/fluctuating response to L-3, 4-dihydroxyphenylalanine (L-Dopa) with long-term administration of this agent (Marsden et al., 1982). The causes for this declining therapeutic efficacy are still uncertain. Loss of efficacy of L-Dopa may be due to alterations in the synthesis, storage, and release of dopamine, linked to further degeneration, with progressing disease, of the nigrostriatal nerve terminals (Markham and Diamond, 1981). Accordingly, positron emission tomography (PET) studies revealed reduced [18F]fluoro-L-Dopa uptake in the basal ganglia (BG) of PD patients (Leenders et al., 1986), more marked with advanced disease. Regarding the role of alterations of postsynaptic striatal dopamine receptors, postmortem (Guttman et al., 1986; Reisine et al., 1977) and in vivo PET studies (Hagglund et al., 1987; Rutgers et al., 1987) reported contrasting results. However, evidence exists that changes at the postsynaptic site may influence the therapeutic response of PD patients (Brooks et al., 1992; Rinne et al., 1980).

    G. Pizzolato et al.

We used single photon emission tomography (SPET) with the D2 ligand (S)-(−)-3-iodo-2-hydroxy-6-methoxy-N-(1-ethil-2-pyrrodinyl)methyl-benzamide ([123I]-IBZM) (Kung et al., 1989) to investigate if changes of striatal D2 receptors' densities could contribute to an altered response to L-Dopa in PD patients. To this end, we determined D2 receptor densities in striatal regions in a group of PD patients who were untreated until SPET examination and in groups of patients separated on the basis of their clinical response to L-Dopa.

Materials and methods

Patient selection

Twenty-nine patients diagnosed as suffering from idiopathic PD were included in the study. Their main characteristics are summarised in Table 1. The control group comprised 9 subjects (mean age: 58.2 ± 10.6 years, range: 43 to 72 years) who were checked at our neurological department for minor subjective symptoms and who were found free of neurological disease and had normal CT and/or MRI findings. Informed consent was obtained from each subject after detailed explanation of the nature, purposes, and possible consequences of the study.

According to the aim of our study, we evaluated three groups of PD patients, separated on the basis of their exposure and response to L-Dopa. Their main character-

Table 1. Subject characteristics

	Controls	PD patients
Number (Sex)	9 (3M/6F)	29 (10M/19F)
Age (yrs) mean	58.2 ± 10.6	58.4 ± 11.9
range	43–72	34–76
Disease duration (yrs) mean	N.A.	5.9 ± 4.4
range	N.A.	1–15
Disease onset (yrs) mean	N.A.	52.5 ± 11.9
range	N.A.	27–71
Hoehn-Yahr score	N.A.	2.1 ± 0.8

Numbers represent mean ± SDM. *N.A.* not appliable

Table 2. Characteristics of the PD patient groups: response to therapy

	UNTR-PD	RESP-PD	COMPL-PD
Number	8	13	8
Age (yrs)	59.0 ± 8.9	53.7 ± 12.9	65.6 ± 5.2*
Duration of disease (yrs)	2.0 ± 1.4	8.0 ± 4.5#	6.0 ± 4.0
Onset of disease (yrs)	56.6 ± 9.0*	45.6 ± 13.2	59.6 ± 5.1*
Hoehn-Yahr score	1.6 ± 0.5	2.1 ± 0.5	2.6 ± 1.1#

Numbers represent mean ± SD. * significantly different from the RESP-PD group ($p < 0.05$). # significantly different from the UNTR-PD group ($p < 0.05$). *UNTR* untreated; *RESP* stable response to L-Dopa; *COMPL* complicated response to L-Dopa

istics are depicted in Table 2. The first group comprised eight recently diagnosed patients who were untreated until SPET study (UNTR-PD group). The other two groups comprised PD patients who were on chronic L-Dopa therapy, but the therapeutic response varied among patients. Thirteen patients (RESP-PD group) had a stable and sustained response to L-Dopa therapy after years of treatment, whereas eight patients (COMPL-PD group) showed a complicated/fluctuating response to L-Dopa, with short periods of motility and long "off" periods. Noteworthy, the average daily doses of L-Dopa were not significantly different in these two groups of patients. Antiparkinsonian therapy was kept constant for at least two weeks before SPET, and was withdrawn 18 to 24 hours before scanning procedure.

Scanning procedure

Subjects were in resting conditions in a quiet room when they received the tracer (185 MBq of [123I]-IBZM) i.v. The acquisition began 2 hours thereafter, with a single-head rotating gamma-camera (GE Starcam 400 AC), provided with a LEAP collimator, the energy window being centred around the photopeak of ^{123}I. At this time the ratio between striatal specific (D2 receptors) binding vs. non-specific (cerebellar) binding is at a maximum. The correct positioning of the head was controlled by a laser device to define the orbitomeatal line and axial alignment of the patient. Data were collected on 360° rotation, recording 64 views 40 sec each, on a 128 × 128 matrix. Reconstruction of transaxial (along the orbitomeatal plane), coronal, and sagittal images was made by filtered back-projection algorithm, using a Ramp filter, and after pre-filtering raw data by Butterworth filter with cut-off 0.5 cycles/cm power 10, after attenuation correction ($0.12\,\mathrm{cm}^{-1}$). The thickness of the reconstructed slices was 1.2 cm. The system had an in-slice resolution (FWHM) of 12–15 mm.

Data analysis

For regions of interest (ROI) placement, four transaxial slices in the orbitomeatal plane were considered. Two contiguous ROIs were placed over the BG regions of each hemisphere: a circular one (2 × 2 pixels) anterior, corresponding to the anatomical location of the head of the caudate nucleus, and one elliptical (2 × 3 pixels) posterior, over the lenticular nucleus. Since BG regions were visible on two slices (in the OM + 2.4 cm and OM + 3.2 cm planes), the slice with the highest activity on BG regions was chosen for ROI placement. Because cerebellum is almost devoid of dopamine receptors (Fields et al., 1977), the activity over the cerebellar hemispheres (CER) was determined as index of aspecific binding. Therefore, specific D2 receptor activity on striatal regions was calculated as the ratio of mean count densities in BG regions to mean activity over the cerebellar hemispheres. Cerebellar ROIs were positioned on the OM – 1.2 cm plane and had a size of 3 × 4 pixels.

A two-tailed Student's test with Bonferroni's correction for multiple comparisons was used to evaluate the statistical significance of the differences between groups of subjects. The correlation between clinical parameters and BG/CER tracer uptake ratios was determined by Pearson product-moment correlation coefficients. The criterion of significance was set as $p < 0.05$.

Results

The [123I]-IBZM SPET images showed a selective uptake of the radioligand in the BG regions that stood up as the more evident structure in the brain

Table 3. Striatal [123I]-IBZM uptake in Parkinson's disease

	Controls (9)	PD patients (29)	%change from controls
BG/CER ratio	1.68 ± 0.09	1.58 ± 0.14*	−15%

The number of subjects in each group is shown in parentheses. Numbers represent mean ± SD. *significantly different from the Controls group (p < 0.05)

Table 4. Striatal [123I]-IBZM uptake in PD patients groups: response to therapy

	UNTR-PD (8)	RESP-PD (13)	COMPL-PD (8)
BG/CER ratio	1.65 ± 0.09	1.63 ± 0.10	1.41 ± 0.09*#

The number of subjects in each group is shown in parentheses. Numbers represent mean ± SD. *significantly different from the Controls group (p < 0.05). #significantly different from the previous PD patient groups (p < 0.05). *UNTR* untreated; *RESP* stable response to L-Dopa; *COMPL* complicated response to L-Dopa

Table 3 shows mean striatal uptake ratios in controls and in the group of all examined PD subjects. In our PD patients group, we found a significant reduction of BG [123I]-IBZM uptake from controls: mean BG/CER ratio was 1.58 ± 0.14, with a percent change of striatal specific binding of −15% from mean control values. However, the BG/CER ratio was less than 1.50 (2 SD below control mean) in a minority of PD patients. Hence, the reduction of BG [123I]-IBZM activity for the whole group of PD subjects likely reflects heterogeneous changes in different subgroups of patients.

We were, therefore, mostly interested to evaluate the relative contribution of different clinical characteristics of subgroups of PD patients to reduced striatal D2 receptors potential. We first evaluated [123I]-IBZM SPET results in 3 groups of PD patients, separated on the basis of their exposure and response to L-Dopa therapy. As shown in Table 4, the mean [123I]-IBZM BG activity ratios in the UNTR-PD patients group and in the RESP-PD group were not significantly different from controls (−4% and −7% reductions from control mean, respectively), and were very similar to each other. On the contrary, significant reductions of striatal tracer uptake were found in the group of patients with a poor and fluctuating response to L-Dopa, as compared both with the controls (−40% decrease from control mean) and with the mean values of the UNTR-PD and RESP-PD subjects. This reduction does not conceivably represent receptor downregulation due to chronic therapy because BG activity was almost the same in UNTR-PD and RESP-PD groups.

Table 5. Striatal [123I]-IBZM uptake in PD patient groups: other clinical characteristics

	BG/CER ratio (mean ± SDM)	% change from controls (specific binding)
— Age		
<45 years (4)	1.68 ± 0.14	−0%
<65 years (17)	1.58 ± 0.13	−15%
⩾65 years (8)	1.53 ± 0.15	−22%*
— Age at onset		
<45 years (8)	1.65 ± 0.10	−4%
<60 years (11)	1.56 ± 0.17	−18%
⩾60 years (10)	1.53 ± 0.11	−22%*
— Duration of disease		
1–3 years (12)	1.63 ± 0.13	−7%
4–9 years (10)	1.53 ± 0.14	−22%
10–15 years (7)	1.57 ± 0.14	−16%
— Severity of disease (Hoehn-Yahr score)		
1–1.5 (8)	1.64 ± 0.12	−6%
2–2.5 (15)	1.58 ± 0.13	−15%
3–4 (6)	1.48 ± 0.14	−29%[#]

The number of subjects in each group is shown in parentheses. * significantly different from the Controls group (p < 0.05). [#] significantly different from the previous PD patient groups (p < 0.05)

Concerning [123I]-IBZM uptake in the BG of groups of PD patients separated in accord with other relevant clinical features (Table 5), the duration of the disease did not significantly affect striatal [123I]-IBZM binding. In contrast, striatal activity was significantly reduced in patients with more severe disease, as scored at the Hoehn and Yahr scale, as compared to less impaired patients. With regard to the age of the patients at time of the SPET study and age at onset of symptoms, there was a tendency for older patients to have reduced BG tracer uptake (significant reductions from control values), but differences between groups were not statistically significant.

The issue of the influence of age on striatal D2 receptor binding potential is crucial, since our group of COMPL-PD patients was older (all were aged sixty years or older) than the RESP-PD group. In Fig. 1 the BG [123I]-IBZM activity ratio for each PD patient is plotted against subject's age. The BG/CER activity ratios showed a significant negative correlation with patients' age (r = −0.46; p = 0.04). We were not able to show the same correlation in our control subjects group, possibly due to the low number of subjects. However, previous studies showed a consistent decline with age of striatal D2 receptors number in normal subjects (Brucke et al., 1991; Severson et al., 1982). Therefore, we interpret our results as the mainly effect of normal aging in a disease population. However, we do believe that age does not represent the main cause for the decline of D2 receptor binding potential in our PD patients. In fact, when we evaluated the BG/CER ratios in the COMPL-PD and in the RESP-PD patients aged sixty years or more, we found a significant difference between the BG/CER ratios of these two groups of patients (t = 3.04, p = 0.012, t test), being significantly lower in the former group.

118   G. Pizzolato et al.

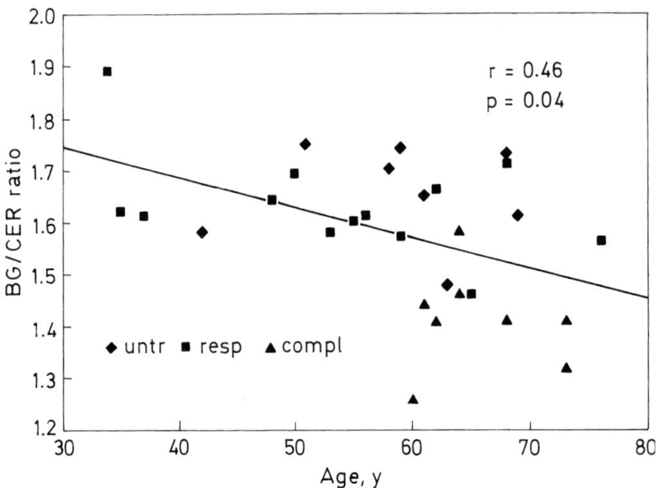

Fig. 1. Correlation between [123I]-IBZM specific activity in basal ganglia regions in parkinsonian patients and their age at the moment of SPET study. BG/CER RATIO for the whole group of patients showed a significant inverse correlation with age

In addition, we performed factor analysis to evaluate the relative influence of the various clinical characteristics to the observed BG/CER ratios in all patients. When four factors were chosen, the variables age and age at onset, duration of the disease, severity of the disease, respectively, showed the main loading contribution to the first three factors. Interestingly, only the fourth factor contained the relevant contribution of BG [123I]-IBZM uptake together with response to therapy. It appears, therefore, that response to therapy in PD patients alone is the clinical parameter that is linked to the reduced D2 receptors binding potential.

Discussion

In PD patients, we found a significant decline of basal ganglia [123I]-IBZM uptake, as compared to control subjects. These findings are in accord with previous pathological (Quik et al., 1979; Reisine et al., 1977) and PET (Brooks et al., 1992; Wienhard et al., 1990) reports in which decreased D2 receptor densities in striatum have been observed in treated PD patients. In this study, 21 out of the 29 examined patients had been exposed to chronic L-dopa therapy. On the other hand, postmortem and in vivo studies (Brooks et al., 1992; Guttman and Seeman, 1986) showed normal or moderately increased striatal D2 binding potential in untreated PD patients. The first question is, therefore, whether such changes may represent receptor downregulation due to therapy.

Results from previous studies have been interpreted as evidence that chronic L-Dopa treatment may cause down-regulation of striatal dopamine receptors in PD patients (Brucke et al., 1991, Reisine et al., 1977). Indeed, experimental studies suggest that chronic exposure to L-Dopa or dopamine agonists can result in striatal D2 receptors down-regulation (Mishra et al.,

1978; Reches et al., 1984). However, such changes likely represent a subacute and transient adaptive response to drug treatment (Fuxe et al., 1981). Furthermore, Guttman and Co-workers (1986), in their analysis of 36 parkinsonian patients, found that the duration of L-Dopa treatment had no effect on caudate and putamen [³H]spiperone binding sites. Consequently, from their findings, the authors suggest that the L-Dopa down-regulation of D2 receptors occurs very early in the treatment and further reduction in number does not occur with length of treatment or duration of disease. In addition, we do believe that our data indicates that reduced striatal [123I]-IBZM in our PD patients is not due to chronic L-Dopa therapy. In fact, mean striatal [123I]-IBZM activity was almost the same in our group of drug-naive PD patients as well as in the group of patients with a sustained response to chronic L-Dopa treatment. Second, both the COMPL-PD and the RESP-PD groups, in which we found significantly different striatal [123I]-IBZM activities, were exposed to chronic L-Dopa therapy, which was not different both in duration and dose administered.

In this study, we found that only the group of PD patients with a poor, fluctuating response to L-Dopa showed a significant decrease of BG tracer uptake ratios. These findings, therefore, suggest that loss of dopamine receptors in the striatum contributes to the development of an altered response to therapy in PD patients. They may be of relevance from a clinical and therapeutic point of view. The mechanisms involved in the development of a fluctuating/complicated response to L-Dopa during prolonged therapy are currently unknown.

Changes in peripheral pharmacokinetic factors do not appear to be the main determinant. Therefore, central pharmacodynamic factors, that is loss of synthesis or storage capacity for dopamine within the nigro-striatal axis, have been implied (Chase et al., 1986). Accordingly, PET studies demonstrated significant declines of striatal [18F]fluoro-L-Dopa (Leenders et al., 1986) or [11C]nomifensine (Tedroff et al., 1990) activity in PD, due to loss of mesostriatal dopamine nerve terminals. The accumulation of [18F]fluoro-L-Dopa was further reduced in the striatum of patients with fluctuating response to therapy.

Changes taking place at the striatal dopamine receptor sites are still controversial. However, our results agree with tissue receptor studies showing that alterations of BG dopamine receptors take place in PD patients with a deteriorating response to L-Dopa. Rinne et al. (1980) in their pathological study found that PD patients with a sustained response to L-Dopa had normal striatal [³H]-spiperone binding, whereas the number of D2 receptors was reduced in the fluctuating group. Ahlskog et al. (1991) found caudate D2 receptors reduced by 40% in specimens obtained at the time of cerebral transplantation from a clinically homogeneous group of 8 fluctuating responders patients. Finally, Brooks et al. (1992), using PET with the D2 ligand [11C]-raclopride, showed up to a 40% reduction of striatal/cerebellar uptake ratios in PD patients with a fluctuating response to L-Dopa. As the Authors notice, these patients "would fit into the second category of Rinne and co-workers".

We found a significant correlation between reductions of BG/CER ratios in our PD patient group and increasing age. Decline in striatal dopamine D2 receptors during normal aging has been previously found (Brucke et al., 1991; Severson et al., 1982). With regard to PD, in the majority of the studies there was a tendency for older patients to have reduced receptors binding sites (Brooks et al., 1992; Guttman and Seeman, 1986). In any case, the possible influence of loss of striatal D2 receptors with age must be considered. In our opinion, the reduction of striatal [^{123}I]-IBZM activity in the COMPL-PD group cannot be explained by differences in mean age between groups of patients. In fact, we found a significant difference between the BG/CER ratios of the COMPL-PD group and the RESP-PD patients aged sixty years or more. In addition, factor analysis segregated age and age at onset, duration of the disease, severity of the disease as the main loading variables to the first three factors, whereas the fourth factor contained the contribution of BG [123I]-IBZM uptake together with response to therapy. Finally, it should be pointed out that Severson et al. (1982) estimated a decrease of [^{3}H]spiperone binding sites in human striatum of about 2.5% per decade. Therefore, the effect of age appears marginal for the average age differences of our groups of patients.

In conclusion, in vivo imaging of the D2 receptors using [123I]-IBZM SPET confirms previous postmortem and in vivo studies showing alterations of BG dopamine receptors in PD patients associated with the development of a complicated/fluctuating response to L-Dopa. Whereas the literature has been confusing in determining the effects of the disease and its treatment on the receptor density, in our opinion such alterations do not represent receptors' down-regulation due to chronic L-Dopa therapy. On the other hand, the significant effect of disease severity on striatal [123I]-IBZM activity suggests that such changes may be linked to the progression of the disease.

The evolution of motor oscillations in PD patients during chronic treatment, and their underlying physiopathological mechanisms would be best evaluated by longitudinal studies in individual patients over many years.

References

Ahlskog JE, Richelson E, Nelson A (1991) Reduced D2 dopamine and muscarinic cholinergic receptor densities in caudate specimens from fluctuating responders. Ann Neurol 30: 185–191

Brooks DJ, Ibanez V, Sawle GV, Playford ED, Quinn N, Mathias CJ, Lees AJ, Marsden CD, Bannister R, Frackowiak RSJ (1992) Striatal D2 receptor status in patients with Parkinson's disease, striatonigral degeneration, and progressive supranuclear palsy, measured with ^{11}C-raclopride and positron emission tomography. Ann Neurol 31: 184–192

Brucke T, Podreka I, Angelberger P, Wenger S, Topitz A, Kufferle B, Muller Ch, Deeke L (1991) Dopamine D2 receptor imaging with SPECT: studies in different neuropsychiatric disorders. J Cereb Blood Flow Metab 11: 220–228

Chase TN, Juncos J, Serrati C, Fabbrini G, Bruno G (1986) Fluctuation in response to chronic levodopa therapy: pathogenetic and therapeutic considerations. Adv Neurol 45: 477–480

Fields JZ, Reisine TD, Yamamura HI (1977) Biochemical demonstration of dopaminergic receptors in rat and human brain using [^{3}H]spiroperidol. Brain Res 136: 578–584

Fuxe K, Agnati LF, Kohler C (1981) Characterisation of normal and supersensitive dopamine receptors: effects of ergot drugs and neuropeptides. J Neural Transm 51: 3–37

Guttman M, Seeman P (1986) Dopamine D2 receptor density in parkinsonian brain is constant for duration of disease, age, and duration of L-DOPA therapy. Adv Neurol 45: 51–57

Guttman M, Seeman P, Reynold GP, Riederer P, Jellinger J, Tourtellotte WW (1986) Dopamine D2 receptor density remains constant in treated Parkinson's disease. Ann Neurol 19: 487–492

Hagglund J, Aquilonius S-M, Eckernas S-A, Hartvig P, Lundqvist H, Gullberg P, Langstrom B (1987) Dopamine receptor properties in Parkinson's disease and Huntington's chorea evaluated by positron emission tomography using 11C-N-methyl-spiperone. Acta Neurol Scand 75: 87–94

Hoehn MM, Yahr MD (1967) Parkinsonism: onset, progression and mortality. Neurology 17: 427–442

Kung HF, Pan S, Kung MP, Billings J, Kasliwal R, Reilley J, Alavi A (1989) In vitro and in vivo evaluation of [123I]-IBZM: a potential CNS D-2 dopamine receptor imaging agent. J Nucl Med 30: 88–92

Leenders KL, Palmer AJ, Quinn N, Clark JC, Firnau G, Garnett ES, Nahmias C, Jones T, Marsden CD (1986) Brain dopamine metabolism in patients with Parkinson's disease measured with positron emission tomography. J Neurol Neurosurg Psychiatry 49: 853–860

Markham CH, Diamond SG (1981) Evidence to support early levodopa therapy in Parkinson's disease. Neurology 31: 125–131

Marsden CD, Parkes JD, Quinn N (1982) Fluctuations of disability in Parkinson's disease: clinical aspects. In: Marsden CD, Fahn S (eds) Movement disorders. Butterworth, London, pp 106–108

Mishra RK, Wonk YW, Varmuza SL, Tuff L (1978) Chemical lesion and drug induced supersensitivity and subsensitivity of caudate dopamine recptors. Life Sci 23: 443–446

Pizzolato G, Dam M, Borsato N, Saitta B, Da Col C, Perlotto N, Zanco G, Ferlin G, Battistin L (1988) [99mTc]-HM-PAO SPECT in Parkinson's disease. J Cereb Blood Flow Metab 8: S101–S108

Reches A, Wagner H, Jackson-Lewis V (1984) Chronic levodopa or pergolide administration induces down-regulation of dopamine receptors in denervated striatum. Neurology 34: 1208–1212

Reisine T, Fields J, Yamamura H (1977) Neurotransmitter receptor alterations in Parkinson's disease. Life Sci 21: 335–344

Rinne UK, Koskinen V, Lonnberg P (1980) Neurotransmitter receptors in the parkinsonian brain. In: Rinne UK, Kringler M, Stamm G (eds) Parkinson's disease. Current progress, problems and management. Elsevier, Amsterdam, pp 93–107

Rutgers AWF, Lakke JPWF, Paans AMJ, Vaalburg W, Korf J (1987) Tracing of dopamine receptors in hemiparkinson with positron emission tomography. J Neurol Sci 80: 237–248

Schwarz J, Tatsch K, Arnold G, Gasser T, Trenkwalder C, Kirsch CM, Oertel WH (1992) [123I]-iodobenzamide-SPECT predicts dopaminergic responsiveness in patients with de novo parkinsonism. Neurology 42: 556–561

Severson JA, Marcusson J, Winblad B, Finch CE (1982) Age-correlated loss of dopaminergic binding sites in human basal ganglia. J Neurochem 39: 1623–1631

Tedroff J, Aquilonius S-M, Laihinen A, Rinne U, Hartvig P, Andersson J, Lundqvist H, Haaparanta M, Solin O, Antoni G, Gee AD, Ulin J, Langstrom B (1990) Striatal kinetics of [11C]-(+)-nomifensine and 6-[18F]fluoro-L-dopa in Parkinson's disease measured with positron emission tomography. Acta Neurol Scand 81: 24–30

Wienhard K, Coenen HH, Pawlik G (1990) PET studies of dopamine receptor distribution using [18F]fluoroethylspiperone: findings in disorders related to the dopaminergic system. J Neural Transm 81: 195–213

Authors' address: G. Pizzolato, M.D., Department of Neurology, University of Padova, via Giustiniani 5, I-35128 Padova, Italy.

J Neural Transm (1995) [Suppl] 45: 123–131
© Springer-Verlag 1995

PET studies of the striatal dopaminergic system in Parkinson's disease (PD)

P. Piccini*, N. Turjanski, and **D. J. Brooks**

MRC Clinical Medical Centre, Hammersmith Hospitals, London, United Kingdom

Summary. Positron emission tomography (PET) is a functional imaging technique which allows detection of biochemical and pharmacological dysfunction of the nigrostriatal dopaminergic system and provides the opportunity to investigate living patients with PD.

This paper reviews the contribution of PET studies to the understanding of neurochemical changes underlying Parkinson's disease.

Introduction

Endogenous dopamine is synthesised in the substantia nigra pars compacta from the aminoacid tyrosine, via levodopa by the enzyme tyrosine hydroxylase and then by the enzyme aromatic amino acid decarboxylase. Dopamine is then stored and concentrated in vesicles within the dopaminergic nerve terminals until released. Dopamine is metabolised by the enzymes monoamine oxidase B and catechol-O-methyl transferase to its main metabolites, homovanilic acid (HVA) and dihydroxyphenylacetic acid (DOPAC) respectively.

Post synaptic dopamine receptors are located on spiny striatal neurons which project via the globus pallidus and thalamus to cortical areas. D1 receptors are thought to be located on striatal neurons projecting to the internal globus pallidum and substantia nigra pars reticulata, while D2 receptors are present on striatal neurons projecting to the external globus pallidus. Recently genes encoding D1, D2, D3, D4 and D5 receptors have been cloned (Bunzow et al., 1988; Dearry et al., 1990; Solokoff et al., 1990; Van-Tol et al., 1991). These receptors may be considered as "D1 like" or "D2 like" on the basis of their pharmacological properties. The "D1 like" receptors include D1 and D5 receptors, while the "D2 like" includes D2, D3 and D4 receptors. D1, D2 and D3 receptors are most densely represented in the striatum, but dopamine receptors are also found in cortical and limbic areas of the brain (Strange, 1993).

---

*On leave of absence from the Institute of Clinical Neurology, University of Pisa, Italy

The neuronal degeneration of the nigrostriatal pathway which characterises PD is accompanied by corresponding biochemical changes. Markers of biochemical dysfunction include decreases in dopamine (nigral ventral cells are targeted, resulting in a greater dopamine loss in the putamen than caudate) (Bernheimer et al., 1973; Bokobza et al., 1984; Hornykiewicz and Kish, 1986; Perry et al., 1990) tyrosine hydroxylase (Hornykiewicz and Kish, 1986; Goto et al., 1989) tyrosine hydroxylase mRNA (Agid et al., 1987), dopa decarboxylase (Hornykiewicz and Kish, 1986), dopamine metabolites (Bernheimer et al., 1973; Hornykiewicz and Kish, 1986; Perry et al., 1990; Bobozka et al., 1984), and the dopamine transporter (Pimoule et al., 1983; Janowsky et al., 1987; Pearce et al., 1990). The effect of nigrostriatal deafferentation on striatal postsynaptic dopamine receptors is unclear. Post-mortem studies have shown conflicting results with both unchanged and changed postsynaptic receptor binding in the striatum of PD patients (Lee et al., 1978; Rinne et al., 1981; Bobozka et al., 1984; Guttman et al., 1986; Pierot et al., 1988).

PET assessment of nigrostriatal function in PD

PET measurements are performed by administering a tracer labelled with short-lived positron emitting isotopes (Phelps et al., 1982) Using appropriate modelling, tracer uptake can be shown to be proportional to the biochemical integrity of the system studied. As regard to the study of nigrostriatal function there are PET ligands available to investigate the function of both presynaptic and postsynaptic component of the dopaminergic system.

Pre-synaptic studies

Garnett et al. (1983) first reported the in vivo use of L-6-[^{18}F]-fluorodopa to visualise the nigrostriatal dopaminergic system.

After intravenous administration ^{18}F-dopa is transported across the blood-brain barrier by the neutral amino acid carrier (Leenders et al., 1986a) and then converted by aromatic aminoacid decarboxylase (AAD) to ^{18}F-dopamine (Firnau et al., 1987; Melega et al., 1990). Striatal ^{18}F-dopamine is then metabolised to ^{18}F-DOPAC and to ^{18}F-HVA by monoamine oxidase B and catechol-O-methyltransferase.

Kinetic analysis of striatal ^{18}F-dopa uptake is complex because of its peripheral and central metabolism. Fortunately, over the 90 minutes following tracer administration, little metabolite loss from striatum occurs, as a consequence ^{18}F-dopa uptake can be regarded as irreversible. Striatal ^{18}F-dopa uptake is usually described as an influx constant, Ki, which reflects both the free striatal ^{18}F-dopa pool and the rate constant for decarboxylation of ^{18}F-dopa into ^{18}F-dopamine. The striatal Ki value therefore reflects striatal uptake of exogenous ^{18}F-dopa rather than endogenous dopamine production.

The original reports of Garnett et al. (1984) and Nahmias et al. (1985) in hemiparkinsonian subjects demonstated bilateral reductions in putamen ^{18}F-dopa uptake with normal caudate uptake, confirming previous pathological observation of greater involvement of nigro-putamen than nigro-caudate projections in PD. Subsequently a number of PET studies have shown a good correlation between severity of disability and decrease in ^{18}F-dopa uptake in PD (Leenders et al., 1986b; Brooks et al., 1990; Martin et al., 1989; Otsuka et al., 1991). Patients with sustained response to levodopa therapy show greater striatal ^{18}F-dopa accumulation than those with a fluctuating response (Leenders et al., 1986b). On average putamen ^{18}F-dopa Ki values are reduced to 40–50% of normal in PD (Brooks et al., 1990). This reduction in putamen fluorodopa is comparable with the 60% reduction in striatal aromatic amino acid decarboxylase activity, observed in post-mortem studies (Nagatsu et al., 1979; Goto et al., 1989).

Recent studies (Vingerhoets et al., 1994; Morrish et al., in press) have also been showed the potential of ^{18}F-dopa in measuring disease progression in PD. These results indicate that nigral lesion in PD occurs at a rate more rapid than that in the normal population, although the rate of PD progression in the two studies is considerably different (1.7% per annum vs 18% per annum respectively). Differences in methodological procedure could account for the discrepancy between the two studies. As quoted above, previous PET studies on PD have demonstrated a decrease in putamen F-dopa uptake with relative sparing of the caudate. Morrish and co-workers used for their analysis separate caudate and putamen regions. The use of large ROIs, encompassing caudate and putamen, by Vingerhoets et co-authors, inevitably dilutes the effects of change in either structure and it may contribute to an understimation of the rate of the PD progression.

[18]F-dopa PET measurement has proven useful in the interpretation of the contribution of genetic factors to the aetiology of PD. Mjones (1949) was the first to suggest that PD might be a familial condition. Following this, clinical twin studies were interpreted as showing no evidence of a genetic contribution (Ward et al., 1983) and the consensus view was that inherited factors play a minor role in the aetiology of PD; recently the tables have turned again with a reconsideration of previous data (Johnson et al., 1990), together with new clinical-pathological data (Degl'Innocenti et al., 1989; Golbe et al., 1990) and PET studies of large kindred with familial PD (Sawle et al., 1992a) and twins (Burn et al., 1992; Holthoff et al., 1994). More recent ^{18}F-dopa PET data obtained at this Unit (Piccini et al., 1995) showed a 38% prevalence of dopaminergic dysfunction in relatives of cases with familial PD, far higher than the 15% prevalence normally reported for positive familial history of PD. Our results also suggest that the concordance for nigral pathology in PD twins (27% in the MZ and 25% in the DZ pair) is higher than previously realized.

Striatal transplantation of foetal mesenephalic tissue has been advocated as a treatment for Parkinson's disease. PET can provide quantitative data regarding dopaminergic function within grafted and ungrafted tissue. Sequential ^{18}F-dopa scans in PD patients (Sawle et al., 1992b; Morrish et al., 1994) have provided evidence for survival and growth of the grafted dopamine neurons as well as for disease progression, suggested by reduced uptake of ^{18}F-dopa in parts of the striatum outside the graft (Sawle et al., 1992b).

Recent evidence suggests that striatal fluorodopa uptake may not be a reliable index of the ability of the striatal neuronal tissue to decarboxylate levodopa. In fact experimental reports indicate that although striatal levodopa decarboxylation is a process controlled by AADC it does not appear to be exclusively confined to nigrostriatal neurons: other neural cells, and also glial cells, can express AADC and metabolise L-dopa (Opacka-Juffry and Brooks, in press). Taking these facts into account, striatal ^{18}F-dopa uptake may overestimate residual nigrostriatal function in PD and so lead to an underestimation of the severity of the disease, particularly at advanced stages.

What kind of a ligand would then be more appropriate as a dopamine PET tracer? In theory a positron emitting analogue of tyrosine would give information on the endogenous synthesis of dopamine. However, the extensive conversion of tyrosine to protein in the brain, as well as dopamine, would yield only a poor striatal to background ("signal-to-noise") ratio.

Alternatively, PET and SPECT ligands binding to dopamine re-uptake sites have been developed as markers of dopamine terminal integrity.

The dopamine transporter is a membrane-bound protein that mediates reuptake of dopamine into pre-synaptic nerve terminals following its release.

Nomifensine is a reversible mono amine reuptake site inhibitor. [11C]Nomifensine like ^{18}F-dopa provides a measure of the functional integrity of nigro-striatal terminals (Salmon et al., 1990). Mean putamen uptake of [11C]Nomifensine is reduced by 50% in PD while caudate uptake is less affected. Striatal uptake of [11C]Nomifensine and ^{18}F-dopa are correlated in PD patients (Salmon et al., 1990; Tedroff et al., 1990) and putamen [11C]Nomifensine binding falls with increasing severity of the disease. However unwanted labelling of adrenergic and serotonergic uptake sites by [11C]Nomifensine limited accurate quantification of dopamine transporter binding.

Recently a series of cocaine analogues have been developed with very high affinity for the dopamine transporter and some have been labelled with positron emitting isotopes to permit imaging by PET (Scheffel et al., 1992; Dannals et al., 1993; Fowler et al., 1993; Volkow et al., 1994) A recent PET study with the cocaine analogue [11]WIN35428 (Frost et al., 1993) in healthy volunteers and PD subjects showed a reduction by 78% in posterior putamen binding in the patients with PD; the authors were able to obtain a high specific striatal signal and could also detect mid brain activity, presumably from dopamine transporter in the substantia nigra (Frost et al., 1993).

Recent developments, using PET-MRI coregistration, have offered further possibilities in the use of [18F]dopa tracer. This technique allows to define anatomical regions on an MRI scan, then transfer them to similar coordinates on a functional [18F]dopa PET image. Image coregistration is able to identify dopa uptake in the midbrain and a difference in nigral uptake between PD patients and normal volunteers (Morrish et al., in press). This preliminary data indicates that this technique may allow study of function in any region of the brain that can be clearly defined by MRI, and offers a significant advance in the application of [18F]dopa PET.

Postsynaptic studies

D2 receptors

The first PET images of dopamine receptors in man were achieved using the high affinity irreversibly bound D2 antagonist [^{11}C]methylspiperone (Wagner et al., 1983). Other spiperone tracers include [^{18}F]fluspiperone, [^{18}F]fluoroethylspiperone, and [^{76}Br]bromospiperone. Because the spiperone family of drugs have significant affinity for HT2-receptors, radiolabelled analogues of the benzamide family have been prepared as PET ligands. [^{11}C]raclopride is a positron labelled benzamide which is reversibly bound and highly selective and specific for the D2 receptor. However, its affinity for the D2 receptor is weaker than the irreversibly bound antagonists, and cannot distinguish between changes in receptor density and receptor occupancy. Bmax and Kd of striatal D2 receptors have been measured using [^{11}C]raclopride following displacement by cold tracer. However in most clinical studies separate values of Bmax and Kd are not evaluated. The binding potential (Bmax/Kd) has proved to be a useful clinical measure of specific receptor binding.

Using ^{11}C-raclopride, two PET studies have shown that in untreated PD there is relative upregulation of putamen D2 binding sites contralateral to the more affected limbs (Rinne et al., 1990; Sawle et al., 1990). Absolute levels of putaminal D2 binding sites in untreated PD have been reported either normal or mildly increased (Leenders et al., 1992; Brooks et al., 1992). Caudate nucleus D2 site density appears to be unchanged. Where putamen ^{18}F-dopa and ^{11}C-raclopride uptake have both been measured in individual dopa-naive patients an inverse correlation between the binding of the two tracers has been found (Sawle et al., 1990).

Treated PD patients showed normal (Hagglund et al., 1987; Shinotoh et al., 1993) or reduced (Leenders et al., 1991; Wienhard et al., 1990; Brooks et al., 1992) striatal level of D2 receptor binding. The reduction was more pronounced in the caudate nucleus than in the putamen (Wienhard et al., 1990; Brooks et al., 1992) and it occurred particularly in chronically treated cases who had developed a fluctuating response to levodopa therapy (Brooks et al., 1992).

D1 receptors

PET studies on the localisation of the D1 receptors have been limited by the lack of D1 selective compounds until the development of the reversible antagonist ^{11}C-SCH23390. In untreated PD patients striatal ^{11}C-SCH23390 uptake was similar to those of normal subjects (Shinotoh et al., 1993) and no side-to-side difference was found in hemiparkinsonian patients (Rinne et al., 1990) suggesting that in spite of striatal deafferentation there is no compensatory upregulation of D1 sites in PD.

In treated patients striatal D1 receptor binding was found unchanged (Shinotoh et al., 1993) or decreased (Turjanski et al., 1994). In the paper of

Turjanski et al. the reduction of striatal D1 and caudate D2 receptors observed in PD patients did not correlate with the presence or absence of long-term levodopa-induced dyskinesia. This result suggests that levodopa-induced dyskinesia may not be determined at the dopaminergic site and that the decrease of striatal dopamine receptors in these patients may be the result either of long-term exposure to non physiological levels of exogenous levodopa or disease progression itself.

Conclusion

In summary functional imaging has been used to demonstrate the selective pattern of disruption of striatal dopaminergic system associated with Parkinson's disease.

PET can also detect the presence of subclinical functional abnormalities in at-risk subjects, such as relatives of patients with Parkinson's disease, it can provide a means of monitoring the therapeutic effects of engraftment and in the future may help to establish the role of neuroprotective agents and nerve growth factors in the treatment of Parkinson's disease and other neurodegenerative factors.

References

Agid Y, Javoy-Agid F, Ruberg M (1987) Biochemistry of neurotransmitters in Parkinson's disease. In: Marsden CD, Fahn S (eds) Movement disorders 2. Butterworths, London, pp 166–230

Bernheimer H, Birkmayer W, Hornykiewicz O, et al (1973) Brain dopamine and the syndromes of Parkinson and Huntington. Clinical, morphological, and neurochemical correlations. J Neurol Sci 20: 415–455

Bokobza B, Ruberg M, Scatton B, et al (1984) [^{3}H]spiperone binding, dopamine and HVA concentration in Parkinson's disease and supranuclear palsy. Eur J Pharmacol 99: 167–175

Brooks DJ, Ibanez V, Sawle GV, et al (1990) Differing patterns of striatal ^{18}F-dopa uptake in Parkinson's disease, multiple system atrophy and progressive supranuclear palsy. Ann Neurol 28: 547–555

Brooks DJ, Ibanez V, Sawle GV, et al (1992) Striatal D2 receptor status in Parkinson's disease, striatonigral degeneration, and progressive supranuclear palsy, measured with ^{11}C-raclopride and PET. Ann Neurol 31: 184–192

Bunzow JR, Van Tol HHM, Grandy DK, et al (1988) Cloning expression of a rat D2 dopamine receptor cDNA. Nature 336: 783–787

Burn DJ, Mark MH, Playford ED, et al (1992) Parkinson's disease in twins studied with ^{18}F-dopa and positron emission tomography. Neurology 42: 1894–1900

Dannals RF, Neumeyer JL, Milius RA, et al (1993) Synthesis of a radiotracer for studying dopamine uptake sites in vivo using PET: 2beta-carbomethoxy-3beta-(4-flourophenyl-o-[N-^{11}C-methyl]-tropane ([^{11}C]-WIN35428). J Label Compounds Radiopharmacol 33: 147–152

Dearry A, Gingrich JA, Falardeau P, et al (1990) Molecular cloning and expression of the gene for a human D1 dopamine receptor. Nature 347: 72–75

Degl'Innocenti F, Maurello MT, Marini P (1989) A parkinsonian kindred. Ital J Neurol Sci 10: 307–310

Firnau G, Sood S, Chirakal R, et al (1987) Cerebral metabolism of ^{18}F-fluoro-L3,4-dihydroxyphenylalanine in the primate. J Neurochem 48: 1077–1082

Fowler JS, Volkow ND, Wolf AP, et al (1993) Mapping cocaine binding sites in human and baboon brain in vivo. Synapse 4: 371–377

Frost JJ, Rosier AJ, Reich SG, et al (1993) Positron emission tomographic imaging of the dopamine transporter with ^{11}C-WIN 35,428 reveals marked declines in mild Parkinson's disease. Ann Neurol 34: 423–431

Garnett ES, Firnau G, Nahmias C (1983) Dopamine visualised in the basal ganglia of living man. Nature 305: 137–138

Garnett ES, Nahmias C, Firnau G (1984) Central dopaminergic pathways in hemyparkinsonism examined by positron emission tomography. Can J Neurol Sci 11 [Suppl 1]: 174–179

Golbe LI, Di Iorio G, Bonavita V, et al (1990) A large kindred with autosomal dominant Parkinson's disease. Ann Neurol 27: 276–282

Goto S, Hirano A, Matsumoto S (1989) Subdivisional involvement of nigrostriatal loop in idiopathic Parkinson's disease and striatonigral degeneration. Ann Neurol 26: 766–770

Guttman M, Seeman P, Reynolds GP, et al (1986) Dopamine D2 receptor densitity remains constant in treated Parkinson's disease. Ann Neurol 19: 487–492

Hagglund J, Aquilonius SM, Eckernas SA, et al (1987) Dopamine receptor properties in Parkinson's disease and Huntington's chorea evaluated by positron emission tomography using ^{11}C-N-methyl-spyperone. Acta Neurol Scand 75: 87–94

Holthoff VA, .Vieregge P, Kessler J, et al (1994) Discordant twins with Parkinson's disease: positron emission tomography and early signs of impaired cognitive circuits. Ann Neurol 36: 176–182

Hornykiewiccz O, Kish SJ (1986) Biochemical pathophysiology of Parkinson's disease. Adv Neurol 45: 19–34

Janowsky A, Vocci F, Berger P, et al (1987) ^{3}H]GBR-12935 binding to the dopaminergic transporter is decreased in the caudate nucleus in Parkinson's disease. J Neurochem 49: 617–621

Johnson WG, Hodge SE, Duvoisin R (1990) Twin studies and the genetics of Parkinson's disease. A reappraisal. Mov Dis 5: 187–194

Lee T, Seeman P, Rajput A, et al (1978) Receptor basis for dopaminergic supersensitivity in Parkinson's disease. Nature 273: 59–61

Leenders KL, Poewe WH, Palmer AJ, et al (1986a) Inhibition of L-6-[^{18}F]Fluorodopa uptake into human brain by amino acids demonstrated by positron emission tomography. Ann Neurol 20: 258–262

Leenders KL, Palmer AJ, Quinn N, et al (1986b) Brain dopamine metabolism in patients with Parkinson's disease measured with positron emission tomography. J Neurol Neurosurg Psychiatry 49: 853–860

Leenders KL, Antonini A, Schwartz J, et al (1992) Brain dopamine D2 receptors in "de novo" drug-naive parkinsonian patients measured using PET and 11C-raclopride. Mov Dis 7 [Suppl 1]: 1992

Martin WRW, Palmer MR, Patlak CS, Calne DB (1989) Nigrostriatal function in humans studied with positron emission tomography. Ann Neurol 26: 535–542

Melega WP, Luxen A, Perlmutter MM, et al (1990) Comparative in vivo metabolism of 6-[^{18}F]fluoro-L-dopa and [^{3}H]L-dopa in rats. Biochem Pharmacol 39: 1853–1860

Mjones H (1949) Paralysis agitants. A clinical genetic study. Acta Psychiatr Neurol Scand 25 [Suppl 54]: 1–95

Morrish PK, Sawle GV, Brooks DJ, et al (1994) One year follow up by ^{18}F-dopa positron emission tomography (PET) scanning of fetal mesencephalic grafting for Parkinson's disease in one patient with unilateral putamen and one patient with unilateral caudate and putamen graft. Mov Dis 9 [Suppl 1]: 113

Morrish PK, Sawle GV, Brooks DJ (1995) The rate of progression of Parkinson's disease: a longitudinal ^{18}F-dopa PET study. Adv Neurol (in press)

Morrish PK, Sawle GV, Brooks DJ (1995) Imaging the midbrain in Parkinson's disease using ^{18}F-dopa positron emission tomography. Neurology (in press)

Nagatsu T, Kato T, Nagatsu I, et al (1979) Cathecolamine related-enzymes in the brains of patients with parkinsonism and Wilson's disease. Adv Neurol 24: 283–292

Nahmias C, Garnett ES, Firnau G, Lang A (1985) Striatal dopamine distribution in parkinsonian patients during life. J Neurol Sci 69: 223–230

Opacka-Juffry J, Brooks DJ (1995) L-dopa and its decarboxylase- new ideas on their neuroregulatory roles. Mov Dis (in press)

Otsuka M, Ichiya Y, Hosokawa S, et al (1991) Striatal blood flow, glucose metabolism, and ^{18}F-dopa uptake: difference in Parkinson's disease and atypical parkinsonism. J Neurol Neurosurg Psychiatry 54: 898–904

Pearce RKB, Seeman P, Jellinger K, Tourtellotte WW (1990) Dopamine uptake sites and dopamine receptors in Parkinson's disease and schizophrenia. Eur Neurol 30 [Suppl 1]: 9–14

Perry TL, Wright JM, Berry K, et al (1990) Dominantly inherited apathy, central hypoventilation, and Parkinson's syndrome: clinical, biochemical, and neuro-pathological studies of 2 new cases. Neurology 40: 1882–1887

Phelps ME, Mazziotta JC, Huang SC (1982) Study of cerebral function with positron computed tomography. J Cereb Far Blood Flow Metab 2: 113–162

Piccini P, Burn D, Sawle GV, et al (1995) Dopaminergic function in relatives of Parkinson's disease patients: a clinical and PET study. Neurology 45 [suppl 4]: 203

Pierot L, Desnos C, Blin J, et al (1988) D1 and D2-type dopamine receptors in patients with Parkinson's disease and progressive supranuclear palsy. J Neurosci 86: 291–306

Pimoule C, Schoemaker H, Javoy-Agid F, et al (1983) Decrease in [3H]cocaine binding to the dopaminergic transporter in Parkinson's disease. Eur J Pharmacol 95: 145–146

Rinne UK, Koskinen V, Lonnberg P (1981) Dopamine receptors in the parkinsonian brain. J Neural Transm 51: 97–106

Rinne UK, Laiehinen A, Rinne OJ, et al (1990) Positron emission tomography demon-strates dopamine D2 receptors supersensitivity in the striatum of patients with early Parkinson's disease. Mov Dis 5: 55–59

Salmon EP, Brooks DJ, Leenders KL, et al (1990) A two-compartment description and kinetic procedure for measuring regional cerebral [11C]nomifensine uptake using positron emission tomography. J Cereb Blood Metab 10: 307–316

Sawle GV, Brooks DJ, Ibanez V, Frackowiak RSJ (1990) Striatal D2 receptor density is inversely proportional to dopa uptake in untreated hemi-Parkinson's disease. J Neural Neurosurg Psychiatry 53: 170–177

Sawle GV, Wroe SJ, Lees AJ, et al (1992a) The identification of presymptomatic parkinsonism: clinical and ^{18}F-dopa positron emission tomography studies in an Irish kindred. Ann Neurol 32: 609–617

Sawle GV, Bloomfield PM, Bjorklund A, et al (1992b) Transplantation of fetal dopamine neurons in Parkinson's disease: PET [^{18}F]6-L-fluorodopa studies in two patients with putaminal implants. Ann Neurol 31: 166–173

Scheffel U, Dannals RF, Wong DF, et al (1992) Dopamine transporter imaging with novel selective cocaine analogues. Neurol Rep 3: 969–972

Shinotoh H, Hirayama K, Tateno Y (1993) Dopamine D1 and D2 receptors in Parkinson's disease and striatonigral degeneration determined by PET. Adv Neurol 60: 488–493

Solokoff P, Giros B, Martres MP, et al (1990) Molecular cloning and characterisation of a novel dopamine receptor (D3) as a target for neuroleptic. Nature 347: 148–151

Strange P (1993) Dopamine receptors in the basal ganglia: relevance to Parkinson's disease. Mov Dis 8: 263–270

Tedroff J, Aquilonius SM, Laihinen A, et al (1990) Striatal kinetics of [11C]-(+)-Nomifensine and 6-[^{18}F]fluoro-L-dopa in Parkinson's disease measured with positron emission tomography. Acta Neurol Scand 81: 24–30

Turjanski N, Lees AJ, Brooks DJ (1994) Striatal D1 and D2 receptor status in L-Dopa treated Parkinson's disease patients with or without dyskinesia. A PET study. Mov Dis 9 [Suppl 1]: 151

Van-Tol HHM, Bunzow JR, Guan HC, et al (1991) Cloning of the gene for a human dopamine D4 receptor with high affinity for the antipsycothic clozapine. Nature 350: 610–616

Vingerhoets FJG, Snow BJ, Lee S, et al (1994) Longitudinal fluorodopa positron emission tomographic studies of the evolution of idiopathic parkinsonism. Ann Neurol 36: 759–764

Volkow ND, Fowler JS, Wang GL, et al (1994) Decreased dopamine transporters with age in healthy human subjects. Ann Neurol 36: 147–152

Wagner HN, Burns HD, Dannals RF, et al (1993) Imaging dopamine receptors in the human brain by positron emission tomography. Science 221: 1264–1266

Ward CD, Duvoish RC, Ince SE, et al (1983) Parkinson's disease in 65 pairs of twins and in a sets of quadruplets. Neurology 19: 815–824

Wienhard K, Coenen HH, Pawlik G, et al (1990) PET studies of dopamine receptor distribution using [18F]fluoroethylspiperone: findings in disorders related to the dopaminergic system. J Neural Transm 81: 195–213

Authors' address: P. Piccini, MD, MRC Cyclotron Unit, Hammersmith Hospital, Ducane Rd, London W12 ONN, United Kingdom.

J Neural Transm (1995) [Suppl] 45: 133–136
© Springer-Verlag 1995

Apomorphine continuous stimulation in Parkinson's disease: receptor desensitization as a possible mechanism of reduced motor response*

R. Maggio, P. Barbier, and **G. U. Corsini**

Istituto di Farmacologia, Scuola Medica, Università di Pisa, Italy

Summary. Apomorphine is a potent nonselective agonist at D1 and D2 dopamine receptors. The utility of apomorphine in Parkinson's disease (PD) is well asserted but its clinical use is reduced because of its short half-life and numerous side-effects. The disabling "on-off" fluctuations are among the most frequent and troublesome complications of chronic levodopa therapy in PD. Apomorphine is effective to reverse refractory L-dopa induced "off" periods, but a reduced motor response after repeated administrations has also been described with this drug. The loss of response to apomorphine, when the drug is administered repeatedly, is well fitted by the processes of receptor phosphorylation and down regulation. Elucidation of the molecular bases of dopaminergic receptors desensitization may lead to a better understanding of the mechanisms of dopaminergic regulation, and to a more appropriate treatment of PD.

Apomorphine (10,11-dihydroxyaporphine) was first synthesized in 1869 (Mathiessen and Wright). Soon after its discovery the emetic, antimanic and antispasmodic effects in man, and the ability to induce stereotyped behavior in experimental animals, were reported (Gee, 1869). Apomorphine was initially tried in a large variety of medical disorders, but it was not until the discovery of its mechanism of action that a rational use of the drug began (Ernst, 1967; Anden et al., 1967).

Apomorphine is a potent nonselective agonist at D1 and D2 dopamine receptors. It has a rapid onset of action after subcutaneous injection (time to peak plasma concentration: 8 minutes) and a short half-life (34 minutes) (Gancher et al., 1989). The drug has proved to have an antipsychotic effect (Corsini et al., 1977; Tamminga et al., 1978), and a further reevaluation study revealed useful properties on schizoaffective patients (Del Zompo et al., 1986). The utility of apomorphine in Parkinson's Disease (PD) has been reported since 1951 by Schwab et al., but the drug has not had a large clinical use on account of its short half-life and because of its numerous side-effects (Cotzias

---

*Supported by grant 93-1563 from Biomed

et al., 1976) In the late 1980s, apomorphine has presented a renewed interest in the management of PD, since the emetic action was circumvented by using a peripheral dopamine receptor blocker domperidone (Corsini et al., 1979).

The disabling "on-off" fluctuations are among the most frequent and troublesome complications of chronic levodopa therapy in PD. Daily fluctuations of motor performance occur in more than 50% of patients after 3–5 years of treatment (Marsden and Parkers, 1976). The development of a tolerance has been evocated to explain this phenomenon (Sweet et al., 1976; Weiner et al., 1980). Apomorphine is effective to reverse refractory L-dopa induced "off" periods in PD (Yahr et al., 1982; Hardie et al., 1984) but a reduced motor response after repeated administrations has also been described with this drug (Grandas and Obeso, 1989); and the loss of response is greater when drug administration is prolonged (Gancher et al., 1992).

Instead of peripheral pharmacokinetics explanations, the occurence of motor fluctuations may involve particularities in the central metabolism of L-dopa, and/or pharmacodynamic factors, since the peripheral metabolism of levodopa does not exhibit significant differences between de novo, stable, and fluctuating patients (Gancher et al., 1987; Fabbrini et al., 1987). Others studies (Gancher et al., 1992; Grandas et al., 1992) have also shown that alterations in the peripheral pharmacokinetics could not be an explanation for the tolerance observed with apomorphine. A reduction in the motor response after repeated and closely spaced doses of apomorphine in patients with PD has been shown (Grandas and Obeso, 1989). The interval between doses seems to be a critical determinant of motor response as the duration of the effect is reduced by 40% after apomorphine injections at 2-hour intervals whereas the motor improvement is of equal duration when the doses are given at 4-hour intervals (Grandas et al., 1992). Gancher et al. (1992) have also demonstrated that a decrement in response to apomorphine is significantly more accentuated after longer periods of drug exposure, this pattern being consistent with the development of drug tolerance. Then, an hypothesis implicating a time-dependent decrease in dopaminergic sensitivity in relation with the physiopathology of motor fluctuations in the PD could be proposed. In the striatum of parkinsonian patients, postsynaptic dopaminergic receptors sensitivity following pulsatile stimulation could be altered by a tolerance phenomenon, without sufficient recovery when the injections are performed too soon one to another.

Dopaminergic receptors are members of the G-protein receptor family. Five dopaminergic receptors have been characterized by molecular cloning (for review see: Seemann and Van Tol, 1994; O'Dowd, 1993). Based on their functional activity they are divided in D1- and D2-like receptors. The D1-like receptors (D1 and D5) induce cAMP accumulation, while D2-like receptors (D2, D3 and D4) reduce cAMP level. The physiological regulation of G protein-coupled receptors is determined by multiple processes. Receptor stimulation by agonist elicits not only a rapid modulation of a second messenger response but also palmitoylation, internalization, phosphorylation and desensitization of the receptor itself. Stimulation of dopaminergic D1 receptors for at least 30 minutes with high concentration of dopamine ($10\,\mu M$) results in a broad pattern of receptor desensitization that appears to involve an increase in phosphorylation level (Ng et al., 1994). In analogy to D1 receptors, D2 receptors as well can be modified by phosphorylation (Ng et al., 1994). Thus, an increase in phosphorylation appears to be involved in the overall process of receptor desensitization.

Consensus sequence for cAMP-dependent protein kinase phosphorylation are present in the primary structure of the dopamine D1 receptors (O'Dowd, 1993), and also serine and threonine residues which could serve as potential sites for receptor specific kinase such as β-adrenergic-receptor kinase, are present in the carboxy tail of the dopamine D1 receptors. Since these kinases are known to contribute to the desensitization of the β-adrenergic receptors, they could play also a role in the desensitization of the dopaminergic receptors.

Agonist treatment of cells expressing the dopamine D1 receptor induces a rapid redistribution of the surface dopamine D1 receptors. This response is consistent with a rapid agonist induced sequestration of dopamine receptors. It is suggested that uncoupled and phosphorylated receptors are rapidly sequestered away from the cell surface and are dephosphorylated and returned to the surface in an active form (Perkins et al., 1990). Down regulation of receptors is a complex process that occurs more slowly than sequestration and leads to the irreversible loss of receptors from the plasma membrane. The rate of receptor loss is greatest during the first four hours of agonist stimulation (Bouvier et al., 1989). Within 24 hours, the process usually approaches steady state. This process has been studied accurately for the β-adrenergic receptors (Kobilka, 1992). The early phase appears to require protein-kinase A mediated receptor phosphorylation. It is likely that, following prolonged agonist exposure accelerated degradation of the total number of receptors undergoing to the continuous turnover of phosphorylation and dephosphorylation can contribute to the overall process of receptor desensitization. The later phase of down regulation, which extends from 4 to 24 hours, is apparently due to a reduction in new receptor biosynthesis.

The loss of response to apomorphine when the drug is administered repeatedly, is well fitted by the processes of receptor phosphorylation and down regulation. Moreover, the occurrence of motor fluctuations "on-off phenomena" after chronic levodopa therapy could be partially explained by an altered regulation of receptor desensitization. It is possible that after apomorphine administration striatal dopaminergic receptors are rapidly phosphorylated. If a repeated challenge with apomorphine occurs, receptor down regulation takes place with a marked reduction of motor response. Vice versa, the suspension of the apomorphine therapy or the increase of the interval between doses might consent to restore a normal receptor sensitivity. Further elucidation of the molecular bases of desensitization, and of factors influencing dopaminergic responsiveness, may lead to a better understanding of the mechanism of dopaminergic regulation, and to a better treatment of PD.

References

Anden NE, Rubenson A, Fuxe K, Hokfelt T (1967) Evidence for dopamine receptor stimulation by apomorphine. J Pharm Pharmac 19: 627–629
Bouvier M, et al (1989) Two distinct pathways for cAMP-mediated down-regulation of the β2-adrenergic receptor. J Biol Chem 264: 16786–16792

Corsini GU, et al (1979) Therapeutic efficacy of apomorphine combined with an extracerebral inhibitor of dopamine receptors in Parkinson's disease. Lancet i: 954–956

Corsini GU, et al. (1977) Sedative, hypnotic, and antipsychotic effects of low doses of apomorphine in man. Adv Biochem Psychopharmacol 16: 645–648

Cotzias GC, Papavasiliou PS, Tolosa ES, Mendez JS, Bell-Midura M (1976) Treatment of Parkinson's disease with apomorphine. N Engl J Med 294: 567–572

Del Zompo M, Bocchetta A, Piccardi MP, Corsini GU (1986) Dopamine agonists in the treatment of schizophrenia. Prog Brain Res 65: 41–48

Ernst AM (1967) Mode of action of apomorphine and dexamphetamine on gnawing compulsion in rats. Psycopharmacologia 10: 316–323

Fabbrini G, et al (1987) Levodopa pharmacokinetic mechanisms and motor fluctuation in Parkinson's disease. Ann Neurol 21: 370–376

Gancher ST, Nutt JG, Woodward WR (1987) Peripheral pharmacokinetics of levodopa in untreated, stable, and fluctuating parkinsonian patients. Neurology 37: 940–944

Gancher ST, Nutt JG, Woodward WR (1992) Time course of tolerance to apomorphine in parkinsonism. Clin Pharmacol Ther 52: 504–510

Gancher ST, Woodward WR, Boucher B, Nutt JG (1989) Peripheral pharmacokinetics of apomorphine in humans. Ann Neurol 26: 232–238

Gee S (1869) On the action of a new organic base, apomorphia. Tr Clin Soc Lond ii: 166–169

Grandas F, Obeso JA (1989) Motor response following repeated apomorphine administration is reduced in Parkinson's disease. Clin Neuropharmacol 12: 14–22

Grandas F, et al (1992) Time interval between repeated injections conditions the duration of motor improvement to apomorphine in Parkinson's disease. Neurology 42: 1287–1290

Kobilka B (1992) Adrenergic receptors as models for G protein-coupled receptors. Annu Rev Neurosci 15: 87–114

Hardie RJ, Lees AJ, Stern GM (1984) On-off fluctuations in Parkinson's disease. A clinical and neuropharmacological study. Brain 107: 487–506

Marsden CD, Parkers JD (1976) "On-off" effects in patients with Parkinson's disease on chronic levodopa therapy. Lancet i: 292–296

Matthiesson A, Wright CRA (1869) III. Researches into the clinical constitution of the opium bases, part I. On the action of hydrochloric acid on morphia. Proc Roy Soc Lond Ser B 17: 455–460

Ng GYK, et al (1994) Desensitization, phosphorylation and palmitoylation of the human dopamine D1 receptor. Eur J Pharmacol 267: 7–19

Ng GYK, et al (1994) Phosphorylation and palmitoylation of the human D2L dopamine receptor in Sf9 cells. J Neurochem 63: 1589–1595

O'Dowd BF (1993) Structures of dopamine receptors. J Neurochem 60: 804–816

Perkins JP, et al (1990) Mechanisms of ligand-induced desensitization of the β-adrenergic receptor. In: Perkins JP (ed) The β-adrenergic receptor. Human Press, New York

Schwab RS, Amador LV, Lettvin JY (1951) Apomorphine in Parkinson's disease. Trans Am Neurol Assoc 76: 251–253

Seeman P, Van Tol HHM (1994) Dopamine receptor pharmacology. TIPS 15: 264–270

Sweet RD, Lee JE, Spiegel HE, McDowell FH (1976) Enhanced response to low doses of levodopa after withdrawal from chronic treatment. Neurology 22: 520–525

Tamminga CA, Schaffer MH, Smith RC, Davis JM (1978) Schizophrenic symptoms improve with apomorphine. Science 200: 567–568

Weiner WJ, Koller WC, Perlik S, Nausieda PA, Klawans HL (1980) Drug holiday and management of Parkinson's disease. Neurology 30: 1257–1261

Yahr MD, Clough CC, Bergman KJ (1982) Cholinergic and dopaminergic mechanism in Parkinson's disease after long-term levodopa administration. Lancet ii: 709–710

Authors' address: Dr. R. Maggio, Institute of Pharmacology, Medical School, University of Pisa, Via Roma 55, I-56100 Pisa, Italy.

J Neural Transm (1995) [Suppl] 45: 137–141

Pharmacokinetics of apomorphine in Parkinson's disease

S. Gancher

Department of Neurology, Oregon Health Sciences University,
Portland, Oregon, U.S.A.

Summary.   The pharmacokinetic properties of apomorphine in patients with Parkinson's disease are described. Apomorphine is lipophilic; it has a large volume of distribution and is rapidly cleared from plasma, with an elimination half life of 33 minutes. It is rapidly absorbed following subcutaneous injection, with peak levels achieved within 5–10 minutes in most patients. There is a large variation in absorption between patients but is more constant within patients following repeated dosing. Apomorphine rapidly equilibrates between plasma and brain. Like levodopa, the response tends to be largely "all or none"; larger doses produce a longer duration of effect within a 30–90 minute range.

Apomorphine may be administered intranasally and sublingually; of these routes, the former is more quickly and completely absorbed. Other routes of administration, including rectally, are not as well absorbed but may also be used effectively.

Introduction

Apomorphine is a potent short acting dopaminergic agonist used in the treatment of Parkinson's disease. It was discovered in 1869 that morphine, when heated, yielded a compound that induced running and stereotypic movements in animals and exhibited potent sedating and emetic properties in humans, as reviewed by Neumeyer et al. (1981). A rearrangement product of morphine, it is a polycyclic molecule which has a dopamine-like moiety as part of the structure. Until the last decade, it was widely used in the emergency treatment of poisoning and is still used to induce emesis in veterinary applications.

Stability

Apomorphine is soluble to over 10 mg/ml in aqucous solution. It auto-oxidizes in solution, forming turquoise-colored reaction products, but may be stabilized by protection from light and oxygen and by the addition of antioxidants. It is supplied either in tablet form intended for parenteral use soon after dissolution or in light-protected vials containing benzoic acid or sodium metabisulfite.

Absorption

Apomorphine is poorly absorbed following oral administration. In early studies, Cotzias et al. (1976) described that effective doses of orally administered apomorphine were in a range of 750–1,500 mg/day, in contrast to typical injected doses of 1–4 mg. This poor oral bioavailability, estimated at 5% (Gancher et al., 1991), is not due to poor absorption but instead reflects a very rapid, nearly complete first-pass hepatic metabolism (Campbell et al., 1980) to form glucuronidated and methylated products (Colpaert et al., 1976).

We have measured the absorption of apomorphine following subcutaneous and intravenous injection (Gancher et al., 1989). Apomorphine is quickly absorbed following subcutaneous injection, with peak levels achieved in 3–5 min in most patients. The speed of absorption varies regionally according to blood flow. Faster peak levels are achieved following subcutaneous injection into the abdominal wall as compared to the upper arm, an area with poorer blood flow. Cooling the site of injection slows the time to peak level and lowers the apparent amount of drug absorbed; this latter observation likely is due to simultaneous hepatic clearance.

There is significant variation in the peak plasma levels between patients, with nearly 5–10 fold differences measured. Absorption within individual patients following repeated dosing is more reproducible, varying 25% or less in most patients.

Apomorphine is rapidly absorbed following subcutaneous infusion, with little regional retention of drug. After discontinuing a subcutaneous infusion, plasma levels begin to fall within 5 min and decay at a rate comparable to intravenous infusion. With chronic use, though, subcutaneous nodules tend to develop in the infusion sites and may present a mechanical barrier toward drug infusion (Stibe et al., 1987; Gancher et al., 1994).

Other routes of administration

Apomorphine may also be administered by intranasal, sublingual, and rectal routes. The intranasal route produces the fastest and most complete absorption. Using a nebulized spray, apomorphine is rapidly absorbed, and has been observed to produce peak plasma levels (Kapoor et al., 1990) and clinical effects comparable to subcutaneous injection (Kleedorfer et al., 1991; van Laar et al., 1992). Nasal stuffiness and crusting, however, may occur and may limit its practical use in some patients.

Apomorphine may also be administered by the sublingual route. It is less well absorbed, though; absorption is slow and bioavailability is less than 20% (Gancher et al., 1991). Consequently, doses of 3–10 times the subcutaneous dose are required (Panegyres et al., 1991; Montastruc et al., 1991; Deffond et al., 1993). Although some of the delay in effect is due to time needed for dissolution of solid tablets, sublingual administration even of a concentrated solution still results in delays of nearly 30–45 minutes in some patients (Panegyres et al., 1991). Like the intranasal route, irritation of the oral mucosa have been noted in some patients (Montastruc et al., 1991); however, other patients (Hughes et al., 1991) have been treated for up to 8 months without severe mucosal irritation.

A third route that has been examined in two acute studies is rectal administration. Although this route is impractical for individual "off" periods, suppository preparations of apomorphine may provide prolonged effect and may be useful in patients with nocturnal impairments that are refractory to other agonists (Hughes et al., 1991).

Pharmacokinetics and distribution

Apomorphine is rapidly cleared from plasma and has a short half-life, approximately 30 minutes. It rapidly equilibrates between plasma and tissue compartments, with a lag of 5 min or less. Although highly lipophilic, apomorphine is not retained in the brain. In a study in which the clearance rates of apomorphine from plasma and different brain regions were measured, there was no evidence for storage or retention of apomorphine in any region; striatum, cerebellum, cortex, and other brain regions all exhibited a clearance rate similar to plasma (Bianchi et al., 1986).

Apomorphine is highly bound to plasma proteins, possibly as high as 95% protein bound. Cisternal CSF levels, which generally reflect drug concentrations in the unbound fraction, are 10% that of plasma in monkeys (Gancher et al., 1990).

The pharmacokinetics of apomorphine do not change in most patients following chronic treatment. Chronic treatment studies utilizing apomorphine have not reported any requirement to increase doses (Obeso et al., 1987; Stibe et al., 1988; Frankel et al., 1990). In fact, selected patients are able to reduce the infusion rate over time, particularly those patients able to discontinue oral dopamine agonists. Interestingly, we have observed individual patients who exhibit higher plasma apomorphine levels and decreased clearance rates achieved after chronic treatment (Gancher et al., 1994). Although the reasons for these changes are not clear, some patients are able to discontinue oral dopamine agonists and it is possible that discontinuation of oral dopamine agonists could reduce hepatic enzyme clearance mechanisms used by both oral agonists and apomorphine.

Pharmacological observations

Like L-DOPA, apomorphine's effects are largely "all or none". Increasing doses of apomorphine produce a longer duration of effect but produce effects of similar magnitude than do small doses (Fig. 1). These properties of

                    S. Gancher

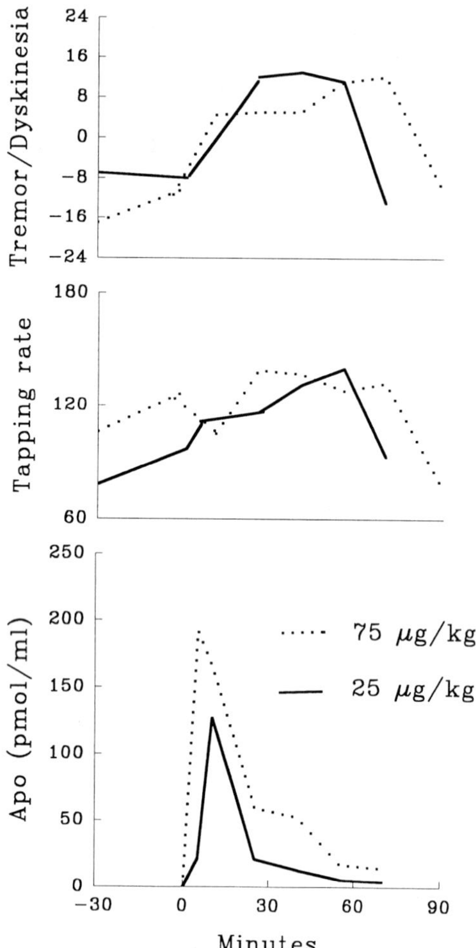

Fig. 1. A patient with Parkinson's disease received two different doses of apomorphine (IV infusion over 10 min on different days). The duration of response was longer with the larger dose but the magnitude of motor response, as measured by changes in a timed tapping task and induction of dyskinesia, was similar

apomorphine have two clinical implications. First, doses used to reverse "off" periods should be chosen to be well above a minimal threshold level; if doses just at threshold level are chosen, dose failures may occur. Second, the effects closely resemble those of L-DOPA; apomorphine may be used as a diagnostic test of L-DOPA responsiveness (Hughes et al., 1990). Therefore, patients in which the qualitative response to L-DOPA is poor are not good candidates for apomorphine treatment; instead, patients in whom the duration of L-DOPA effects are inadequate but who respond well to L-DOPA are more likely to respond will and improve functionally.

References

Bianchi G, Landi M, Garattini S (1986) Disposition of apomorphine in rat brain areas: relationship to stereotypy. Eur J Pharmacol 131: 229–236
Campbell A, Kula NS, Jeppson B, Baldessarini RJ (1980) Oral bioavailability of apomorphine in the rats with a portocaval venous anastomosis. Eur J Pharmacol 67: 139–142

Colpaert FC, Van Bever WFM, Leysen JEM (1976) Apomorphine: chemistry, pharmacology, biochemistry. Int Rev Neurobiol 19: 225–268

Cotzias GC, Papavasilious PS, Tolosa ES, Mendez J, Bell-Midura M (1976) Treatment of Parkinson's disease with aporphines. N Engl J Med 294: 567–572

Deffond D, Durif F, Tournilhac M (1993) Apomorphine in treatment of Parkinson's disease: comparison between subcutaneous and sublingual routes. J Neurol Neurosurg Psychiatry 56: 101–103

Frankel JP, Lees AJ, Kempster PA, Stern GM (1990) Subcutaneous apomorphine in the treatment of Parkinson's disease. J Neurol Neurosurg Psychiatry 53: 96–101

Gancher ST, Woodward WR, Boucher B, Nutt JG (1989) Peripheral pharmacokinetics of apomorphine in humans. Ann Neurol 26: 232–238

Gancher ST, Woodward WR, Gliessman P, Boucher B, Nutt JG (1990) The short-duration response to apomorphine: implications for the mechanism of dopaminergic effects in parkinsonism. Ann Neurol 27: 660–665

Gancher ST, Nutt JG, Woodward WR (1991) Absorption of apomorphine by various routes in parkinsonism. Mov Disord 6: 212–216

Gancher ST, Nutt JG, Woodward WR (1995) Apomorphine infusional therapy in Parkinson's disease: clinical utility and lack of tolerance. Mov Disord 10: 37–43

Hughes AJ, Lees AJ, Stern GM (1990) Apomorphine test to predict dopaminergic responsiveness in parkinsonian syndromes. Lancet 336: 32–34

Hughes AJ, Bishop S, Lees AJ, Stern GM, Webster R, Bovingdon M (1991) Rectal apomorphine in Parkinson's disease. Lancet 337: 118

Hughes AJ, Webster R, Bovington M, Lees AJ, Stern GM (1991) Sublingual apomorphine in the treatment of Parkinson's disease complicated by motor fluctuations. Clin Neuropharmacol 14: 556–561

Kapoor R, Turjanski N, Frankel J, Kleedorfer B, Lees A, Stern GM (1990) Intranasal apomorphine: a new treatment in Parkinson's disease. Lancet 53: 1015

Kleedorfer B, Turjanski N, Ryan R, Lees AJ, Stern GM (1991) Intranasal apomorphine in Parkinson's disease. Neurology 41: 761–762

Montastruc JL, Rascol O, Senard JM, Gualano V, Bagheri H, Houin G, Lees A, Rascol A (1991) Sublingual apomorphine in Parkinson's disease: a clinical and pharmacokinetic study. Clin Neuropharmacol 14: 432–437

Neumeyer JL, Lal S, Baldessarini RJ (1981) Historical highlights of the chemistry, pharmacology, and early clinical uses of apomorphine. In: Gessa GL, Corsini GU (eds) Apomorphine and other dopaminomimetics, vol 1. Basic pharmacology. Raven Press, New York, pp 1–17

Obeso JA, Grandas F, Vaamonde J, Luquin MR, Martinez-Lage JM (1987) Apomorphine infusion for motor fluctuations in Parkinsons disease. Lancet 1: 1376–1377

Panegyres PK, Graham SJ, Williams BK, Higgins BM, Morris JGL (1991) Sublingual apomorphine solution in Parkinson's disease. Med J Aust 155: 371–374

Stibe CM, Kempster PA, Lees AJ, Stern GM (1988) Subcutaneous apomorphine in parkinsonian on-off oscillations. Lancet 1: 403–406

van Laar T, Jansen ENH, Essink AWG, Neef C (1992) Intranasal apomorphine in parkinsonian on-off fluctuations. Arch Neurol 49: 482–484

Author's address: S. Gancher, M.D., Department of Neurology, Oregon Health Sciences University, 3181 SW Sam Jackson Park Road, Portland, Oregon 97201, U.S.A.

J Neural Transm (1995) [Suppl] 45: 143–155

Injection of apomorphine — a test to predict individual different dopaminergic sensitivity?

A. Surmann and **U. Havemann-Reinecke**

Psychiatric Hospital, University of Göttingen, Göttingen,
Federal Republic of Germany

Summary. Male rats, treated with apomorphine (APO; 2 mg/kg s.c.) in an Animex-Motility-Meter, showed individually different motility patterns, each expressed by oral stereotyped behaviour and enhanced locomotor activation reproducible in a second test 4 days later. One group of the rats showed stereotyped sniffing with an increased locomotor activation, S(L,G)-rats, beeing predominantly "mesolimbic active" rats. The other groups could be classified as mainly licking or gnawing rats, L(S,G)-rats or G(L,S)-rats, with less increase of locomotor activation, resembling predominantly "nigrostriatal active" rats. The G(L,S)-rats seemed to be mostly "nigrostriatal active".

In this study the different types of rats were treated with neuroleptic drugs in presence of APO. Haloperidol (HAL; 0.2 and 0.4 mg/kg i.p.) had a clear dose dependent antagonizing effect on APO-induced stereotypies and locomotor activity: a pronounced effect on the L(S,G)- and G(L,S)-rats and less on S(L,G)-rats, In contrast, clozapine (CLO; 10 and 15 mg/kg i.p.) did not antagonize the stereotyped behaviour in the rats tested but showed a characteristic shift in the S(L,G)- and G(L,S)-rats: the predominant stereotypy of these rats, quantified by scoring, changed to licking. In the L(S,G)-rats the predominant licking stereotypy was not changed and the locomotor activity, which was completely antagonized in the S(L,G)- and G(L,S)-rats at both CLO-doses, was affected by 15 mg/kg, only. Furthermore, after the combined treatment with APO and HAL or APO and CLO these rat-types also differed in their amount of ACTH and corticosterone release.

DA-1/DA2 and/or DA-1/DA3 receptor mechanisms may be involved in these individually different motility patterns and endocrine reactions. In summary, pretesting of rats with APO and measuring the motility and endocrine parameters may give us information on a preexisting different sensitivity of individuals to react to DAergic stimulation.

Introduction

Apomorphine(APO)-induced responses frequently have been used in clinical tests to evaluate dopaminergic function or activity in physiological processes or neuropsychiatric disorders (for review see Lal, 1988). The results of these clinical pretests are still in discussion, least of all due to the difficulty to find appropriate measurement parameters. For this reason we decided to do basic studies on the effect of APO in dopaminergic function and neuroendocrinology.

It is well known, that APO injected in rats in postsynaptically active doses (0.5–5.0 mg/kg s.c.) produces stereotyped behaviour and an increase of locomotor activation. These effects are presumed to be mediated by the stimulation of postsynaptically located dopamine (DA) receptors (Ernst, 1967; Anden et al., 1967), especially of DA-2 receptors. The existence of DA-3 receptors recently has been shown by Sokoloff et al. (1990). Furthermore, these authors showed that APO binds to DA-2- and DA-3-receptors with a similar potency. The role of DA-3 receptors for motility changes, however, is still unknown. APO was also found to have some affinity to DA-4 receptors (Seeman and Van Tol, 1993), the role of which is still unclear, too. In addition, several authors point to the role of DA-1 receptors in mediating DA related behaviour (for reviews see Clark and White, 1987; Waddington, 1989). The meaning of the more recently described DA- receptors for the problems of clinically pretesting with APO is not defined, yet.

In previous studies we developed an animal model to evaluate individual different DAergic activity in rats. Male rats, treated with 2 mg/kg of APO, showed individually different motility patterns, each expressed by oral stereotyped behaviour and enhanced locomotor activation and reproducible in a second test 4 days later (Havemann et al., 1986; Havemann, 1988; Havemann-Reinecke, 1992). One group of rats predominantly showed stereotyped sniffing with an increased locomotor activation, called S(L,G)-rats. The other two groups could be classified as mainly licking or gnawing rats, the L(S,G)-rats and G(L,S)-rats, with less increase of locomotor activation.

In this study we treated these groups of rats with the classical neuroleptic haloperidol (HAL) and the atypical neuroleptic clozapine (CLO) in presence of APO in order to find, if the individual different APO-induced DAergic response of these different rat-groups is influenced in a different way after pretreatment with these two anti-DAergic drugs, which are well known to have very different receptor affinities and action profiles (see discussion, for reviews see Tamminga and Gerlach, 1987; Coward, 1992).

Additionally, in another series of experiments we tested if the different DAergic activation of rats is reflected in endocrine parameters, too. On the level of the nucleus periventricularis in the hypothalamus the release of ACTH and subsequently of corticosterone is regulated by CRH. Beside noradrenaline, serotonine and acetylcholine also DA might play a regulating role in CRH-release (for review see Moore, 1987). Therefore, in this study we measured the secretion of the stress hormones ACTH and corticosterone after injection of APO alone or in combination with CLO or HAL.

Materials and methods

Male albino Wistar rats (TNO/W70, F. Winkelmann, Borchen, FRG) weighing 220–240 g were used. All experiments of this study were performed according to the same schedule between 9 a.m. and 4 p.m.: On the first day the rats were tested upon their sensitivity to DAergic stimulation with APO as described by Havemann et al. (1986). Three days later (4th day) the rats were injected with HAL, CLO or saline one hour before the injection of APO. Immediately after the administration of APO the animals were put into the activity meter and the recording of motility was started. The recording periods lasted for 10 min (0–10, 30–40 and 60–70 min after injection of APO). Between the recording intervals the rats were always kept in their home cages.

During all recording periods the rats were carefully observed and categorized according to their predominant pattern of stereotyped behaviour as described below. Additionally, in a series of experiments blood samples were taken to determine the ACTH and corticosterone secretion of the rats.

1. Automatic recording of motility

The automated recording of motility was performed by using an Opto-Varimex-3 Activity Meter (Columbus Instruments, Columbus, Ohio, USA) as described by Havemann et al. (1986). The activity was recorded in an open plexiglas cage ($40 \times 40 \times 20$ cm), the bottom of which was equipped with a sheet of paper covered with chaff and faces. The motility of the rats was discriminated by infrared light beams into one horizontal and two vertical components. Simultaneously, horizontal movements were recorded by using a xy-plotter. The Opto-Varimex-3 Activity Meter was connected via an interface to an Apple-II-Europlus computer registering and storing all data seperately in relation to time.

In addition, a computer program written by O. Kurre and U. Havemann-Reinecke, calculated the counts of the horizontal and both vertical actions and the distance run by the animals. In this study we will focus on two variables, which were defined as follows:

Horizontal activity: The horizontal movements were recorded by sensors 3 cm above the floor and represent the locomotor activity plus non-locomotor activity (head movements, oral stereotypies etc.) of the rats.

Total distance: Distance run by each animal, representing the locomotor part of motility (running activity).

2. Scoring of stereotyped behaviour

The stereotyped behaviour of the rats was scored by observation according to the definition of oral stereotypies by Lewis et al. (1985) and Havemann et al. (1986). A special scoring-system was used to quantify the stereotypy data. The 10 min observation periods were devided into 30 sec intervals. If a certain stereotypy-pattern, e.g. licking, continuously occurred during this interval for at least 10 sec, it was scored. The stereotypy which got the most scores within the 10 min observation period was classified as the predominant behaviour pattern and the animals were classified as S(L,G)-rats (predominant stereotypy: sniffing), L(S,G)-rats (predominant stereotypy: licking) or G(L,S)-rats (predominant stereotypy: gnawing).

3. Blood sampling and hormon analysis

In groups of all rat-types pretested with APO (1st day) blood samples were taken in the second test by a jugular vein catheter implanted under ether-anaesthesia the day before. The blood samples were collected throughout the whole experiment in 10–20 min intervals.

Serum ACTH and Corticosterone were measured by RIA (charcoal-assay) in the laboratory of Prof. W. Wuttke (Dept. Clinical and Experimental Endocrinology, University of Göttingen).

4. Statistics

The quantified recording in the activity meter (horizontal activities and total distance) are presented as mediane values and were compared between the different groups of rats by Mann-Whitney U-tests. The stereotypy-scores counted within the second observation period are presented as median values and are compared between the 1st and the 4th day by Wilcoxon Sign-test.

The time course of corticosterone and ACTH blood levels was used to calculate AUC values. The mean AUC values of the different rat groups, drug-treated and saline treated, were compared by ANOVA followed by Student's t-Test.

5. Drugs

Apomorphine(APO)hydrochloride (kindly donated by Woelm Pharma GmbH, Eschwege, FRG) was dissolved in saline immediately before each experiment. Haloperidol (HAL, kindly donated by Janssen, Beerse, Belgium) was dissolved in 1% lactic acid and adjusted to pH 5 with 1 N-NaOH. Clozapine (CLO, kindly donated by Sandoz, Basel, Switzerland) was dissolved in a few drops 5% lactic acid, filled up with saline and adjusted to pH 5–6 with 1 N-NaOH. APO was injected s.c., HAL and CLO were injected i.p.

Results

1. Individual effect of APO on motility

All rats used were pretested upon their sensitivity to a single dose of APO (2 mg/kg s.c., 1st day) and were discriminated into three groups with significantly different behavioural reactions to DAergic stimulation. About 30% of the rats tested predominantly showed stereotyped sniffing with an increased locomotor activation and were called S(L,G)-rats ("sniffing" rats). The other two groups of rats showed a significantly less increase of locomotor activation in combination with predominantly licking or gnawing stereotypies and were classified as L(S,G)-rats ("licking" rats, 24%) or G(L,S)-rats ("gnawing" rats, 46%).

2. Effects of HAL on APO-induced motility

Three days later (4th day) the "APO-test" was repeated in presence of HAL (0.2 and 0.4 mg/kg i.p.). Pretreatment with HAL had a clear dose dependent effect on APO induced stereotypies *and* locomotor activity. Figure 1 (a,b) shows the horizontal activity of S(L,G)- and L(S,G)-rats after injection of

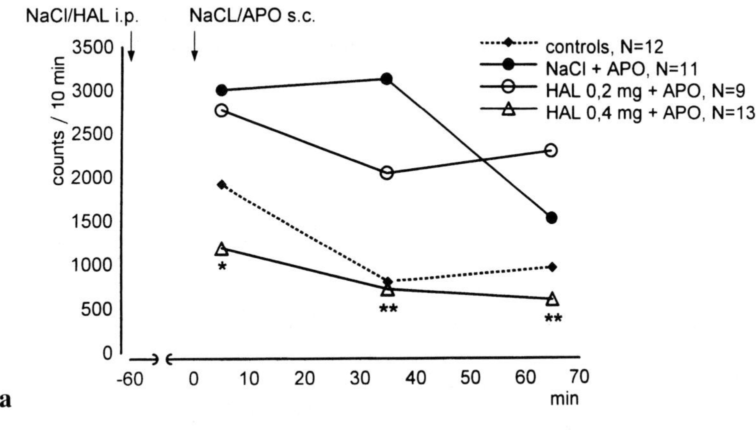

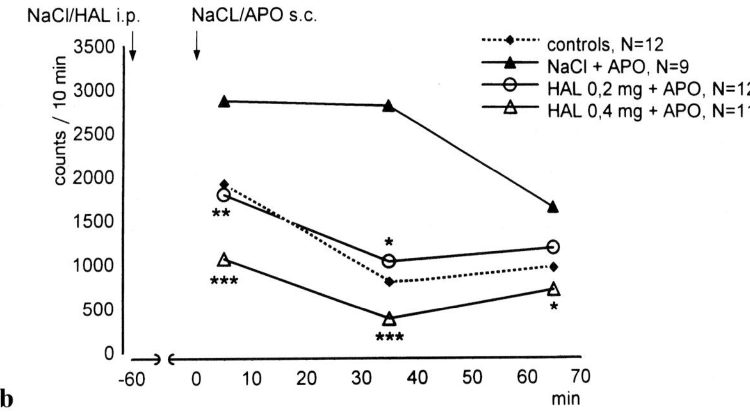

Fig. 1. Horizontal activity of S(L,G)-rats (**a**), L(S,G)-rats (**b**) in the Motility-Meter after injection of APO (2 mg/kg s.c.) with or without HAL (0.2 and 0.4 mg/kg i.p.) and of controls (saline s.c.) Abscissa: time (min) after injection of the drugs. Ordinate: horizontal counts/10 min. *N* number of rats. Median values: *p < 0.05, **p < 0.01, ***p < 0.002. Mann Whitney U-test

saline i.p. and s.c. (controls), saline i.p. and APO (2 mg/kg) s.c. and HAL (0.2 and 0.4 mg/kg) i.p. and APO (2 mg/kg) s.c.. In L(S,G)-rats the APO-induced horizontal activity was completely antagonized by pretreatment with both HAL dosages, whereas in S(L,G)-rats 0.4 mg/kg of HAL had a clear antagonizing effect, only. In this rats 0.2 mg/kg of HAL merely had a small effect on the APO-induced motility pattern. The G(L,S)-rats showed a similar reaction with regard to stereotypies and locomotor activation than the L(S,G)-rats upon the combined treatment with HAL and APO (data not shown).

3. Effects of CLO on APO-induced motility

In these series of experiments APO-pretested rats were injected with saline i.p. and s.c. (controls), saline i.p. and APO (2 mg/kg) s.c. and CLO (5, 10 and

                A. Surmann and U. Havemann-Reinecke

total distance: S(L,G)-rats

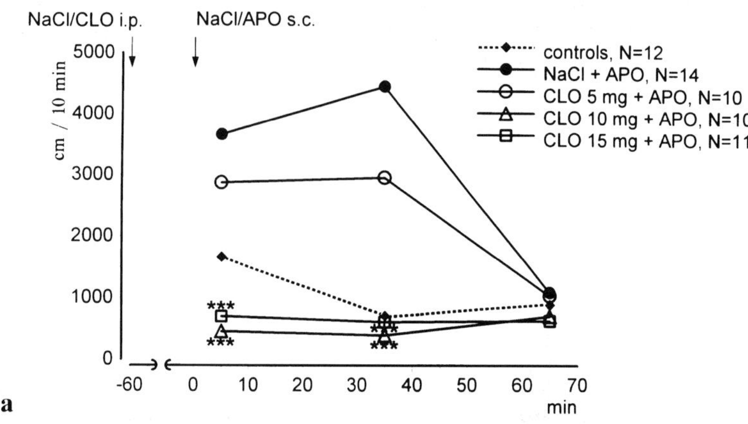

total distance: L(S,G)-rats

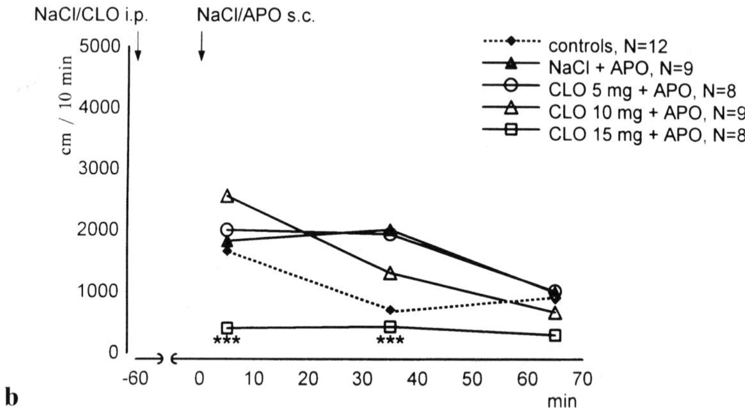

total distance: G(L,S)-rats

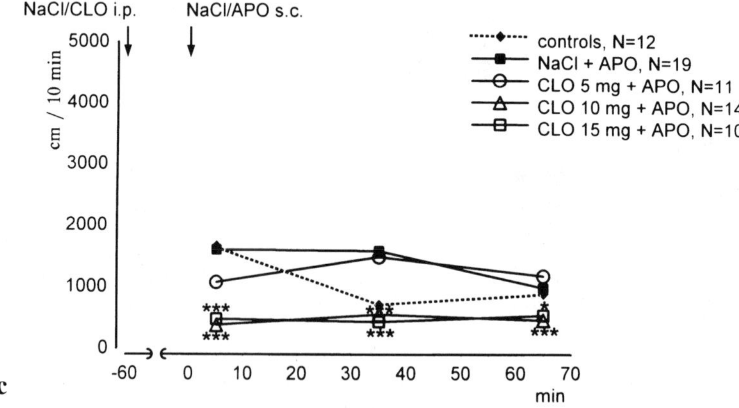

Fig. 2. Total distances run by S(L,G)-rats(**a**), L(S,G)-rats (**b**) and G(L,S)-rats(**c**) in the Motility-Meter after injection of APO (2 mg/kg s.c.) with or without CLO (5, 10 and 15 mg/kg i.p.) and of controls (saline s.c.). Abscissa: time (min) after injection of the drugs. Ordinate: cm/10 min for the distance run by the rats (cm). *N* number of rats. Median values: *p < 0.05, **p < 0.01, ***p < 0.002. Mann Whitney U-test

15 mg/kg) i.p. and APO (2 mg/kg) s.c. on the 4th day. Since CLO did not influence stereotypies and locomotor activity in the same way, the effects on locomotor activation (total distance, Fig. 2) and on stereotyped behaviour (Fig. 3) are presented separately.

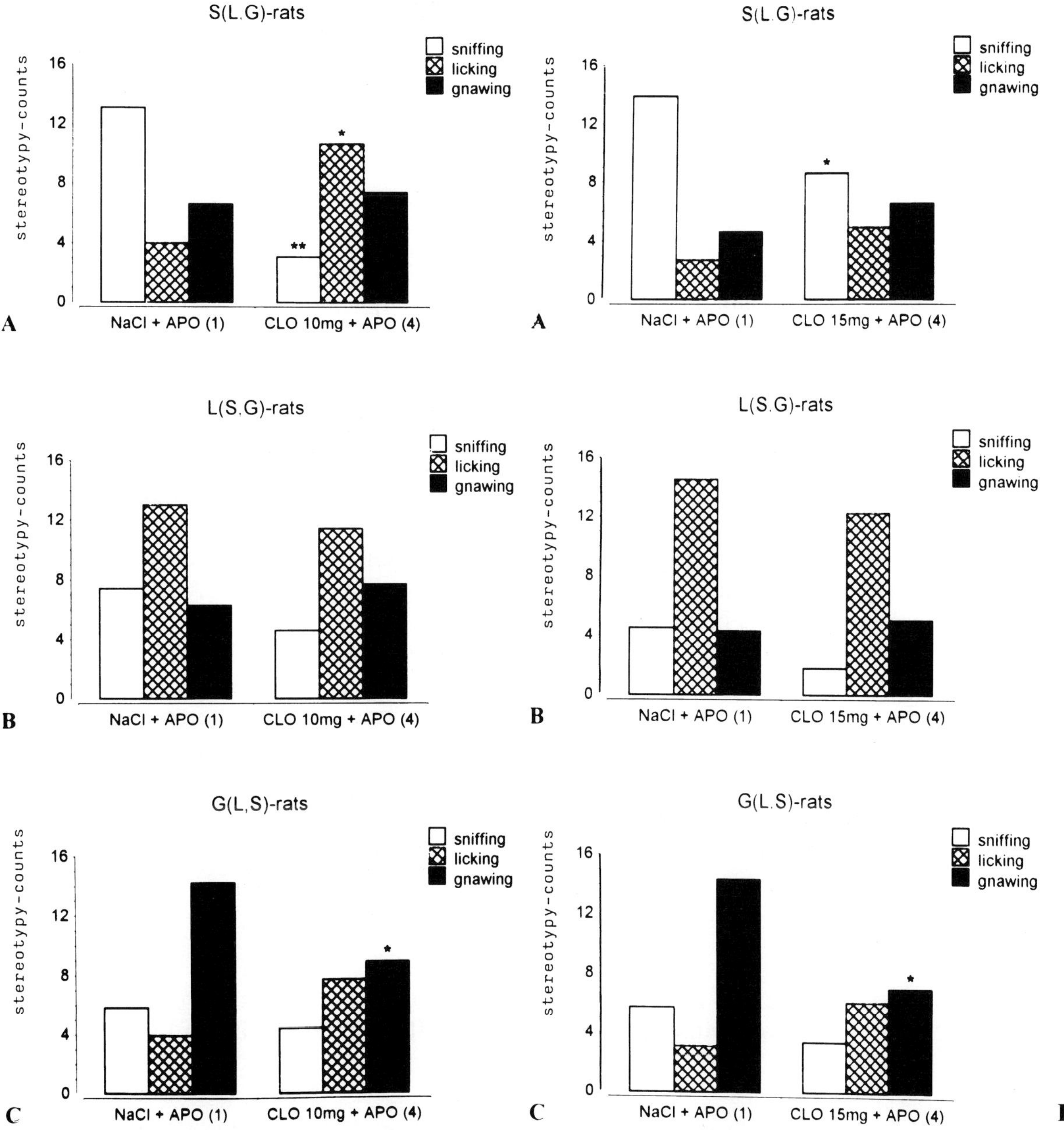

Fig. 3. Stereotypy-scores of S(L,G)-rats (**A**), L(S,G)-rats (**B**) and G(L,S)-rats (**C**) after injection of APO (2 mg/kg s.c.) and saline i.p. on the 1st day and of APO (2 mg/kg s.c.) and CLO (10 mg/kg i.p.) on the 4th day (a) and after injection of APO (2 mg/kg s.c.) and saline i.p. on the 1st day and of APO (2 mg/kg s.c.) and CLO (15 mg/kg i.p.) on the 4th day (b) Median values of scores noted during the second observation period. *p < 0.05, **p < 0.01, Wilcoxon Sign test. Each of the predominant stereotypies (1st day vs. 4th day) were compared

In contrast to HAL CLO did not antagonized the APO-induced stereotyped behaviour in all rats tested. In L(S,G)-rats the predominant licking stereotypy was not affected by administration of CLO, 10 and 15 mg/kg, at all (Fig. 3a+b,B). However, in S(L,G)- and G(L,S)-rats pretreatment with CLO, especially at the dose of 10 mg/kg, sgnificantly changed the predominant sniffing (S(L,G)) or gnawing behaviour (G(L,S)) to licking (Fig. 3a+b,A,C).

In addition, the locomotor activation caused by APO was completely antagonized in S(L,G)- and G(L,S)-rats by pretreatment with 10 and 15 mg/kg of CLO (Fig. 2a+c). However, in L(S,G)-rats only 15 mg/kg of CLO completely blocked the running activity, whereas 10 mg/kg of CLO had no effect at all (Fig. 3b).

4. ACTH and corticosterone secretion after administration of APO with and without neuroleptic pretreatment

After administration of APO (2 mg/kg s.c.) the ACTH and corticosterone secretion was significantly increased in all types of rats compared to controls. The ACTH and corticosterone levels both were influenced in the same way by DAergic stimulation.

Surprisingly, pretreatment with HAL (0.2 mg/kg i.p.) did not antagonize the APO-induced ACTH and corticosterone increase but caused a further elevation, especially in licking rats and much lesser in sniffing and gnawing rats. On the other hand HAL, injected alone, showed no effect on ACTH and corticosterone levels in all types of rats (Fig. 4a+c).

In contrast to HAL the single administration of CLO (10 mg/kg i.p.) caused a clear ACTH and corticosterone increase in S(L,G)-, L(S,G)- and G(L,S)-rats, similar to the effect of APO. In analogy to HAL the combined administration of CLO and APO was followed by a further increase of ACTH and corticosterone, but to a more pronounced degree compared to HAL. However, in licking rats this increase was significantly less marked than in S(L,G)- and G(L,S)-rats (Fig. 4b+d).

Discussion

In this study different APO-induced motility patterns of rats were used to select groups of rats with an interindividual different sensitivity to DAergic

Fig. 4. Serum ACTH (**a+b**) and corticosterone (**c+d**) of S(L,G)-rats, L(S,G)-rats and G(L,S)-rats and of controls. Blood samples were taken over a time course of 140 min, beginning 45 min after i.p.-injection (saline i.p., 10 mg/kg CLO i.p. or 0.2 mg/kg HAL i.p.) and 15 min before s.c.-injection (2 mg/kg APO s.c. or saline s.c.) and ending 125 min after s.c.-injection. Mean values ± SEM of AUCs (area under the curve). N number of rats. *p < 0.5, **p < 0.002, drug-treated rats vs controls. [+]p < 0.5, [++]p < 0.01, S(L,G) and G(L,S)-rats vs L(S,G)-rats. [#]p < 0.5, [##]p < 0.01, rats after NaCl [+] APO (a) and CLO/HAL + saline (c) vs rats after CLO/HAL + APO (b). ANOVA followed by Student's t-test

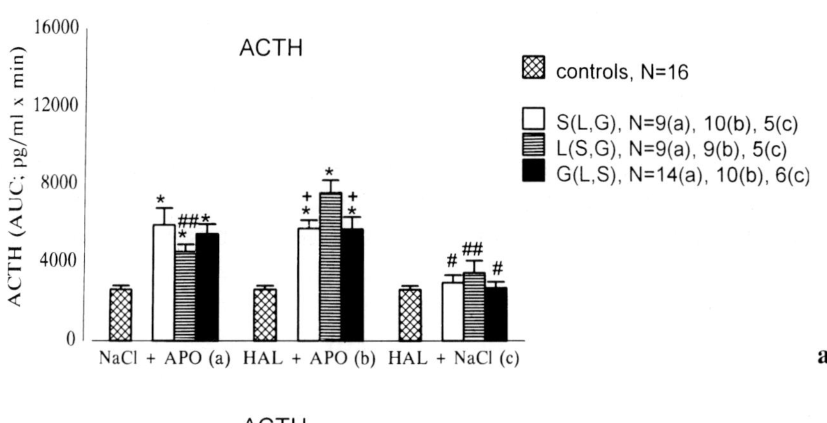

a

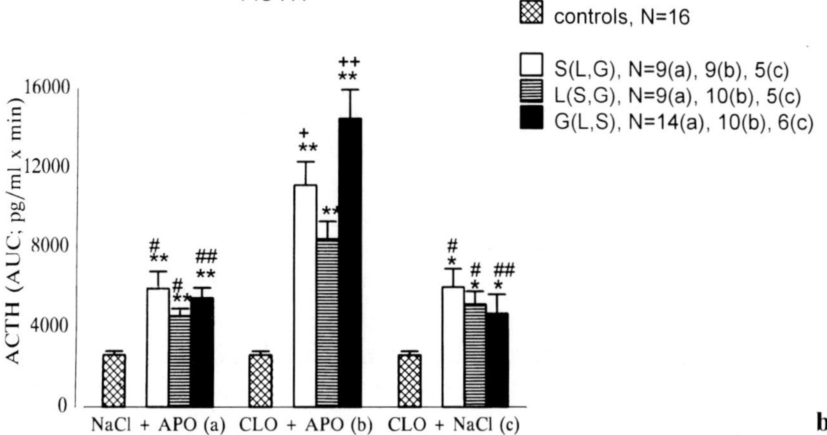

b

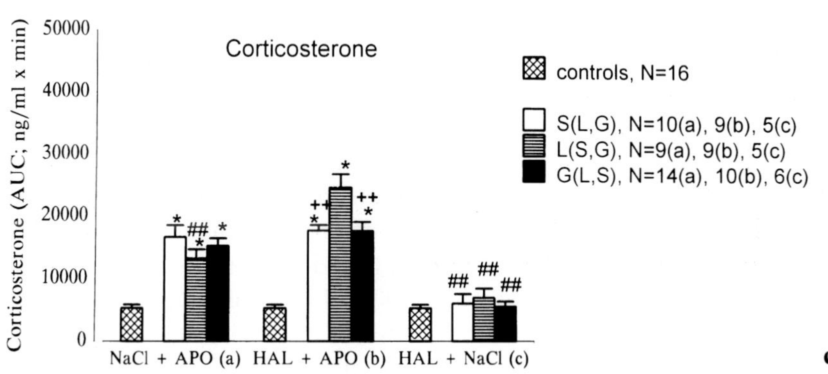

c

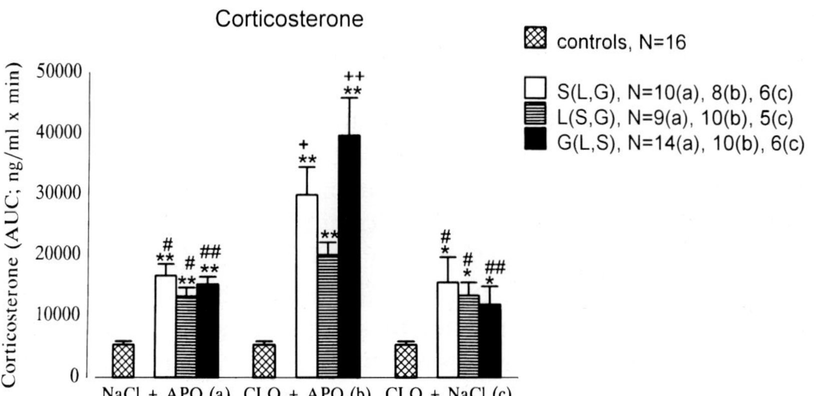

d

stimulation as described by Havemann et al. (1986). The so-called S(L,G)-rats predominantly showed stereotyped sniffing with an increased locomotor activation, whereas in L(S,G)- and G(L,S)-rats licking and gnawing stereotypies predominated, respectively. In addition, the former two groups of rats showed a significantly lesser increase of locomotor activation compared to S(L,G)-rats. According to Ljungberg and Ungerstedt (1977, 1978) and Havemann (1988) APO-induced changes of motility are mediated by topographically different DAergic systems in the brain. An increase of locomotor activity is obviously due to an activation of the mesolimbic DAergic system, whereas oral stereotypies shall be due to an activation of the nigrostriatal DAergic system. Following these results, the S(L,G)-rats seemed to be predominantly "mesolimbic DAergic active" rats, the L(S,G)-rats predominantly "nigrostriatal DAergic rats" and the G(L,S)-rats seemed to be most intensively "nigrostriatal DAergic active". The interindividual different APO-induced motility patterns obviously are mediated by *postsynaptically* located DAergic mechanisms, since the DAergic neuronal activity (DOPAC/DA-quotient) in striatum and nucleus accumbens is not different in these three rat-types after injection of APO (Surmann and Havemann-Reinecke, in preparation).

From literature APO is known to have similar affinity to DA-2 and DA-3 receptors in vitro (Sokoloff et al., 1990). In addition, several authors showed a functional interaction of DA-1 and "DA-2 like"-receptors in mediating DA related behaviour (for reviews see Clark and White, 1987; Waddington, 1989). As described below, our own results point also to a possible role of DA-3 receptors in mediating APO-induced behaviour, so that we suggest that postsynaptically located mechanisms on the level of DA-1/DA-2 receptors and DA-1/DA-3 receptors, respectively, may be responsible for the interindividual different sensitivity of rats to DAergic stimulation and inhibition.

This hypothesis is based on the effects of neuroleptic pretreatment upon the APO-induced motility patterns of the rats. After pretreatment with HAL the motility of L(S,G)- and G(L,S)-rats was antagonized at both HAL-doses used whereas in the S(L,G)-rats the higher dose had an antagonizing effect, only. According to Sokoloff et al. (1990) HAL has a nearly 20 fold higher affinity to DA-2 than to DA-3 receptors in vitro. The same authors reported a predominantly location of DA-3 receptors in mesolimbic brain areas (e.g. nucleus accumbens, tuberculum olfactorium, islands of calleja), whereas DA-2 receptors were found in high concentrations in striatum and to a lesser degree in mesolimbic areas, too. The obviously different affinity of HAL to DA-2 and DA-3 receptors may be a reason for the stronger effect on the predominantly "nigrostriatal active" licking and gnawing rats than on the predominantly "mesolimbic active" sniffing rats.

In comparison to HAL, pretreatment of the rats with CLO led to quite different results. The APO-induced locomotor activity of S(L,G)- and G(L,S)-rats was completely blocked by CLO (10 and 15 mg), whereas in the L(S,G)-rats the locomotor activity was affected by the higher dose, only. The APO-induced stereotyped behaviour was not antagonized in any of the rats tested. These results are in agreement with observations of Ljungberg and

Ungerstedt (1978, 1985), who also found CLO to antagonize APO- or amphetamine-induced locomotion but not APO-induced stereotyped behaviour. However, in S(L,G)- and G(L,S)-rats a remarkably shift in the pattern of stereotypies was seen, especially after pretreatment with 10 mg CLO: the originally predominant sniffing (S(L,G)-rats) and gnawing (G(L,S)-rats) stereotypies changed to licking in both types of rats. In L(S,G)-rats the predominant licking stereotypy did not change.

One reason for the different effects of HAL and CLO on the individual APO-induced motility may be the different receptor affinities of these two drugs. In contrast to HAL, CLO has a weaker affinity to DA receptors and binds to several other receptor subtypes like serotonine(5-HT)-1C, 5-HT-2, α-1 adrenergic, acetylcholinergic and Histamin(H-1) receptors (Tamminga and Gerlach, 1987; Coward, 1992). Van Tol et al. (1991) recently reported CLO to have a high affinity to DA-4 receptors, the role of which for behaviour is still unknown.

A different action profile of CLO and HAL on the three rat-types was also found in *neuroendocrine* parameters. After injection of APO the release of ACTH and corticosterone was stimulated in all rats to nearly the same degree. Differences in the stimulated levels of ACTH and corticosterone produced by APO in the three types of rats were evident after neuroleptic pretreatment, only. Pretreatment with HAL surprisingly led to a further increase of serum ACTH and corticosterone, especially in licking rats. HAL injected alone did not have an increasing effect on serum ACTH and corticosterone. The failure of HAL to block the APO-induced elevation of ACTH and corticosterone may be due to its weak affinity to DA-3 receptors, which were found in much higher concentrations in hypothalamic brain areas than DA-2 receptors (Sokoloff et al., 1990; Bouthenet et al., 1991). Obviously the APO induced increase of ACTH and corticosterone release might be induced especially via DA-3-receptors.

Pretreatment with CLO, however, increased the ACTH and corticosterone levels to a more pronounced degree in all rat-types, but less in licking rats. After the injection of CLO alone a similar increase of ACTH and corticosterone was seen than after the single injection of APO. Therefore the high increase of ACTH and corticosterone after APO combined with CLO may be an additive effect of both drugs. For the effect of CLO other than DAergic mechanisms may be responsible.

HAL and CLO act in a contradictionary way on the ACTH and corticosterone levels in the licking (L(S,G)-rats, but not in the other types of rats. Generally, the L(S,G)-rats seem to have an exceptional position: The APO-induced licking stereotypies and the locomotor activity were antagonized in these rats by low doses of HAL, but not by CLO. In licking rats CLO caused merely a slight further increase of the APO-stimulated ACTH and corticosterone release, in contrast to sniffing and gnawing rats. Additionally, in licking rats but not in sniffing and gnawing rats the injection of HAL in presence of APO caused a further stimulation of serum ACTH and corticosterone. The mechanisms leading to this exceptional position of licking rats are still unclear. *To conclude*, pretesting of rats with APO and measuring the motility and endocrine parameters may give us information on a preexisting different sensitivity of individuals to react to DAergic stimulation. Obviously a genetic predisposition seems to be involved (Cools et al., 1990), but also other factors like early life experiences or early stress factors may be responsible for interindividual different DAergic sensitivities.

Further basic studies are necessary, for example with selective DA-agonists and antagonists or with 5-HT-substances, to improve the "APO-test" for the clinical use. Probably, a combination test (APO + neuroleptic drug) might be useful for the clinical practice.

Acknowledgements

We thank Prof. Dr. W. Wuttke and Dr. H. Jarry, Department of Clinical and Experimental Endocrinology of the University of Göttingen, for helpful advice and support in measuring ACTH and corticosterone.

References

Anden NE, Rubensson A, Fuxe K, Hökfelt T (1967) Evidence of dopamine receptor stimulation by apomophine. J Pharm Pharmacol 19: 627–629

Bouthenet M-L, Souil E, Martres M-P, Sokoloff P, Giros B, Schwartz J-C (1991) Localization of dopamine D_3 receptor mRNA in the rat brain using in situ hybridization histochemistry: comparison with dopamine D_2 receptor mRNA. Brain Res 564: 203–219

Clark D, White FJ (1987) D-1 dopamine receptor — the search for a function: a critical evaluation of the D-1/D-2 dopamine receptor classification and its functional implications. Synapse 1: 347–388

Cools AR, Brachten R, Heerden D, Willemen A, Ellenbroek B (1990) Search after a neurobiological profile of individual-specific features of Wistar-rats. Brain Res Bull 24(1): 49–69

Coward DM (1992) General pharmacology of clozapine. Br J Psychiatry 160(17): 5–11

Ernst AM (1967) Mode of action of apomorphine and dexamphetamine in gnawing compulsions in rats. Psychopharmacology 10: 316–323

Havemann U (1988) Does individually different sensitivity to dopaminergic stimulation determine the degree of tolerance and dependence to opioids? Pharmacopsychiatry 21: 314–316

Havemann U, Magnus B, Möller HG, Kuschinsky K (1986) Individual and morphologic differences in the behavioural response to apomorphine in rats. Psychopharmacology 90: 40–48

Havemann-Reinecke U (1992) Individuelle Prädisposition und Konditionierungsphänomene bei der Entwicklung von Abhängigkeit. In: Gaebel W, Laux G (eds) Biologische Psychiatrie. Synopsis 1990/1991. Springer, Berlin Heidelberg New York Tokyo, pp 22–34

Lal S (1988) Apomorphine in the evaluation of dopaminergic function in man. Prog Neuropychopharmacol Biol Psychiatry 12: 117–164

Lewis MH, Baumeister AA, McCorkle DL, Mailman RB (1985) A computer supported method for analyzing behavioral observations: studies with stereotypy. Psychopharmacology 85: 204–209

Ljungberg T, Ungerstedt U (1977) Different behavioural patterns induced by apomorphine: evidence that the method of administration determines the behavioural response to the drug. Eur J Pharmacol 46: 41–50

Ljungberg T, Ungerstedt U (1978) Classification of neuroleptic drugs according to their ability to inhibit apomorphine induced locomotion and gnawing: evidence for two different mechanisms of action. Psychopharmacology 56: 239–247

Moore KE (1987) Hypothalamic dopaminergic neuronal systems. In: Meltzer HY (ed) Psychopharmacology: the third generation of progress. Raven Press, New York, pp 127–139

Seeman P, Van Tol HHM (1993) Dopamine D_4 receptors bind inactive (+)aporphines, suggesting neuroleptic role. Sulpiride not stereoselective. Eur J Pharmacol 233(1): 173–174

Sokoloff P, Giros B, Martres M-P, Bouth M-L, Schwartz J-C (1990) Molecular cloning and characterization of a novel dopamine receptor (D_3) as a target for neuroleptics. Nature 347: 146–151

Tamminga CA, Gerlach J (1987) New neuroleptics and experimental antipsychotics in schizophrenia. In: Meltzer HY (ed) Psychopharmacology: the third generation of progress. Raven Press, New York, pp 1129–1140

Van Tol HHM, Bunzow JR, Guan H-C, Sunahara RK, Seeman P, Niznik HB, Civelli O (1991) Cloning of the gene for a human dopamine D_4 receptor with high affinity for the antipsychotic clozapine. Nature 350: 610–614

Waddington JL (1989) Functional interactions between D-1 and D-2 dopamine receptor systems: their role in the regulation of psychomotor behaviour, putative mechanisms, and clinical relevance. J Pharmacol 3(2): 54–63

Authors' address: Dr. U. Havemann-Reinecke, Psychiatric Hospital, University of Göttingen, von-Siebold-Strasse 5, D-37075 Göttingen, Federal Republic of Germany.

J Neural Transm (1995) [Suppl] 45: 157–161
© Springer-Verlag 1995

Sublingual apomorphine: a new pharmacological approach in Parkinson's disease?

J. L. Montastruc[1], O. Rascol[1], J. M. Senard[1], G. Houin[2], and A. Rascol[3]

[1] Laboratoire de Pharmacologie Médicale et Clinique, INSERM U317, Faculté de Médecine, Toulouse, and [2] Unité de Pharmacocinétique, and [3] Service de Neurologie, Centre Hospitalier Universitaire, Hôpital Purpan, Toulouse, France

Summary. Apomorphine, a potent dopamine agonist with mixed D1 and D2 properties, has long been recognized to have antiparkinsonian effect. Its oral administration is limited by both its hepatic first pass metabolism and adverse side effects (nausea, vomiting, azotemia). It is now widely used by subcutaneous route for the treatment of severe "off" periods seen with levodopa treatment. However, the use of penjects can be difficult in some patients with severe tremor or akineto-rigid symptoms during "off" periods. Our group has recently investigated the effect of sublingual administration of apomorphine in patients suffering from Parkinson's disease. Sublingual apomorphine was shown to reduce extrapyramidal symptoms. The main characteristics of the pharmacodynamic effects of sublingual apomorphine in parkinsonians and the relationship between pharmacodynamic and pharmacokinetic effects are discussed. Sublingual apomorphine has the advantage of being easier to administer than subcutaneous injection. For the moment, the long-term use of sublingual apomorphine is limited by two major problems: first, time for dissolution and switch "on" (which is longer than after subcutanous route) and secondly, the occurrence of local side effects (stomatitis). Further clinical studies using either more efficient (tablets with faster dissolution) and better tolerated sublingual formulations or other dopamine agonists should be carried on before recommending this approach in the treatment of Parkinson's disease.

Introduction

Apomorphine, a potent dopamine agonist with mixed D1 and D2 properties has long been recognized to have antiparkinsonian effects (Cotzias et al., 1976; Lal, 1988; Lees, 1993). Its long-term oral administration is limited by both its hepatic first pass metabolism and adverse side effects (nausea, vomiting, azotemia) (Cotzias et al., 1976; Lees, 1993). In contrast, it is now widely demonstrated that subcutaneous (SC) injection of apomorphine, associated with oral domperidone, is a safe treatment for severe "off" periods seen with levodopa treatment (Frankel et al., 1990; Lees, 1993; Stibe et al., 1988). Recent studies from our group (Lees et al., 1989) have also indicated that apomorphine can be effectively absorbed by the sublingual (SL) route and that acute sublingual administration is able to reduce extrapyramidal symptoms.

The aim of the present study was to compare pharmacokinetic parameters of sublingual and subcutaneous apomorphine in order to be able to select appropriate doses of SL apomorphine in future studies. Preliminary results of a long-term pilot study of SL apomorphine in the treatment of severe "off" periods will be also presented.

Materials and methods

1. Pharmacokinetic study

Six patients with idiopathic Parkinson's disease and severe refractory motor fluctuations were included in this study after giving their informed consent. The protocol was approved by the local ethical committee. Patients' mean age was 69 (56–78) years, mean duration of the disease 8 years (1–15 years), mean duration of levodopa therapy 6 years (1 to 10 years), mean daily dose: 720 mg, stage 2 to 4 on Hoehn and Yahr scale. All the patients were known to respond to SC apomorphine. After 48 hours of oral domperidone pretreatment (60 to 90 mg daily), the first 3 patients received, when fasting, 30 mg (i.e. 10 tablets containing 32 mg each) SL apomorphine (Lab. Chabre, France) on day 1, and 3 mg SC apomorphine (Lab. Aguettant, France) on day 2. The 3 other patients were treated with the inverse sequence (day 1: SC, day 2: SL). Antiparkinsonian drugs were stopped 12 hours before each study. Baseline assessment using a modified Webster scale and tapping test (Kempster et al., 1989) were carried out and repeated every 10 min. Plasma samples were performed at time 5 min every 10 min and levels of apomorphine measured using HPLC with electrochemical detection (Bianchi and Landi, 1985; Nicolle et al., 1993).

2. Pilot study

Eight patients with idiopathic Parkinson's disease were treated with SL apomorphine. They were all suffering from disabling "on-off" fluctuations in motor performance despite many changes and adaptations in levodopa and/or dopamine agonists. Their mean age was 66 years (51–71 years) and the mean duration of the disease 11 years (6–16 years). They received levodopa for 10 years (4–16 years). Their mean stage of Hoehn and Yahr when "off" was 3.4 (2–4). All patients were admitted to hospital for pretreatment assessment (using a daily chart) and education in the use of SL apomorphine. After 4 to 5 days without change in baseline treatment, SL apomorphine was introduced. All the patients received oral domperidone (20–30 mg t.i.d.) to avoid peripheral side effects of SL apomorphine.

3. Statistical analysis

Results are presented as mean values ± SEM and statistical analysis was made using the Wilcoxon signed rank test.

Results

1. Pharmacokinetic study

The magnitude of the motor responses (evaluated by tapping and walking tests and maximal changes in Webster scale) to 30 mg SL and 3 mg SC apomorphine was similar. However, latent periods were longer than after SC apomorphine, since most of the patients switched "on" 30 min after SL vs 10–20 min after SC administration. Side effects were sedation (3 patients with SC and 2 patients with SL apomorphine), 1 yawning (with SL apomorphine) and 1 nausea (with SC apomorphine). The pharmacokinetic analysis indicated that 3 mg SC and 30 mg SL apomorphine were bioequivalent: no significant difference was observed between AUC ($1{,}000 \pm 174\,\text{ng·ml}^{-1}\text{·min}$) and Cmax ($30.1 \pm 5.7\,\text{ng/ml}$ vs $32.4 \pm 10.8\,\text{ng/ml}$) values. However, Tmax was shorter after SC ($23 \pm 6\,\text{min}$ vs $43 \pm 6\,\text{min}$, $p < 0.05$).

2. Pilot study

Patients remained on similar doses of levodopa (866 mg/day) combined with same doses of bromocriptine (59 mg/day). The first patient was treated with relatively low doses of SL apomorphine (6 mg × 5/day). This dose had little or not effect. The 7 other patients received higher doses. Patients were instructed to use SL apomorphine in the same way that has been proposed for SC route (3–6), i.e. as soon "off" periods appeared. One patient used 9 mg t.i.d., another 30 mg t.i.d., another 24 mg t.i.d., the 4 others 30 mg t.i.d. respectively. The last patient suffered from two major "off" periods per day. Diary records showed a mean reduction in "off" hours from 5.0 to 2.2 hours ($p < 0.05$) after a mean 4 month (1 to 6 months) follow-up. The mean time for switch "on" after SL apomorphine was 20 to 40 min according to the patients. The duration of effect was about 60 to 90 min. No tolerance was observed except in one patient in whom 30 mg SL apomorphine progressively lost its efficacy after 5 months. Adverse reactions were stomatitis with ulcerations of buccal mucosae in 4 patients. This side effect (associated with loss of taste) appeared after 2 to 6 months of treatment and disappeared after stopping SL apomorphine (after 1 month of withdrawal) and the local side effect reappeared leading to permanent stoppage of the drug. No change in routine laboratory investigations was observed.

Discussion

This study allows three conclusions to be made:

1. SL administration of apomorphine is able to reduce extrapyramidal symptoms. This conclusion agrees with the findings of several other groups (Deffond et al., 1993; Durif et al., 1993; Hughes et al., 1991).

2. 30 mg SL apomorphine are equivalent to 3 mg SC apomorphine in terms of both pharmacodynamics (magnitude and duration of action) and pharmacokinetics (AUC, Cmax) parameters. However, Tmax values were shorter after SC administration. This observation is in agreement with the relatively long latent period to switch "on" observed after SL apomorphine. These clinical and pharmacokinetic differences can probably be explained by the time necessary for dissolution. Durif's group has recently compared the clinical efficacy and pharmacokinetic parameters of two dosages (0.3 and 0.6 mg/kg) of SL apomorphine. These authors found that Cmax values and bioavailability of 0.6 mg/kg were higher than those of 0.3 mg/kg. They also found a clear relationship between improvement of motor score and apomorphine plasma levels (Durif et al., 1993).

3. These preliminary results could suggest that SL apomorphine might be of value in some levodopa-treated patients suffering from severe "off" periods. It has the advantage of being easier to administer than SC injection. However, for the moment, its long-term use is limited by two major problems: first, time for dissolution and switch "on" and secondly, the occurrence of local side effects (stomatitis). This side effect was also described by others (Deffond et al., 1993). Hughes et al. (1991) found that 3 of their 10 patients complained of an unpleasant taste. Further clinical studies using more efficient (tablets with faster dissolution) and better tolerated sublingual formulations of apomorphine or other dopamine agonists should be carried on before recommending this approach in the treatment of Parkinson's disease.

References

Bianchi G, Landi M (1985) Determination of apomorphine in rat plasma and brain by high-performance liquid chromatography with electrochemical detection. J Chromatogr 338: 230–235

Cotzias GC, Papavasiliou PS, Tolosa ES, Mendez JS, Bell-Midura MD (1976) Treatment of Parkinson's disease with apomorphines. N Engl J Med 294: 567–572

Deffond D, Durif F, Tournilhac M (1993) Apomorphine in treatment of Parkinson's disease: comparison between subcutaneous and sublingual routes. J Neurol Neurosurg Psychiatry 56: 101–103

Durif F, Paine M, Deffond D, Eschalier A, Dordain G, Tournilhac M, Lavarenne J (1993) Relation between clinical efficacy and pharmacokinetic parameters after sublingual apomorphine in Parkinson's disease. Clin Neuropharmacol 16: 157–166

Frankel JP, Lees AJ, Kempster PA, Lees AJ (1990) Subcutaneous apomorphine in the treatment of Parkinson's disease. J Neurol Neurosurg Psychiatry 53: 96–101

Gancher ST, Nutt JG, Woodward WR (1991) Absorption of apomorphine by various routes in Parkinsonism. Mov Disord 6: 212–216

Hughes AJ, Webster R, Bovingdon M, Lees AJ, Stern GM (1991) Sublingual apomorphine in the treatment of Parkinson's disease complicated by motor fluctuations. Clin Neuropharmacol 14: 556–561

Kempster PA, Frankel JP, Bovingdon M, Webster R, Lees AJ, Stern G (1989) Levodopa peripheral pharmacokinetics and duration of motor response in Parkinson's disease. J Neurol Neurosurg Psychiatry 52: 718–723

Lal S (1988) Apomorphine in the evaluation of dopaminergic function in man. Prog Neuropsychopharmacol 12: 117–164

Lees AJ (1993) Dopamine agonists in Parkinson's disease: a look at apomorphine. Fundam Clin Pharmacol 7: 121–128

Lees AJ, Montastruc JL, Turjanski N, Rascol O, Kleedorfer B, Peyro Saint-Paul H, Stern GM, Rascol A (1989) Sublingual apomorphine and Parkinson's disease. J Neurol Neurosurg Psychiatry 52: 1440

Nicolle E, Pollak P, Serre-Debeauvais F, Richard P, Gervason CL, Broussolle E, Gavend E (1993) Pharmacokinetics of apomorphine in Parkinsonian patients. Fundam Clin Pharmacol 7: 245–252

Poewe W, Kleedorfer B, Gerstenbrand F, Oertel W (1988) Subcutaneous apomorphine in Parkinson's disease. Lancet i: 943

Pollak P, Champay AS, Hommel M, Perret JE, Benabid AL (1989) Subcutaneous apomorphine in Parkinson's disease. J Neurol Neurosurg Psychiatry 52: 544

Stibe CMH, Lees AJ, Kempster PA, Stern PA (1988) Subcutaneous apomorphine in parkinsonian on-off fluctuations. Lancet i: 403–406

Authors' address: Prof. J.-L. Montastruc, Laboratoire de Pharmacologie Médicale et Clinique INSERM U317, Faculté de Médecine, 37 allées Jules-Guesde, F-31073 Toulouse Cedex, France.

J Neural Transm (1995) [Suppl] 45: 163–170

Apomorphine SC treatment in parkinsonian patients with long term L-DOPA syndrome during L-DOPA drug holiday

L. Scarzella, M. Delsedime, B. Ferrero, C. Giangrandi, L. Priano, M. Rizzone, and **B. Bergamasco**

Department of Neurology, University of Turin, Italy

Summary. The Long Term Dopa Syndrome (LTDS) is one of the main problems in the management of advanced parkinsonian patients. A transient L-Dopa withdrawal (Drug Holiday, DH) can be useful to improve the drug response after DH, even if this approach presents risks due to patient akinesia. We tried to verify if Apomorphine sc administration during DH (DH with Apomorphine, DHA) can: a) reduce the risks connected with DH; b) maintain the benefits of DH; c) standardize the duration of DH.

Twenty-five parkinsonian patients with LTDS were treated with Apomorphine sc during DH (14 days). No patient had any severe side effects. The follow-up at 180 days, conducted using the Unified Parkinson's Disease Rating Scale, demonstrated a significant improvement in the clinical conditions of about 70% of the patients, allowing a 27.1% reduction in daily L-dopa dosage.

DHA can represent a valid therapeutical approach for parkinsonian patients with LTDS.

Introduction

The onset of motor, autonomic and psychiatric symptoms, representing the so-called "Long-Term Dopa Syndrome" (LTDS), is one of the main problems in the treatment of Parkinson's disease, occurring in a high percentage of patients after some years of L-Dopa therapy (Poewe et al., 1986; Poewe, 1993; Schelosky and Poewe, 1993; Yahr, 1993).

One of the therapeutical approaches in the treatment of parkinsonian patients with LTDS consists of the temporary withdrawal of L-Dopa (Drug Holiday, DH) (Koller et al., 1981; Bermejo et al., 1986; Kaye and Feldman, 1986).

Even though it is still unknown how DH can increase motor responsiveness to L-Dopa, allowing a reduction of its dosage, in a high percentage of patients with LTDS, the rationale of this treatment consists in a temporary restoration of the dopaminergic receptors, followed by a more modulated response to L-Dopa (Sweet et al., 1972; Kaye and Feldman, 1986).

According to the literature in favour of DH, the clinical benefits have a 6–12 month duration (Direnfeld et al., 1980; Koeller et al., 1981; Corona et al., 1991).

The limitations of this treatment are characterized by the severe akinesia that constantly affects parkinsonian patients, greatly compromising the quality of their life and increasing the risk of serious complications such as deep venous thrombosis, bedsores, pulmonary embolisms, malignant hyperthermia (Kaye and Feldman, 1986). For these reasons DH should be reserved for the most severely affected patients, who not do respond to other treatments (modification and fractioning of L-Dopa dosage, reduction of the proteinic dietary content, association with other antiparkinsonian drugs). A standard DH duration has not yet been established, due to the risks described above and poor patient compliance, making the acquisition of homogeneous results impossible.

On the basis of the results obtained from the literature concerning the effects of Apomorphine sc in the off phases of parkinsonian patients (Gancher and Nutt, 1987; Stibe et al., 1988; Steiger et al., 1992), we experimented with this dopamine-agonist during the DH in an attempt to reduce the risks connected with DH, maintaining its benefits and allowing a standardization of its duration.

Subcutaneous Apomorphine, a potent directly acting D1 and D2 receptor agonist, induces a brief, rapid reversal of the off phases motor deficit of parkinsonian patients (Corsini et al., 1979). This dopamine agonist, the side effects (nausea, vomiting, postural hypotension) of which can be controlled by oral administration of a peripheral dopamine antagonist, domperidone, is commonly used today both in the treatment of parkinsonian on-off fluctuations (Frankel et al., 1990; Hughes et al., 1993) and in order to confirm a doubtful diagnosis of idiopathic Parkinson's disease (D'Costa et al., 1991; Gasser et al., 1992; Bonuccelli et al., 1993).

We treated patients with subcutaneous Apomorphine infusion (4.2 hours/day) during DH, calling this approach Drug Holiday with Apomorphine (DHA).

Materials and methods

Twenty-nine parkinsonian patients were tested with Apomorphine sc in order to detect their responsiveness to this drug.

After administering Domperidone (20 mg per so three times a day for five days), and after a 12 hour interruption of L-dopa administration, all the patients, during the critical period of akinesia (off condition), underwent a test consisting of progressively increasing subcutaneous doses of Apomorphine (1.5 mg, 3 mg, 4.5 mg, 30 minutes between each dose), until motor performance improved (positive response) or until side effects forced the test to be stopped. If no response was seen, the test was considered negative.

Twenty-five patients out of 29 showed a positive clinical response to Apomorphine sc, consisting of the recovery of a good motility and autonomy within 5–15 minutes after the administration of this drug; the effect lasted 40–60 minutes on average.

These patients who had a positive response to the test were therefore submitted to the DH with Apomorphine (DHA) (Table 1). All the patients gave their informed consent.

Table 1. Clinical features of 25 parkinsonian patients with LTDS admitted to the study

Patients n°	25	16M–9F
Age, mean	59.7	(42–73)
Disease duration, mean	13.9 y	(4–27)
L-Dopa treatment duration, mean	12.3 y	(3–23)
L-Dopa dose/24 h, mean	601.7 mg	(200–1,100)
HY score, mean	3.4	(2.5–5)
LTDS duration, mean	5.4 y	(1–13)
LTDS principal symptoms	Wearing-Off	22/25
	On-Off	14/25
	Dyskinesias	25/25

The initial daily dose of L-Dopa + DCI was gradually reduced over 5–7 days, up to the total suspension; a gradual reduction and then suspension was also done with any other antiparkinsonian drug. At the same time Domperidone 20 mg three times a day was administered to all the patients.

A daily dose of 25 mg of Apomorphine was subcutaneously administered by means of a microinfusor (Microjet Quark U 40) for the whole period of the DHA, at an infusion speed of 0.10 mg/min. The duration of infusion was 4.2 hours daily. The duration of DHA was 14 days for all the patients. The clinical evaluations, before and during DHA, was performed by the same examiner, at the same hour of the day. The Unified Parkinson's disease Rating Scale was used. The follow-up of patients was planned 30, 90, 180 and 360 days after the end of DH.

Ematochemical and kidney functionality parameters, EKG, and arterial pressure were monitored during the DHA.

Anticoagulant therapy was administered to each patient as prophylaptic purpose.

At the end of the DH the L-dopa therapy was reintroduced gradually until the maximum clinical benefit was obtained.

Results

All the patients treated demonstrated a good clinical response to Apomorphine sc for the whole period of the DHA. During the infusion the patients passed from a complete rigidity phase to a period of good motor performance, being able to perform the normal daily activities of social life.

None of the patients developed tolerance to Apomorphine.

The motor autonomy obtained was about 5 hours a day, allowing all the 25 patients to protract the DHA for 14 days, as planned, without any drop-out.

During such time the quality of life was acceptable for all the patients and none of the side effects associated with the DH described in the literature affected any patients.

The side effects linked to the infusion of Apomorphine sc described in Table 2 resulted readily reversable, and no patients dropped out because of these side effects.

Contrary to instances reported in the literature, no hallucination phenomena occurred. It is to be noticed that 17 of the 25 patients did not present dyskinesias during the infusion of Apomorphine; dyskinesias were instead present before the DHA as a symptom of LTDS.

                          L. Scarzella et al.

Table 2. Side effects associated with the infusion of apomorphine during DH in 25 parkinsonian patients

Patient	Sleepiness	Nausea	Vomiting	Dyskinesias	Renal disturbances
1		*	*	*	*
2	*	*		**	*
3	*				
4	*				*
5	*	*		*	
6		*	*		
7	*			*	*
8	*				*
9	*				*
10	*	*			
11					*
12	*			**	
13		*	*	*	*
14	*	*	*		*
15	*	*			*
16	*				*
17	*				
18		*	*	*	
19					*
20	*				*
21	*	*			
22	*				*
23					*
24	*	*		*	
25	*	*	*		

* = mild; ** = moderate

Seventeen patients out of 25 showed a significant clinical improvement at the end of DHA after restoring L-Dopa therapy (percentage of improvement = 24.1% using the UPDRS, compared to the period pre-DHA, Table 3).

The analysis of the data obtained from this group of 17 patients demonstrated that the improvement of motor conditions reported at 30, 60, 120, 180 days was steady (percentage of improvement = 22% using the UPDRS, at 180 days, compared to the pre-DHA period).

It was furthermore possible to decrease the average dosage of L-Dopa from 660.7 mg/die (pre-DHA) to 482.1 mg/die (in the controls at 180 days), corresponding to a reduction of 27.1% (Table 4).

Due to the lack of data in literature regarding samples of patients with a homogeneous DH duration (14 days), it is not possible to draw a precise comparison between these results and the long term benefits obtained with the traditional DH in previous studies.

From these non-homogeneous studies (Direnfeld et al., 1980; Koeller et al., 1981; Corona et al., 1991), however, the long term benefit seems to be comparable to what we observed in our study.

Table 3

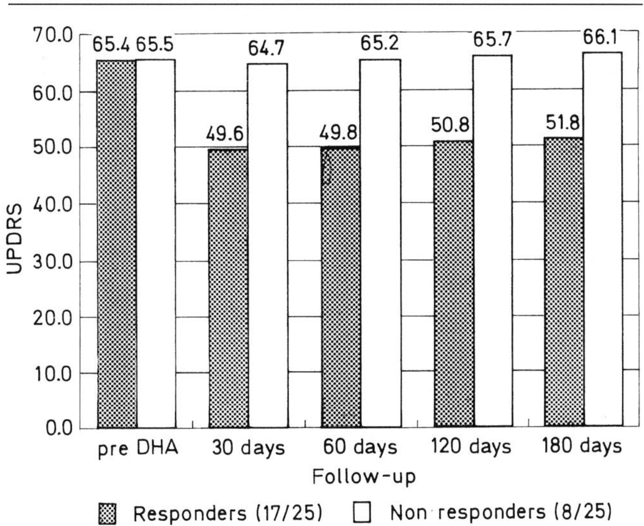

Table 4

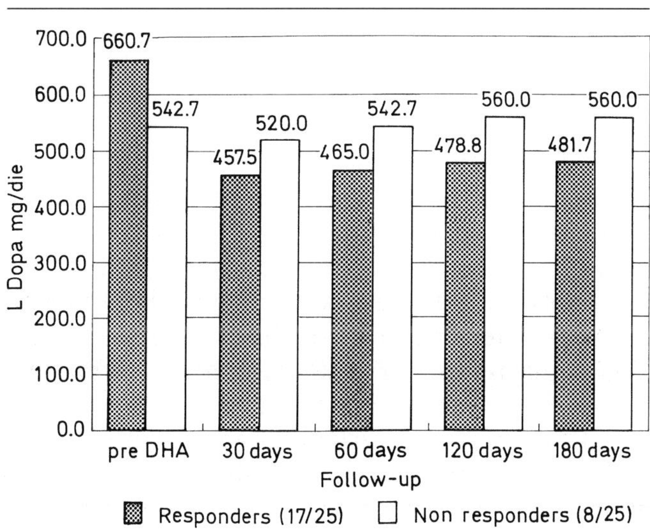

Discussion

In selected parkinsonian patients with LTDS, who are severely affected and
not responsive to any kind of drug adjustment, one of the therapeutical
approaches is represented by the DH, a procedure not to be taken lightly
because of the dramatic worsening of the patients' motor capabilities and
because of its potential complications. It is also for these reasons that the

effectiveness of DH is discussed in literature. Direnfeld and co-workers (1980) underline the importance of the side effects linked to DH, even though they admit its effectiveness in improving the clinical response to L-Dopa.

A further confirmation of the efficacy of DH (as weekly 2- day L-Dopa abstinence periods) comes from Goetz and co-workers (1981). On the other hand Majeux and co-workers (1985), on the basis of the data from a study on 28 patients, do not notice any short or long term improvement with DH, highlighting further the possible complications. Feldman and co-workers (1986) confirm the validity of such treatment, and report an improvement detectable up to 24 months from the end of DH, similarly to what we found in our previous studies (Riccio et al., 1989). Martinez and co-workers (1992) also report on the effectiveness of DH, however underlining the lack of correlation between length of L-Dopa withdrawal and clinical improvement.

Moreover, controversies on the effect of L-Dopa withdrawal also arise from the incertain role of L-Dopa regarding the pathogenesis of LTDS (Chase et al., 1993). Even though peripheral pharmacokinetic factors are included in the pathophysiology of LTDS (Kempster et al., 1989), central mechanisms are probably of greater relevance.

It has been suggested that the improved function of patients after DH could be a result of preventing the ongoing desensitization of the postsynaptic DA receptors caused by chronic L-Dopa administration. Temporary withdrawal of L-Dopa results in reversal of the "downregulated" state (Direnfeld et al., 1978). In a model proposed, the site of abnormal receptor change is presynaptic, so the long-term L-Dopa administration could result in downregulating the DA system by chronic feedback inhibition (presynaptic subsensitization) (Muller and Seemon, 1979).

Another possible mechanism could be connected to the state of postsynaptic receptor supersensitivity that may develop when the postsynaptic site is chronically understimulated by DA. The response would be an increase of postsynaptic receptor densities. Such a mechanism is supposed to play a role in dyskinesias appearing during LTDS (Lee et al., 1978).

These hypotheses concerning the functionality of dopaminergic receptors can probably coexist and, interfering with the evolution of the disease, explain the inconstant and variable response to dopaminergic stimulation.

The results of our study could indicate that a continuous, but limited in time, dopaminergic stimulus does not alter the process of rebalancing of receptor functionality obtained after L-Dopa withdrawal. This hypothesis could be confirmed by the studies on the effects of continuous infusional administration of L-Dopa which is able to rebalance the receptor functionality of PD patients with LTDS (Mouradian et al., 1990).

The administration of Apomorphine sc allowed a standardized duration of the DH (14 days for all cases), with the possibility to compare homogeneous groups of patients.

The absence of severe side effects and the clinical benefits in a good percentage of patients, still present 6 months after the end of DHA, support the hypothesis of a real therapeutic usefulness of the DHA.

In conclusion the results of our study suggest the utilization of Apomorphine sc via continuous infusion during the DH as an effective strategy of intervention in Parkinson's disease with LTDS.

References

Bermejo FP, Calandre LH, Molina JA, Martinez P, De Yebenes JG (1986) Long-lasting drug holiday in Parkinson's disease. Adv Neurol 45: 503–506

Bonuccelli U, Piccini P, Del Dotto P, Rossi G, Corsini GU, Muratorio A (1993) Apomorphine test for dopaminergic responsiveness: a dose assessment study. Mov Disord 8: 158–164

Chase TN, Mouradian MM, Engber TM (1993) Motor response complications and the function of striatal efferent systems. Neurology 43 [Suppl 6]: 23–27

Corona T, Rivera Nava C, Reyes Baez B, Carbajal A (1991) Utilidad de la terapia "holiday" en pacientes con enfermedad de Parkinson de mas de 5 anos de evolucion. Rev Invest Clin 43: 334–337

Corsini GU, Del Zompo M, Gessa GL, Mangoni A (1979) Therapeutic efficacy of apomorphine combined with an extracerebral inhibitor of dopamine receptors in Parkinson's disease. Lancet i: 954–956

D'Costa DF, Abbott RJ, Pye IF, Millac PAH (1991) The apomorphine test in Parkinsonian syndromes. J Neurol Neurosurg Psychiatry 54: 870–872

Direnfeld LK, Feldman RG, Alexander MP, Kelly-Hayes M (1980) Is l-dopa drug holiday useful? Neurology 30: 785–788

Direnfeld L, Spero L, Marotta J, Seeman P (1978) The l-dopa on-off effect in Parkinson's disease: treatment by transient withdrawal and dopamine receptor resensitization. Ann Neurol 4: 573–575

Feldman RG, Kaye JA, Lannon MC (1986) Parkinson's disease: follow-up after "drug holiday". J Clin Pharmacol 26: 662–667

Frankel JP, Lees AJ, Kempster PA, Stern GM (1990) Subcutaneous apomorphine in the treatment of Parkinson's disease. J Neurol Neurosurg Psychiatry 53: 96–101

Gancher ST, Nutt JG (1987) Diurnal responsiveness to apomorphine. Neurology 37: 1250–1253

Gasser T, Schwarz J, Arnold G, Trenkwalder C, Oertel WH (1992) Apomorphine test for dopaminergic responsiveness in patients with previously untreated Parkinson's disease. Arch Neurol 49: 1131–1134

Goetz CG, Tanner CM, Nausieda PA (1981) Weekly drug holiday in Parkinson's disease. Neurology 31: 1460–1462

Hughes AJ, Bishop S, Kleedorfer B, Turjanski N, Fernandez W, Lees AJ, Stern GM (1993) Subcutaneous apomorphine in Parkinson's disease: response to chronic administration for up to five years. Mov Disord 8: 165–170

Kaye JA, Feldman RG (1986) The role of l-dopa holiday in the long-term management of Parkinson's disease. Clin Neuropharmacol 9: 1–13

Kempster PA, Frankel JP, Bovingdon M, Webster R, Lees AJ, Stern GM (1989) Levodopa peripheral pharmacokinetics and duration of motor response in Parkinson's disease. J Neurol Neurosurg Psychiatry 52: 718–723

Koller WC, Weiner WJ, Perlik S, Nausieda PA, Goetz CG, Klawans HL (1981) Complications of chronic levodopa therapy: long-term efficacy of drug holiday. Neurology 31: 473–476

Lee T, Seeman P, Rajput A, Farley IJ, Hornykiewicz O (1978) Receptor basis for dopaminergic supersensitivity in Parkinson's disease. Nature 278: 59–61

Martinez F, Castillo J, Castro A, Lema M, Noja M (1992) Resultados de vacaciones de dopa en la enfermedad de Parkinson. Neurologia 7: 254–259

Mayeux R, Stern Y, Mulvey K, Cote L (1985) Reappraisal of drug holiday in Parkinson's disease. Neurology 35 [Suppl 1]: 200–201

Mouradian MM, Heuser IJ, Baronti F, Chase TN (1990) Modification of central dopaminergic mechanism by continuous levodopa therapy for advanced Parkinson's disease. Ann Neurol 27: 18–23

Muller P, Seeman P (1979) Pre-synaptic subsensitivity as a possible basis for sensitization by long-term dopamine mimetics. Eur J Pharmacol 55: 145–147

Poewe W (1993) Clinical and pathophysiologic aspects of late levodopa failure. Neurology 43 [Suppl 6]: 528–530

Poewe WH, Lees AJ, Stern GM (1986) Low-dose l-dopa therapy in Parkinson's disease: a 6-year follow-up study. Neurology 36: 1528–1530

Riccio A, Gilli M, Chiadò Cutin I, Delsedime M, Dettoni E, Giangrandi C, Rocci E, Zurlo F, Bergamini L (1989) La vacanza terapeutica nel morbo di Parkinson complicato: osservazione su 11 casi. Giornale di Neuropsicofarmacologia 11: 35–36

Schelosky L, Poewe W (1993) Current strategies in the drug treatment of advanced Parkinson's disease — new modes of dopamine substitution. Acta Neurol Scand 87 [Suppl 146]: 46–49

Steiger MJ, Quinn NP, Marsden CD (1992) The clinical use of apomorphine in Parkinson's disease. J Neurol 239: 389–393

Stibe CMH, Lees AJ, Kempster PA, Stern GM (1988) Subcutaneous apomorphine in parkinsonian on-off oscillations. Lancet i: 403–406

Sweet RD, Lee JE, Spiegel HE, McDowell F (1972) Enhanced response to low doses of levodopa after withdrawal from chronic treatment. Neurology 22: 520–525

Yahr MD (1993) Parkinson's disease: new approaches to diagnosis and treatment. Acta Neurol Scand 87 [Suppl 146]: 22–25

Authors' address: Dr. L. Scarzella, Department of Neurology, University of Turin, via Cherasco, 15, I-10126 Turin, Italy.

J Neural Transm (1995) [Suppl] 45: 171–176
© Springer-Verlag 1995

Changes in the amplitude of the N30 frontal component of SEPs during apomorphine test in parkinsonian patients

M. de Mari, L. Margari, P. Lamberti, G. Iliceto, and **E. Ferrari**

Institute of Neurology, University of Bari, Italy

Summary. Somatosensory evoked potentials (SEPs) to median nerve stimulation have been performed before and after apomorphine-test in 10 parkinsonian patients. Latency and amplitude of the P14-N20 parietal complex and of the P20-N30 frontal complex were evaluated.

The N30 amplitude was significantly reduced before apomorphine administration (p < 0.001) with a consequent increase of the N20/N30 amplitude ratio (p < 0.001). Eight patients clinically improved after Apomorphine. Following Apomorphine there was no change in the amplitude of the parietal complex P14-N20. On the other hand the frontal complex P20-N30 showed a significant amplitude potentiation (p < 0.005), with a reduction of the N20/N30 amplitude ratio (ns).

This finding was almost constant among the 8 responder patients. These results suggest the utility of combining clinical and neurophysiological data to assess the responsiveness to dopaminergic treatment.

Introduction

In parkinsonian patients neurophysiological studies have demonstrated a reduction in the amplitude of the frontal component (N30) of median nerve somatosensory evoked potentials (Rossini et al., 1989), which is supposed to arise at the level of the Supplementary Motor Area (SMA) (Desmedt and Cheron, 1981; Mauguiere et al., 1983). Rossini concluded that the N30 amplitude reduction in parkinsonian patients reflects a decreased output of the caudate nucleus to SMA via the globus pallidus and thalamic VL nuclei that could disrupt SMA function with a decrement of its modulation on primary motor cortex excitability (Rossini et al., 1989).

Subcutaneous administration of Apomorphine is now widely used in the treatment of severe fluctuations in parkinsonian patients (Franket et al., 1990) and represents, at the same time, an useful test in diagnosis of Parkinson's disease (PD), and in predicting the response to dopaminergic treatment (Barker et al., 1989).

We studied clinical and neurophysiological effects of a single apomorphine administration in parkinsonian patients in order to verify a possible relationship between clinical and instrumental findings, and to assess an objective method of testing the responsiveness to dopaminergic treatment.

Methods

We studied 10 non demented parkinsonian patients (7M–3F), mean age: 58.6 years (range 36–70), duration of the disease: 7.5 years (range 2–22). Hoehn-Yahr stage was 2.45 (range 2–3). All patients but one were on L-Dopa treatment (duration of L-Dopa therapy was 4.3 years, range 1 month-13 years). 4 patients had motor fluctuations.

Clinical assessment was performed using the Unified Parkinson's disease rating scale (UPDRS), taking into account items for tremor, rigidity and finger tapping, and a patient's global impression scale.

All antiparkinsonian drugs were withdrawn the night before the test. Clinical evaluation and SEPs recordings were performed in the baseline condition and 15, 30 and 60' after subcutaneous administration of a single dose of Apomorphine (mean dosage 3.4 mg, range 2–5 mg). Each patient received the same dosage of Apomorphine which was found to be effective in a previous clinical test. All patients received Domperidone treatment (30 mg daily) during the week before the test.

Median nerve somatosensory evoked potentials were performed according to the American Society Guidelines for Clinical Evoked potentials studies (1984–1986).

The median nerve of the clinically more affected side was stimulated at wrist with a ripetition rate of 2/sec and 0.1 msec duration. Electrical stimulus intensity was adjusted at motor threshold. SEPs were recorded using subcutaneous needle electrodes positioned at the Erb's point (referred to the controlateral Erb's point) and on the scalp 2 cm posterior to C3 or C4 of the 10–20 International System and at FZ (both scalp electrodes were referred to the earlobe controlateral to the stimulated side). A 5–2K Hz filter bandpass was utilized and two averages of 500 responses were superimposed.

Waves were labelled by the Donchin's et al. nomenclature (1977).

The following parameters were evaluated:

— peak latencies of the parietal wave N20 and of the frontal wave N30.
— peak-to-peak amplitude of the parietal wave P14-N20.
— peak-to-peak amplitude of the frontal wave P20-N30.
— the N20/N30 amplitude ratio to correct the wide intersubject variability of the absolute amplitude of the N20 and N30 waves.

EPs patients' data were considered abnormal when they differed by more than 2.5 Standard Deviation (SD) from the normal mean calculated in a control group of 20 age matched healthy volunteers.

Following Apomorphine administration latencies and amplitudes of SEPs were matched against baseline values gathered at "time 0" using the paired Student's t test.

Results

In the baseline condition there was no significant difference between controls and PD patients for the peak latencies of the parietal and frontal waves N20 and N30 (Table 1).

On the other hand both N20 parietal and N30 frontal waves were reduced in amplitude (Table 1). The amplitude reduction was significant for the frontal N30 ($p < 0.001$), as also shown by the increase of the N20/N30 amplitude ratio ($p < 0.001$). In particular the N20/N30 amplitude ratio was increased by more than 2.5 SD from the normal mean in 7/10 PD patients (Fig. 1).

	SEPs amplitude (μv)		
	N20	N30	N20/N30
Controls (20)	3.08 ± 0.66	4.59 ± 1.48	0.71 ± 0.18
PD baseline (10)	2.57 ± 1.40	2.05 ± 0.95*	1.35 ± 1.27*
PD apomorphine (10)	2.77 ± 1.36	2.90 ± 0.87**	0.95 ± 0.42

*p < 0.001 vs controls; **p < 0.005 vs PD baseline

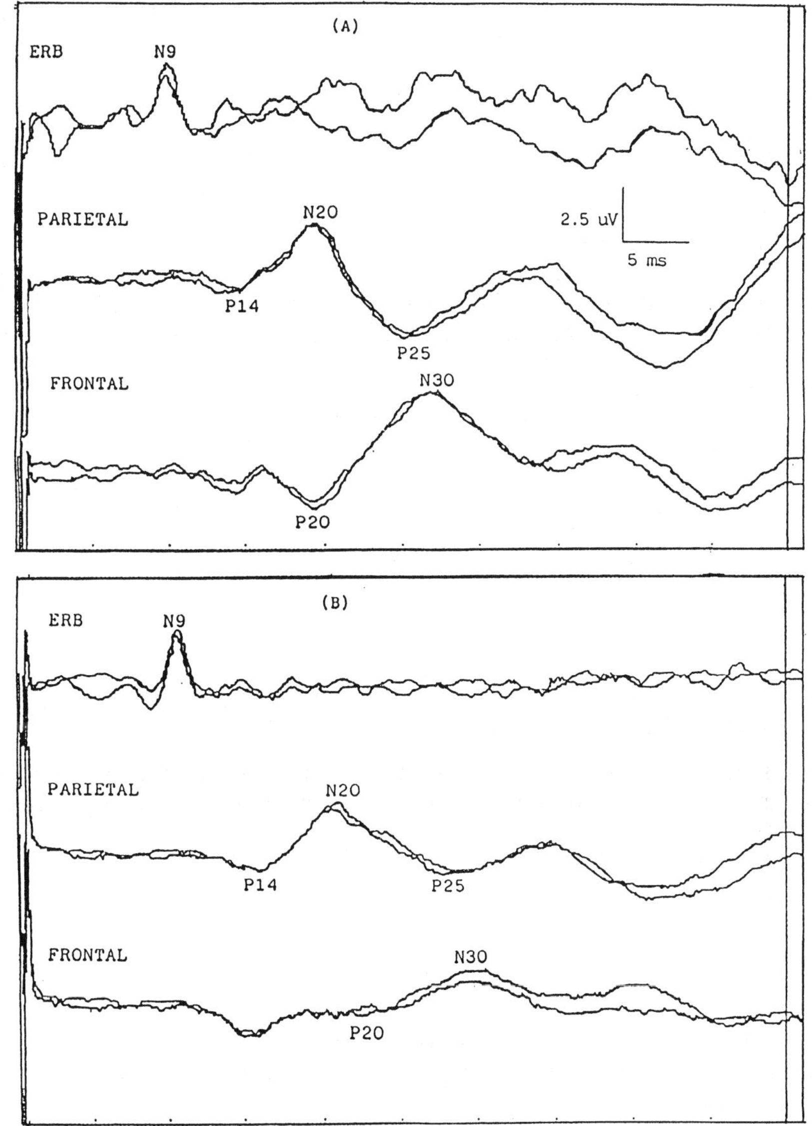

Fig. 1. Median nerve SEPs obtained in a control subject (**A**) and in a parkinsonian patient (**B**). Each recording comprises the N9 wave recorded at the brachial plexus, the N20 parietal and the N30 frontal components. In the PD patient latencies of all these responses are normal. On the other hand there is a marked reduction in the amplitude of the frontal N30 wave with an increased N20/N30 amplitude ratio

From the clinical point of view 8/10 patients had a strong improvement (>30%) of the clinical status in a time lapse comprised between 15 and 30' after Apomorphine administration. In the other 2 patients the clinical response to Apomorphine was absent or very slight even at the maximum dosage (5 mg).

After Apomorphine administration there was a significant potentiation in

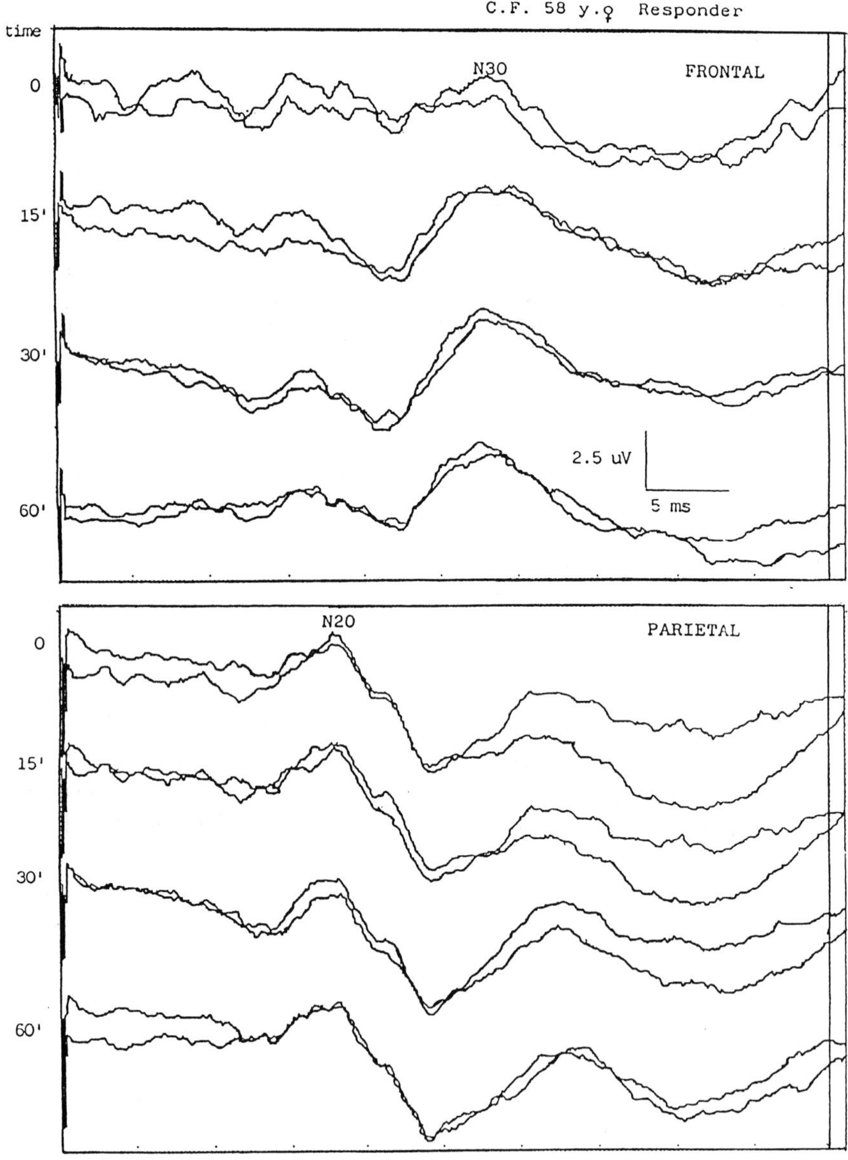

Fig. 2. Median nerve SEPs results obtained in a responder PD patient. In the baseline condition the N30 amplitude is very low with an increased N20/N30 amplitude ratio. After Apomorphine it is evident a progressive amplitude enanchement of the frontal N30 which reachs its maximum value after 30' without any concomitant change in the N20 amplitude

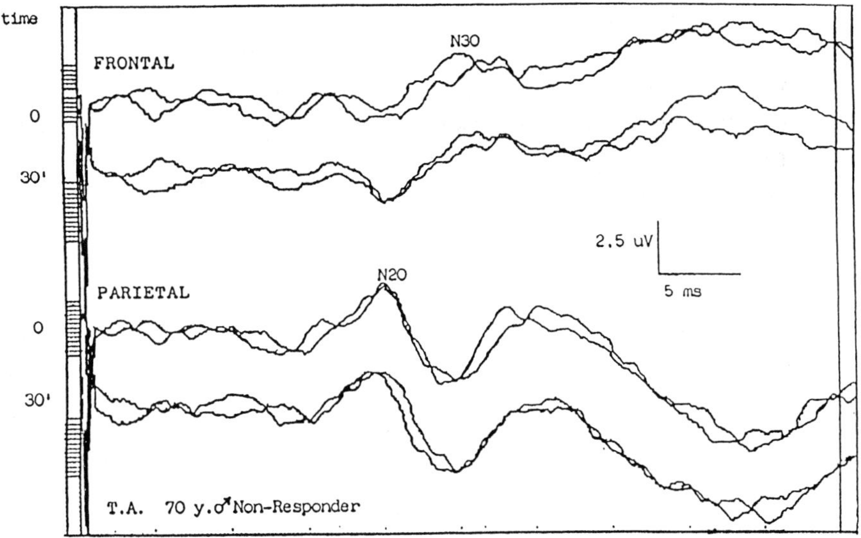

Fig. 3. Median nerve SEPs obtained in a non responder PD patient. In this patient, at time 0, the amplitude of the N30 is very low with an increased N20/N30 amplitude ratio. There is no change in the amplitude of the N30 and N20 waves 30' after the administration of Apomorphine

the amplitude of the frontal N30 ($p < 0.05$), which was more marked after 30'; however the N30 amplitude did not reach the control value (Table 1).

Analysis of individual results showed:

— N20 amplitude potentiation (>20%) in 3/10 patients;
— N30 amplitude potentiation (>20%) in 7/10 patients;
— N20/N30 ratio reduction (>20%) in 6/10 patients.

The N30 amplitude potentiation and the N20/N30 ratio reduction induced by Apomorphine administration were detected only among the responder patients (Fig. 2). In the 2 non responder patients there was no potentiation of the N30 amplitude without any change in the N20/N30 amplitude ratio (Fig. 3).

Discussion

In the last years the use of Apomorphine, a powerful agonist acting on dopamine D1 and D2 postsynaptic receptors, has been utilized in parkinsonian patients in the treatment of severe motor fluctuations (Frankel et al., 1990) and also as a clinical test in order to predict the efficacy of chronic treatment with L-Dopa or dopamine agonists (Barker et al., 1989). At the same time the response to Apomorphine can help in the differential diagnosis between PD and other parkinsonian syndromes such as Multiple System Atrophy and Progressive Supranuclear Palsy. However an instrumental method is desirable in order to obtain a more objective assessment of the response to Apomorphine especially in the early stages of PD when the clinical effect is often very soubtle.

In parkinsonian patients the impairment of the SMA function has been demonstrated by the reduction in the amplitude in the frontal component of SEPs (N30) (Rossini et al., 1989). In addition recent PET studies have demonstrated that the impaired activation of the supplementary motor area in Parkinson's disease is reversed when akinesia is treated with Apomorphine (Jenkins et al., 1992).

In our study, as previously shown by Rossini et al. (1993) the amplitude potentiation of the frontal N30 has been observed only among PD patients clinically responsive to Apomorphine.

These results suggest the utility of combining clinical and neurophysiological data in order to assess an objective method of testing the responsiveness to dopaminergic treatment.

References

Barker R, Duncan J, Lees AJ (1989) Subcutaneous apomorphine as a diagnostic test for dopaminergic responsiveness in parkinsonian syndromes. Lancet i: 1262–1263

Desmedt JE, Cheron G (1981) Non-cephalic reference recording of early somatosensory potentials to finger stimulation in adults or aging man: differentiation of widespread N18 and contralateral N20 from the prerolandic P22 and N30 components. Electroencephalogr Clin Neurophysiol 52: 553–570

Donchin E, Callaway E, Cooper R, Goff WR, Desmedt JE, Hillyard SA, Sutton S (1977) Pubblication criteria for studies of evoked potentials in man. In: Desmedt JE (ed) Attention, voluntary contraction and event-related cerebral potentials. Karger, Basel, pp 1–11 (Prog Clin Neurophysiol, vol 1)

Frankel JI, Lees AJ, Kempster PA, Stern GM (1990) Subcutaneous apomorphine in the treatment of Parkinson's disease. J Neurol Neurosurg Psychiatry 53: 86–101

Jenkins IH, Fernandez W, Playford ED, Lees AJ, Frackowiak RSJ, Pasingham R, Brooks DJ (1992) Impaired activation of the supplementary motor area in Parkinson's disease is reversed when akinesia is treated with Apomorphine. Ann Neurol 32: 749–757

Mauguiere F, Desmedt JE, Courjon J (1983) Astereognosis and dissociated loss of frontal and parietal components of somatosensory evoked potentials in hemispheric lesions. Brain 106: 271–311

Rossini PM, Babiloni F, Bernardi G, Cecchi L, Johnson PB, Malentacca A, Stanzione P, Urbano A (1989) Abnormalities of short latencies somatosensory evoked potentials in parkinsonian patients. Electroencephalogr Clin Neurophysiol 74: 277–289

Rossini PM, Traversa R, Boccasena P, Martino G, Passarelli F, Pacifici L, Bernardi G, Stanzione P (1993) Parkinson's disease and somatosensory evoked potentials: apomorphine-induced transient potentiation of frontal components. Neurology 43: 2495–2500

Authors' address: Prof. P. Lamberti, Institute of Neurology, University of Bari, Ospedale Policlinico, Piazza G. Cesare, I-70124 Bari, Italy.

J Neural Transm (1995) [Suppl] 45: 177–185

N30 wave amplitude of Somatosensory Evoked Potentials from median nerve in Parkinson's disease: a pharmacological study

R. Traversa[1], M. Pierantozzi[2], R. Semprini[2], M. Loberti[2], M. C. Cicardi[3], A. Bassi[2], and P. Stanzione[1,2]

[1] I.R.C.C.S. Clinica S. Lucia, Rome, [2] Clinica Neurologica, "Tor Vergata" University of Rome, and [3] Dipartimento di Psichiatria, Ospedale S. Eugenio, Rome, Italy

Summary. We studied N20 and N30 waves of Somatosensory Evoked Potentials from median nerve stimulation in different pharmacological conditions. N30 wave amplitude was decreased in 33 parkinsonians without therapy in comparison with a group of age-matched normal subjects. In a group of 19 parkinsonians, N30 wave amplitude was significantly augmented during apomorphine infusion and less evidently, but still significantly, during chronic 1-dopa therapy. The administration of an oral dose of haloperidol in 11 normals did not affect significantly the studied parameters. The infusion of apomorphine in 6 psychotic patients with extrapyramidal symptoms secondary to long-term treatment with neuroleptics, determined, together with a clear-cut clinical amelioration, a significant increase of N30 amplitude and N30/N20 ratio. Possible pathophysiological hypothesis of such electrophysiological modifications are discussed.

Introduction

The amplitude of frontal components (N30 wave) of Somatosensory Evoked Potentials (SEPs) have been reported to be decreased in Parkinson's disease (PD) patients (pts) (Rossini et al., 1989) as well as the equivalent anterior negativity in monkeys treated with MPTP (Onofrj et al., 1990). These data raised the question about the relationship between frontal N30 wave and dopaminergic activity. Recently, it has also been reported that the administration of a potent dopamine agonist, apomorphine, can improve N30 wave amplitude in non-treated PD patients (Rossini et al., 1993), suggesting a link between PD physiopathology and N30 wave amplitude decrease. These data strengthen the relationship between N30 amplitude and dopaminergic activity, although they do not clarify its nature. In normal subjects, an amplitude decrease of N30 wave is known to occur during voluntary muscular contraction without any effects on P14 and N20 waves (Cohen and Starr, 1987). Thus, it is not clear whether N30 amplitude decrease in PD is due only to dopamine lack in a cortical-basal ganglia-cortical loop (probably involved in N30 generation), or to the increase of muscle tone due to dopamine lack. In order to relate electrophysiological alterations to dopaminergic lack in PD, a strict relationship should be demonstrated between the use of dopaminergic therapy and the recovery of the electrophysiological alterations. Moreover, the same electrophysiological alterations should be obtained in normals by blocking dopaminergic transmission. Consequently, we planned pharmacological tests in PD pts and in normal subjects while recording SEPs. We studied, in the same group of PD pts, N30 amplitude variations, in basal (untreated) condition, following apomorphine infusion and after chronic 1-dopa treatment. We compared PD pts data with age-matched normals. We also analyzed SEPs variations in normals following the administration of a single oral dose of haloperidol not producing extrapyramidal signs and in psychotic patients affected by extrapyramidal hypertone secondary to long term therapy with high doses of neuroleptics.

Material and methods

Thirty-three PD pts (mean age 62.3 ± 8.6) from the Neurology Department were enrolled in this study and the electrophysiological data obtained from their group without therapy were compared to those obtained from 24 age-matched (65.6 ± 10.7) normals. Nineteen PD pts (mean age 64.4 ± 5.9), out of the previous group, were studied in three conditions: basal control, apomorphine infusion and 1-dopa therapy. Eleven volunteers (mean age 54.0 ± 8.5) were submitted to an acute oral administration of haloperidol. We also studied 6 patients from the Psychiatry Department affected by rigidity due to neuroleptic long-term therapy in basal condition and during apomorphine infusion. All the research protocols were approved by the local Ethics Committee. Apomorphine chloride was given to PD and psychiatric pts through an infusion pump with a dose ranging from 3 to 5 mg/h. The recordings were performed into one session before starting the steady-state infusion and after three hours of it. L-dopa therapy was given orally at a dose ranging between 375 and 750 mg/day producing a clinical improvement of at least 50% of the clinical score. The recordings were performed two hours after the midday dose. Haloperidol was administered orally to normal volunteers at a dose of 0.05 mg/Kg and SEPs recorded 2 hours after drug administration. Electrophysiological data were analyzed by means of ANOVA two-way (eventually corrected by Greenhouse-Gaisser correction). Motor performance of PD pts were evaluated adopting only the motor items for rigidity and bradykinesia only (minimum 0; maximum 24) of the UPDRS scale (Fahn et al., 1987). The mean duration of disease in PD pts was 4.5 ± 5 years. Hoehn and Yahr staging (Hohen and Yahr, 1967) was 2.19 ± 1.03. Median SEPs were recorded via subcutaneous sterile needles positioned at four scalp positions (F3, Fz, F4, C3/C4). A common reference was adopted on the earlobe contralateral to the stimulation. Subjects lay relaxed in supine position. The median nerve was stimulated at the wrist (cathode proximal) with square-wave pulses and an intensity set to the motor threshold for abductor pollicis brevis; interstimulus intervals was 0.99 Hz, bandpass 1–1,000 Hz (−6 dB/Oct), 100 msec the analysis time. Tracings were obtained from 201 artifact-free trials and repeated at least twice to verify their reproducibility. The following measurements were taken: peak latencies of parietal N20 and frontal N30 waves, peak-to-peak amplitudes of N20 (P14-N20) and N30 (P20-N30) waves, N30/N20 amplitude ratio.

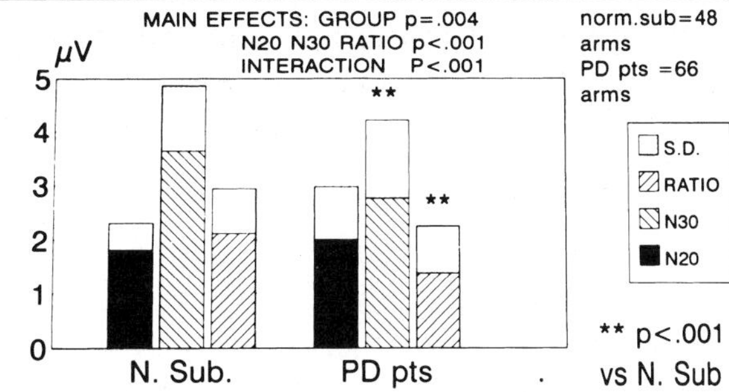

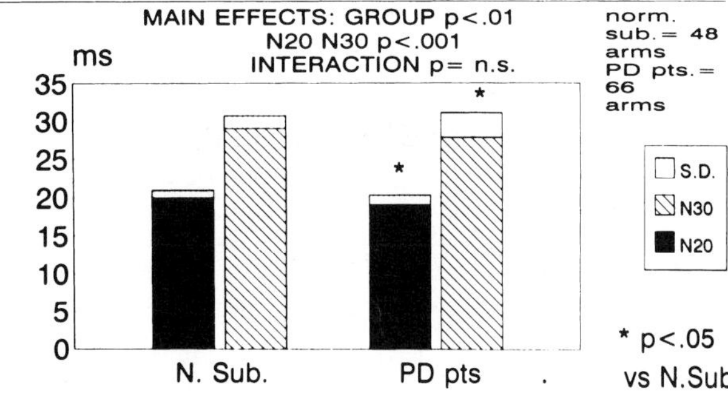

Fig. 1. Statistical analysis of N20 and N30 waves amplitude (upper part) and latency (lower part) with N30/N20 ratio in 24 normal subjects and 33 parkinsonian patients without therapy (basal condition)

Results

Comparison between normal subjects and PD patients without therapy

SEPs N20 and N30 wave latencies, amplitudes and amplitude ratio have been studied in 48 arms of 24 normals and 66 arms of 33 PD pts (Fig. 1). PD pts were "de novo" or in drug holiday from at least 15 days for clinical purposes. The mean H&Y score of PD pts was 2.19. The analysis of N20 and N30 amplitude and N30/N20 ratio, performed by means of an ANOVA two-way (corrected by Greenhouse-Geisser), showed significant effects for both factors "group" (p < 0.005) and "waves" (p < 0.001) and also a significant interaction "group" X "waves" (p < 0.001). The planned comparison in the two groups showed not significant amplitude variation for N20 in the two populations, but there was a significant (p < 0.001) decrease of N30 amplitude in PD pts with a significant (p < 0.001) decrease of N30/N20 ratio. The analysis showed that the main effect "group" was significant and both N20 and N30 latencies were shorter in the PD group, in comparison to normal subjects (Table 1).

Table 1. N20 and N30 waves amplitude and latency with N30/N20 ratio: comparison between 24 normal subjects and 33 parkinsonian patients in basal condition (upper part) and between basal condition, apomorphine infusion and 1-dopa therapy (lower part) in a population of 19 parkinsonians with bradykinesia and rigidity items of UPDRS clinical score

	Normals = 48 arms	PD pts = 66 arms
N20 latency	19.9 ± 0.90 ms	19.3 ± 1.2 ms
N20 amplitude	$1.81 \pm 0.5\,\mu$V	$2.01 \pm 0.9\,\mu$V
N30 latency	29.0 ± 1.7 ms	27.8 ± 3.2 ms
N30 amplitude	$3.64 \pm 1.2\,\mu$V	$2.76 \pm 1.4\,\mu$V
Ratio	2.12 ± 0.8	1.38 ± 0.87

PD pts = 38 arms

	Basal	Apomorphine	L-Dopa
N20 latency	20.1 ± 1.1 ms	19.9 ± 1.0 ms	20.0 ± 1.0 ms
N20 amplitude	$2.17 \pm 1.0\,\mu$V	$2.08 \pm 0.9\,\mu$V	$2.04 \pm 0.8\,\mu$V
N30 latency	28.6 ± 2.8 ms	28.5 ± 2.6 ms	28.1 ± 2.5 ms
N30 amplitude	$2.52 \pm 1.3\,\mu$V	$3.81 \pm 1.4\,\mu$V	$2.72 \pm 0.8\,\mu$V
Ratio	1.30 ± 0.7	2.08 ± 1.0	1.53 ± 0.7
Clin. Score	8.91 ± 4.8	4.30 ± 3.0	6.30 ± 3.3

Variations within parkinsonian patients group following apomorphine or L-DOPA administration

N20 and N30 wave latency and amplitude variations have been studied in 38 arms of 19 PD pts in basal condition, during apomorphine infusion and 1-dopa therapy (Fig. 2 and Table 1). Concerning amplitude variations, the ANOVA two-way analysis (corrected by Greenhouse-Geisser) showed a significant ($p < 0.001$) effect of the factor "treatment" (basal, apomorphine, 1-dopa), of the factor "waves" (N20, N30, N30/N20 ratio) ($p < 0.001$) and an interaction between the two factors ($p < 0.001$). The planned comparison did not show any significant variation of N20 wave amplitude in the three conditions. N30 amplitude increased of a mean of $1.29\,\mu$V from basal to apomorphine conditions ($p < 0.001$) and only of a mean of $0.20\,\mu$V from basal to 1-dopa condition ($p < 0.05$). N30/N20 amplitude ratio significantly increased from 1.30 to 2.08 from basal to apomorphine conditions ($p < 0.001$), while the variation from basal to 1-dopa condition was not significant. The comparison between the values obtained during apomorphine and 1-dopa treatment confirmed the larger electrophysiological effects of apomorphine in comparison to 1-dopa. While N20 amplitude did not vary in a significant way, N30 amplitude was significantly ($p < 0.001$) increased ($1.09\,\mu$V) during apomorphine, as the amplitude ratio was significantly ($p < 0.01$) larger (2.08 vs 1.53) in the same condition. The treatment of PD pts with apomorphine or 1-dopa did not produce any significant variation of latencies. Clinical score variations were also studied in the three conditions (Table 1).

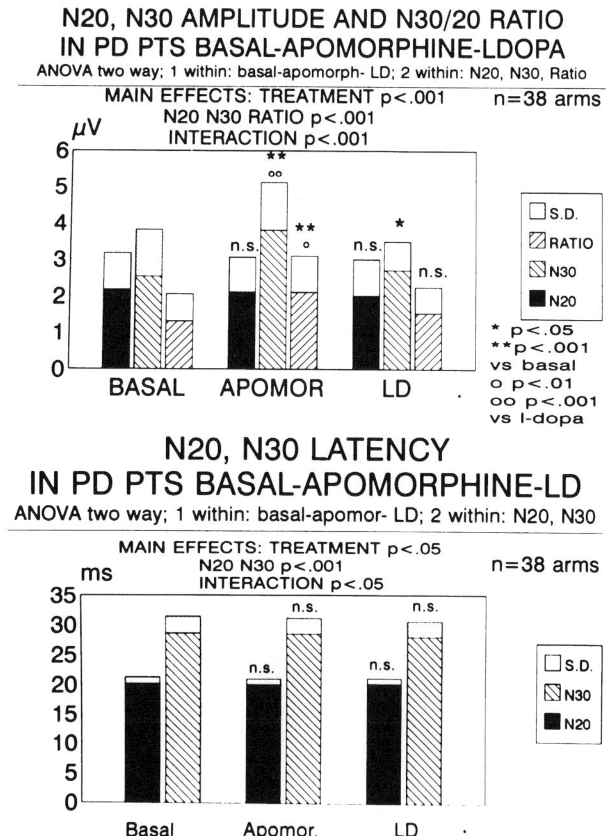

Fig. 2. Statistical analysis of N20 and N30 waves amplitude (upper part) and latency (lower part) with N30/N20 ratio in 19 parkinsonian patients in basal condition, during apomorphine infusion and l-dopa therapy

Effects of neuroleptics in normal subjects and psychotic patients

The effect of haloperidol administration to normal subjects on SEPs waves did not show a significant amplitude or latency change in the considered group (Table 2). We also analyzed the results from 12 arms of 6 psychotic patients with an extrapyramidal hypertone due to neuroleptic treatment (Fig. 3 and Table 2). N20 and N30 latencies were not statistically affected by apomorphine. The ANOVA two-way analysis showed a significant effect of "drug administration" on waves amplitude ($p < 0.001$). The mean N30 amplitude was significantly increased with apomorphine ($p < 0.001$), and so the N30/N20 ratio ($p < 0.01$). There was a marked clinical improvement of rigidity during apomorphine infusion with a return to the basal clinical status after 1 hour from the discontinuation of the drug.

Discussion

The main finding is the large decrease of N30 wave amplitude not related to a N20 amplitude decrease with the decrease of N30/N20 ratio in PD pts. This

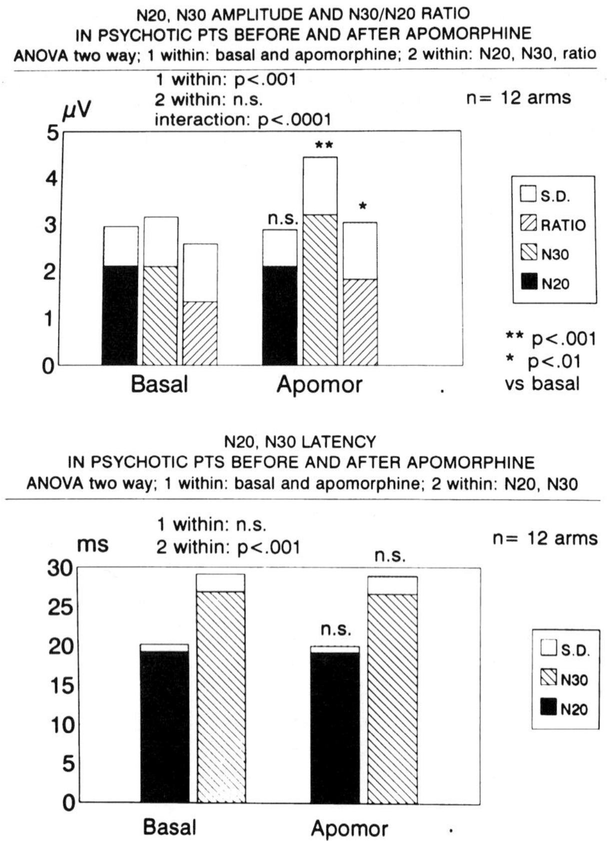

Fig. 3. Statistical analysis of N20 and N30 waves amplitude (upper part) and latency (lower part) in 6 psychotic patients showing extrapyramidal symptoms due to long-term therapy with high doses of neuroleptics. The recordings were analyzed before and during apomorphine infusion

confirms, on a large population of parkinsonians, previous findings (Rossini et al., 1989, 1993). An explanation could be the less efficient activity of a cortico-subcortico-cortical loop constituted by the supplementary motor area, the basal ganglia and the ventrolateral thalamic nuclei probabily involved in N30 generation (Brinkman et al., 1983; Hummelsheim et al., 1988) due to dopamine deficiency in the basal ganglia. A concomitant factor could involve a mechanism due to the sensory afferences produced by the increased muscle tone interfering with N30 wave generation. Many authors report (Jones et al., 1981; Cohen and Starr, 1987; Cheron and Borenstein, 1989, 1991) the phenomenon of "gating" of SEPs amplitude during voluntary contraction, which begins before EMG onset of the target muscle. This finding was explained by Cohen and Starr (1987) as if the gating mechanism were more related to premotor activity than to centripetal sensory volley. However, an interference produced by centripetal sensory inputs originated by rigidity (with a mechanism similar to voluntary contraction) could contribute to the "gating" mechanism at central level.

Table 2. Amplitudes and latencies of N20 and N30 waves with N30/N20 ratio in 11 normal subjects before and after the administration per os of haloperidol (upper part) and in 6 psychotic patients affected by with extrapyramidal hypertone secondary to long-term therapy with neuroleptics (lower part) before and during apomorphine infusion

Normal Subjects N = 11		
	Control	Haloperidol
N20 latency	$19.5 \pm 1.3\,ms$	$19.3 \pm 0.8\,ms$
N20 amplitude	$1.90 \pm 0.5\,\mu V$	$1.84 \pm 0.5\,\mu V$
N30 latency	$27.9 \pm 2.8\,ms$	$27.7 \pm 2.5\,ms$
N30 amplitude	$3.02 \pm 1.2\,\mu V$	$3.09 \pm 1.3\,\mu V$
Ratio	1.63 ± 0.5	1.73 ± 0.6

Psychotic pts = 12 arms		
	Control	Apomorphine
N20 latency	$19.2 \pm 0.9\,ms$	$19.1 \pm 0.8\,ms$
N20 amplitude	$2.10 \pm 0.8\,\mu V$	$2.09 \pm 0.8\,\mu V$
N30 latency	$2.69 \pm 2.2\,ms$	$26.7 \pm 2.3\,ms$
N30 amplitude	$2.09 \pm 1.0\,\mu V$	$3.19 \pm 1.2\,\mu V$
Ratio	1.34 ± 1.2	1.82 ± 1.2

A not expected result is the latency decrease of N20 and N30 waves in PD pts in comparison with age-matched normals. N30 wave complex is constituted by several early and late peaks. An amplitude reduction, mostly involving late components, could produce a different measured peak time. More difficult is to explain N20 latency reduction, although the minimal amount of this reduction (0.636 ms), reduces very much the clinical relevance of this finding. Previous studies on SEPs during voluntary contraction (Cohen and Starr, 1987; Cheron and Borenstein, 1987, 1991) did not report any significant change of N20 latency. This could be related either to the lower number of examined subjects, which reduces the power of the statistical analysis, or to different mechanisms underlying these SEP modifications.

The analysis of PD pts in the three different conditions shows that the main finding is the recovery of N30 wave amplitude during both treatments, much more evident during apomorphine infusion. These data, strictly relate N30 amplitude to the level of dopaminergic activity. N30 wave amplitude has been reported to be decreased in some parkinsonians, in spite of an ongoing dopaminergic therapy able to control the clinical symptoms (Rossini et al., 1989). This finding could suggest that a simple increase of dopaminergic transmission at the basal ganglia level, without complete clinical resolution of rigidity, is not sufficient to restore N30 amplitude. On the contrary, an apomorphine dose adeguate to ameliorate more effectively the rigidity could improve N30 wave amplitude possibly reducing centripetal afferences. Following this line, apomorphine administrated at doses able to produce only a relatively mild clinical improvement in late on-off pts. (5 mg in OFF state and 2.5/3 mg in ON state), as reported by Mauguiere et al. (1993), would not be expected to produce significant electrophysiological modifications.

What is not clear from these results, is whether this relationship imply an improvement of basal ganglia function within the cortical-subcortical-cortical loop only, or whether it is caused also by an indirect effect of dopamine on muscle tone (centripetal input). In this case, it could be possible to hypotesize the importance, on frontal potentials, of muscle tone.

No significant variations of amplitude and/or latency of N20 and N30 waves were found in normal subjects recorded after haloperidol administration. These data could be related to the low dosage utilized, which, although acting at central level, lacks any clinical effect on muscle tone. In fact, in psychotic patients showing an evident hypertonus secondary to high dosage of neuroleptics, we found in the basal condition a depressed amplitude of N30 amplitude with a significant increment, during apomorphine infusion, of N30 and N30/N20 ratio. The electrophysiological data on psychotic patients, coupled with the clinical improvement of rigidity, seems to confirm the importance of muscle tone on N30 amplitude and the major role of dopamine agonists in the cortico-subcortico-cortical circuit involved in the generation of this potential.

References

Brinkman C, Porter R (1983) Motor control mechanisms in health and disease. Raven Press, New York, p 393

Cohen LG, Starr A (1987) Localization, timing and specificity of gating of somatosensory evoked potentials during active movement in man. Brain 110: 451–467

Cheron G, Borenstein S (1987) Specific gating of the early somatosensory evoked potentials during active movement. Electroencephalogr Clin Neurophysiol 67: 537–548

Cheron G, Borenstein R (1991) Gating of the early components of the frontal and parietal somatosensory evoked potentials in different sensory-motor interference modalities. Electroencephalogr Clin Neurophysiol 80: 522–530

Fahn S, Elton RL and the Unified Rating Scale Development Committee (1987) Recent development in Parkinson's disease. MacMillan, New York, p 153

Hoehn MH, Yahr MD (1967) Parkinsoniam: onset, progression and mortality. Neurology 17: 427–442

Hummelsheim H, Bianchetti M, Wiesendanger M, Wiesendanger R (1988) Sensory inputs to agranular motor fields: a comparison between precentral, supplementary motor and premotor areas in the monkey. Exp Brain Res 69: 289–298

Jones SJ, Halonan JP, Shawkat F (1989) Centrifugal and centripetal mechanisms involved in the "gating" of cortical SEPs during movement. Electroencephalogr Clin Neurophysiol 74: 36–45

Mauguiere F, Broussolle E, Isnard J (1993) Apomorphine-induced relief of the akinetic-rigid syndrome and early median nerve somatosensory evoked potentials (SEPs) in Parkinson's disease. Electroencephalogr Clin Neurophysiol 88: 243–254

Onofrj M, Ghilardi MF, Basciani M, Martinez-Tica J, Glover A (1990) Attenuation of the early anterior negativity of median nerve somatosensory evoked potential in the MPTP-treated monkey. Clin Neurophysiol 20: 283–293

Rossini PM, Babiloni F, Bernardi G, Cecchi L, Johnson PB, Malentacca A, Stanzione P, Urbano A (1989) Abnormalities of short-latency somatosensory evoked potentials in parkinsonian patients. Electroencephalogr Clin Neurophysiol 74: 277–289

Rossini PM, Traversa R, Boccasena P, Martino G, Passarelli F, Pacifici L, Bernardi G, Stanzione P (1993) Parkinson's disease and Somatosensory Evoked Potentials: apomorphine-induced transient potentiation of frontal components. Neurology 43: 2495–2500

Authors' address: Prof. P. Stanzione, Universita' degli studi di Roma "Tor Vergata", Clinica Neurologica, Dipartimento di Sanita' Pubblica, via di Tor Vergata 135, I-00133 Roma, Italy.

J Neural Transm (1995) [Suppl] 45: 187–195
© Springer-Verlag 1995

Dopaminergic agonists in the treatment of Parkinson's disease: a review

F. Piccoli and **R. M. Riuggeri**

Institute of Neuropsychiatry, University of Palermo, Italy

Summary. Dopaminergic agonists represent an important class of drugs in Parkinson's Disease, useful: a) in delaying the beginning of L-dopa therapy; b) in supporting it, reducing its dosage and widen the therapeutic window; c) moreover, as the disease advances, in trying to treat motor fluctuations.

Authors describe briefly the problems caused by long term L-dopa therapy, and analize, separately, the characteristics of the most important dopaminergic agonists currently utilized in the treatment of PD.

Levodopa is still considered the major therapeutic agent for the treatment of Parkinson's disease, but it is not the ideal drug for several reasons. As a matter of fact, its efficacy depends on enzymatic conversion to dopamine while the enzyme follows the progressive decline of the population of dopaminergic cells projecting to the striatum, as the disease advances. Moreover the enzymatic decrease has been shown to be predominant in the nigrostriatal system (Hornykiewicz, 1981). The half-life of levodopa is exceedingly short, and at least some of the motor oscillations seen so frequently in patients with advanced Parkinson's disease appear to relate to fluctuations in circulating drug levels (Goetz and Diederich, 1992). Finally, the increased normal metabolism of dopamine, that results from levodopa ingestion, generates hydrogen peroxide and hydroxyl free radicals, which theoretically may contribute to further damage of already compromised cellular function.

Dopamine agonists have been developed in an attempt to overcome several of these levodopa limitations. They act, indipendently of the dopaminergic enzyme system, at the postsynaptic sites; they are highly specific to subpopulations of dopamine receptors and, by lowering the turnover rates of dopamine, can generate less hydrogen peroxide and free radicals, so protecting dopaminergic cells.

However an intriguing question arises when one considers the amount of molecules tested in clinical trials.

This paper will deal with some fifteen drugs showing dopaminergic properties; however, only four of which (bromocriptine, lisuride, pergolide and apomorphine) are available for use in Parkinson's disease current therapy. The mentioned intriguing question seems to be clear at this point: why so many drugs, why so many trials, why so many problems? At the end of this discussion we shall try to give, if possible, an answer.

                                    F. Piccoli and R. M. Riuggeri

Table 1. Dopamine and dopaminergic drugs

Drug	D1	D2	Drug	D1	D2
Dopamine	**	****	Pramipexole		**
Apomorfine	**	***	Quinagolide		**
Bromocriptine	°	***	Ropinirole		***
Cabergoline	*	***	Terguride	°°	**pres.
Lergotrile		**	CY 208 243	**	
Lisuride	*	****	EDM 49980		**
Mesulergine		***	LY 171555		**
Pergolide	*	***	PHNO		***

Site of action * agonist ° antagonist

Dopaminergic drugs: site of action

Multiple subclasses of receptors for the dopamine system have been identified, but to date pharmacologic concerns related to agonists have focused on D_1 and D_2 types (see Table 1). Most of the agonists used so far with success in patient with Parkinson's disease share D_2 agonist properties, the role of D_1 being uncertain, even if drugs as apomorphine, cabergoline, lisuride, pergolide and CY 208 243, show a slight agonist effect on this class of receptors. By contrast, a clear D_1 antagonist profile has been reported for bromocriptine and terguride (Rinne, 1989; Baronti et al., 1992).

We shall refer to the agonists listed on Table 1, summarizing problems, questions and results.

Bromocriptine

Bromocriptine is the most known dopaminergic drug. It has been investigated (U.K.Bromocriptine Research Group, 1982) with the therapeutic goal to correct the long-term complications of levodopa therapy, especially motor fluctuations and abnormal involuntary movements, as well as in monotherapy, in previously untreated patients, with the aim to delay the levodopa therapy. Although bromocriptine has less anti-parkinson effect than levodopa, and many patients experience acute adverse effects, those patients who tolerate chronic bromocriptine monotherapy experience little or no complications as motor fluctuations or dyskinesia (Lieberman and Goldstein, 1985; Hely et al., 1989; Montastruc et al., 1989). Conversely, early combination therapy with low levodopa doses induces a similar motor response to that of levodopa monotherapy but with fewer late complications (Rinne, 1985, 1987, 1989).

Lisuride

When administered orally, lisuride moderately improves all parkinsonian signs (Rinne, 1983). When used as monotherapy in de novo patients, it causes fewer motor fluctuations and dyskinesia than levodopa, but also less improvement (Rinne, 1989). In combination with levodopa it reduces significantly off periods; however, lisuride seems less effective than bromocriptine and pergolide in alleviating end-of-dose akinesia (LeWitt et al., 1982; Lees and Stern, 1981). Side effects are similar to those described for other agonists. Because of its solubility, lisuride is well suited to intravenous or subcutaneous applications, using a mini-infusion pump (Baronti et al., 1992). In spite of dramatic reduction of off time and motor fluctuations, psychiatric sides affects, such as paranoia and hallucinations, and subcutaneous nodules, which may affect drug absorption, developed in most patient, limiting the use of sc lisuride (Obeso et al., 1988).

Pergolide

Pergolide is an ergot-derivative direct-acting dopamine agonist with a long duration of action which is able to reduce disability in Parkinson's disease. The drug possesses a profile of activity and of adverse effects similar to that of bromocriptine. Like bromocriptine, when given concomitantly with levodopa, pergolide may allow a reduction of levodopa doses. Unlike bromocriptine, however, pergolide appears to provide a greater reduction in off time, and with its longer duration of action tend to reduce the wearing-off and end-of-dose effects of levodopa. Long term use of pergolide has produced clinical benefit in some patients for a period up to 7 years (Lieberman et al., 1983; Langtry and Clissold, 1990).

Apomorphine

Apomorphine is the oldest of the available agonists, and it had been proposed as an antiparkinsonian medication more then a century ago (Weill, 1884).

Apomorphine's rapid onset of action provides a rescue strategy for reversing sudden off periods. Using continuous subcutaneous infusion, delivered with a mini-pump in the most severely affected patients, as well as an intermittent bolus injections through a pen-injector in the less severely affected patients, the drug reduces off periods in short time trials, but not when follow-up period was 16 months or more. So far apomorphine may be used as an emergency medicine for the management of the levodopa withdrawal syndrome (Frankel et al., 1990); moreover acute response to apomorphine may become a useful tool in the differential diagnosis of idiopathic Parkinson's disease versus secondary parkinsonian syndromes (Barker et al., 1989). Psychotic episodes, dermatologic disorders (in subjects submitted to continuous infusion) and nausea are the most common side effects, described in 90% to 100% of the treated patients: they are usually temporary and mild (Pollak et al., 1990).

Cabergoline

Cabergoline is an ergoline derivative with a D_2-specific dopaminergic activity. It seems to be more active than other agonists. The elimination half-life of labelled compound is approximately 65 hours (Di Salle et al., 1982). The long-acting effect of cabergoline suggests that it may be efficacious in the treatment of motor fluctuations and loss of efficacy of levodopa therapy in Parkinson's disease patients by providing a continuous stimulation of dopaminergic receptors with once-daily dosing. Recent open studies seem to confirm this hypothesis in combined therapy as well as in dose-ranging studies (Jori et al., 1990; Lera et al., 1990; Obeso et al., 1991). A controlled study confirms reports of the quoted open trials that cabergoline taken once daily, in addition to levodopa, brings about improved efficacy for Parkinson's disease (Hutton et al., 1993).

Pramipexole

Pramipexole is a recently developed dopamine D_2-receptor agonist. Animal studies have shown that the compound has a marked presynaptic effect on both the rate of dopamine synthesis and release (Mierau and Bechtel, 1988). A postsynaptic dopaminergic activity of the compound was observed in dopamine-depleted monkeys (Schingnitz and Mierau, 1991). In adequate individual dosages it produces significant long-lasting antiparkinsonian effects in a single dose study (Albani et al., 1992). It is effective in treating motor fluctuations in advanced Parkinson's disease patients, but side effects (i.e. dyskinesia) can be expected (Molho et al., 1993).

Ropinirole

Ropinirole has been characterized preclinically as a specific dopamine D_2-receptor agonist (Eden et al., 1991). When given in low doses, in combination with levodopa, it has antiparkinsonian activity with a good tolerability (Kapoor et al., 1989). The drug may be as active as levodopa when given alone, showing a clear dose-dependent effect on motor disability (Vidailhet et al., 1990). Ropinirole is able to reverse all motor deficits induced by MPTP in animal model (Eden et al., 1991).

Talipexole

Talipexole is a new type of D_2 dopamine receptor agonist with higher affinity for the presynaptic dopamine receptors than for the postsynaptic ones. However, when the dopaminergic terminals are denervated, it acts as a postsynaptic D_2 agonist. Both open and controlled trials gave positive results in monotherapy as well as in combination with levodopa. A good tolerability has been reported (Mizuno et al., 1992; Zierz et al., 1992; Clarenbach et al., 1992).

Terguride

Terguride is a semisynthetic derivative of lisuride which possesses long acting and partial dopaminergic activity in patients with Parkinson's disease with long terms side effects of levodopa treatment (Baronti et al., 1992; Pacchetti et al., 1992). Terguride's main characteristic is its ability to exert both agonist and antagonist activity on D_2 dopamine receptors (Wachtel et al., 1984). It has been employed in open studies in patients with different neurological or psychiatric diseases (i.e. parkinsonism, Huntington's chorea, tardive dyskinesia and schizophrenia) in which different degrees of striatal dopamine activity and receptor sensitivity are postulated (Pacchetti et al., 1993). Controlled trials indicate that terguride, when added to levodopa therapy, has only a modest additional dopamine agonist action, while does not modify off duration or severity (Pacchetti et al., 1993).

CY 208-243 (Benzergoline)

Benzergoline, a D_1 agonist, produces a significant increase in locomotion in monkeys rendered parkinsonian by MPTP (Gomez-Mancilla et al., 1993). It has no effect on tremor (Gomez-Mancilla et al., 1992), and, when added to chronic bromocriptine treatment, produces an improvement in animal models and exerts a mild antiparkinsonian effect in de novo patients (Gomes-Mancilla et al., 1992; Erme et al., 1992).

EDM 49980

This partial dopamine agonist can ameliorate, in monotherapy, parkinsonian symptoms to a modest yet significant degree (Bravi et al., 1993). It appears to act as a weak dopamine agonist without appreciable dopamine antagonist activity. When administred with levodopa has no effect on parkinsonian and dyskinesia scores. At low doses it is well tolerated (Bravi et al., 1993).

LY 171555 (Quinpirole)

Quinpirole is a D_2 agonist. It shows an antitremor effect when tested in a monkey previously rendered parkinsonian by MPTP. Its effect can be potentiate by the coadministration of a D_1 agonist, benzergoline, which is inactive on tremor when administered alone (Gomez-Mancilla et al., 1992).

Lergotrile, Mesulergine, Phno, Quinagolide

Because of severe side effects (both oncological and hepatic) therapies using these compounds have been abandoned.

Conclusions

The management of Parkinson's disease still represents a major problem. While levodopa is the most effective mean for symptom relief, many Parkinsonians lose the consistency of optimal symptoms control. Several alternative mechanisms at the level of the CNS have been proposed (e.g., a narrowed therapeutical window for receptor-mediated effects, or the loss of storage capability for dopamine in the parkinsonian brain). Dopaminergic agonists have played a major role in improving such problems. They can be extremely usefull for managing problems such as declined efficacy or increased sensitivity to levodopa. While D_2 receptor agonism appears to be a necessary property for most anti-parkinsonian effects, pharmacological characteristics defining the "ideal" drug of this class are not fully known, nor the best strategies for their long-term use along with levodopa. The gradual introduction and titration of these drugs is a key part of their success. Whether their chronic use (alone or as a combination therapy from the start) can lessen the long term risks for dyskinesias and motor fluctuations, or even slow down the disease progression, remains to be clarified.

Different opinions are so far fully justified in such an uncertain field. We report here, without any comment, four conclusive statements from leading scientists on this field.

"The therapeutic efficacy of dopamine agonists alone in the primary treatment of Parkinson's disease is only moderate and significantly less than that of levodopa. Furthermore, only a small proportion of the patients have long-term benefit and tolerance. Thus dopamine agonists alone do not seem to be useful antiparkinsonian agents as the primary treatment for the majority of patients, despite the fact that they produce less fluctuations in disability" (Rinne, 1989).

"The use of dopamine receptor agonists in Parkinson's disease has a compelling logic. These agents are supposed to act indipendently of the dying cells of the substantia nigra directly on the cells of the striatum. Early clinical trials in advanced disease were only mildly impressive. Later they were found to be beneficial in early disease but their effectiveness waned. Their ultimate failure reflect the fact that the majority of current agents do not stimulate D_1 and D_2 receptors in a physiological ratio. The drugs may act presynaptically and with the eventual loss of the anatomic relationships between nigra and striatum the drugs fail" (King, 1992).

"Levodopa sparing strategies designed to minimize the cumulative levodopa dosage employed over the course of the disease seem a rational way to treat Parkinson patients in face of current information. Such a strategy would include the use of dopamine agonists as possible primary symptomatic therapy, the introduction of levodopa as an adjunct when dopamine agonists can no longer sufficiently provide satisfactory clinical control and the use of the lowest dose of levodopa that will provide satisfactory clinical control" (Olanow, 1992).

"The use of early combination therapy with bromocriptine and levodopa in Parkinson's disease is controversial . . . We conclude that there is no justifiable reason to use a combination of bromocriptine and levodopa in early parkinsonian patients' (Factor and Weiner, 1993).

These are the only possible answers to the main question put earlier about the amount of new drugs we have to deal with, in the search of an appropriate therapy of Parkinson's disease.

References

Albani C, Popescu R, Lacher R, Boke-Kuhn K (1992) Single dose response to Pramipexole in patients with Parkinson's disease. Mov Disord 7 [Suppl 1]: 98

Barker R, Duncan J, Lees A (1989) Subcutaneous apomorphine as a diagnostic test for dopaminergic responsiveness in parkinsonian syndromes. Lancet i: 675

Baronti F, Ruggieri S, Stocchi F, et al (1992) Terguride therapy of Parkinson's disease. Mov Disord 7 [Suppl 1]: 98

Baronti F, Mouradian MM, Davis TL, et al (1992) Continuous lisuride effects on central dopaminergic mechanisms in Parkinson's disease. Ann Neurol 32: 776–781

Bravi D, Davis TL, Mouradian MM, Chase TN (1993) Treatment of Parkinson's disease with the partial dopamine agonist EDM 49980. Mov Disord 2: 195–197

Clarenbach P, Ahrens-Kortenbruch D, Zierz S, Gueldenberg V, Boeke-Kuhn K, Herschel M (1992) Talipexole: effects and tolerability in a double-blind, controlled, randomized trial in advanced Parkinson's disease. Mov Disord 7 [Suppl 1]: 99

Di Salle E, et al (1982) FCE21336 (cabergoline): prolactin inhibiting action in the rat compared with pergolide and lisuride and other actions on the endocrine system. Farmitalia Carlo Erba Confidential report n° 204

Eden RJ, Costall B, Domeney AM, et al (1991) Preclinical pharmacology of ropinirole (SK&F 101468-A) a novel dopamine D_2 agonist. Pharmacol Biochem Behav 38: 147–154

Erme M, Rinne UK, Rascol A, Lees A, Agid Y, Lataste X (1992) Effects of a selective partial D_1 agonist, CY 208 243, in de novo patients with Parkinson's disease. Mov Disord 7: 239–243

Factor SA, Weiner WJ (1993) Early combination therapy with bromocriptine and levodopa in Parkinson's disease. Mov Disord 8: 257–262

Frankel JP, Lees AJ, Kempster PA, et al (1990) Subcutaneous apomorphine in the treatment of Parkinson's disease. J Neurol Neurosurg Psychiatry 55: 96–101

Goetz CG, Diederich NJ (1992) Dopaminergic agonists in the treatment of Parkinson's disease. Neurol Clin 10: 527–540

Gomes-Mancilla B, Boucher R, Bédard PJ (1992) Effect of LY 171555 and CY 208 243 on tremor suppression in the MPTP monkey model of parkinsonism. Mov Disord 7: 43–47

Gomes-Mancilla B, Boucher R, Gagnon C, Di Paolo T, Markstein R, Bédard PJ (1993) Effect of adding the D_1 agonist CY 208 243 to chronic bromocriptine treatment. 1°: evaluation of motor parameters in relation to striatal catecholamine content and dopamine receptors. Mov Disord 8: 144–150

Hely MA, Morris JGL, Rail D, et al (1989) The Sydney Multicenter Study of Parkinson's Disease: a report on the first three years. J Neurol Neurosurg Psychiatry 52: 324–328

Hornykiewicz O (1981) Brain neurotansmitters changes in Parkinson's disease. Mov Disord: 41–53

Hutton JT, Morris JL, Brewer MA (1993) Controlled study of the antiparkinsonian activity and tolerability of cabergoline. Neurology 43: 613–616

Jori MC, Franceschi M, Giusti MC, et al (1990) Clinical experience with cabergoline, e new ergoline derivative, in the treatment of Parkinson's disease. In: Streifler MB, Korczyn AD, Melamed E, Youdim MHB (eds) Advances in neurology, vol 53.

Parkinson's disease: anatomy, pathology, and therapy. Raven Press, New York, pp 539–543

Kapoor R, Pirtosek Z, Frankek JP, et al (1989) Treatment of Parkinson's disease with novel dopamine D2 agonist SKF 101468. Lancet ii: 1445–1446

King DB (1992) The place of dopaminergic agonists in the treatment of Parkinson's disease: the view from the trenches. Can J Neurol Sci 19: 156–159

Lees AJ, Stern GM (1981) Pergolide and lisuride for levodopa-induced oscillations. Lancet ii: 557

Lera G, Vaamonde J, Muruzabal J, Obeso JA (1990) Cabergoline: a long-acting dopamine agonist in Parkinson's disease. Ann Neurol 28: 593–594

LeWitt PA, Gopinathan G, Ward CD, et al (1982) Lisuride versus bromocriptine treatment in Parkinson's disease: a double blind study. Neurology 32: 69–72

Lieberman AN, Goldstein M (1985) Bromocriptine in Parkinson's disease. Pharmacol Rev 37: 217–227

Lieberman AN, Neophytides A, Leibowitz M, et al (1983) Comparative efficacy of PERG and BCT in patients with advanced Parkinson's disease. Adv Neurol 37: 95–108

Langtry HD, Clissold SP (1990) Pergolide. A review of its pharmacological properties and therapeutic potential in Parkinson's disease. Drugs 39: 491–506

Mierau J, Bechtel WD (1988) SND 919 Y inhibits dopamine release in vivo and in vitro. Psychopharmacology 96 [Suppl]: 338

Mizuno Y, Kowa H, Yanagisawa N, Nakanishi T (1992) Clinical experience on talipexole dihydrochloride (B-HT 920) in the treatment of Parkinson's disease. Mov Disord [Suppl 1]: 98

Molho S, Factor SA, Weiner WJ, Sanchez-Ramos JR, Singer C, et al (1993) The use of pramipexole, a novel dopamine (DA) agonist, in advanced Parkinson's disease. Neurology 43: 879

Montastruc JL, Rascol O, Rascol A (1989) A randomized controlled study of bromocriptine versus levodopa in previously untreated parkinsonian patients: a 3 year follow up. J Neurol Neurosurg Psychiatry 52: 773–775

Obeso JA, Luquin MR, Vaamonde J, et al (1988) Subcutaneous administration of lisuride in the treatment of complex motor fluctuations in Parkinson's disease. J Neural Transm 27 [Suppl]: 17–25

Obeso JA, Lera G, Vaamonde J, et al (1991) Cabergoline for the treatment of motor complications in Parkinson's disease. Neurology 41 [Suppl 1]: 172

Olanow CW (1992) A rationale for dopamine agonists as primary therapy for Parkinson's disease. Can J Neurol Sci 19: 108–112

Pacchetti C, Martignoni E, Ahfdenmebrinke B, et al (1992) Terguride in fluctuating parkinsonian patients: a double-blind study versus placebo. Mov Disord 7 [Suppl]: 99

Pacchetti C, Martignoni E, Bruggi P, et al (1993) Terguride in fluctuating parkinsonian patients: a double-blind study versus placebo. Mov Disord 8: 463–465

Pollak P, Champay AS, Gaio JM, et al (1990) Administration sous-cutanée d'apomorphine dans les fluctuations motrices de la maladie de Parkinson. Rev Neurol 146: 116–122

Rinne UK (1983) New ergot derivatives in the treatment of Parkinson's disease. In: Calne DB, et al (eds) Lisuride and other dopamine agonists. Raven Press, New York, pp 431–442

Rinne UK (1985) Combined bromocriptine-levodopa therapy early in Parkinson's disease. Neurology 35: 1196–1197

Rinne UK (1987) Early combination of bromocriptine and levodopa in the treatment of Parkinson's disease: a 5-year follow-up. Neurology 37: 826–828

Rinne UK (1989) Early dopamine agonist therapy in Parkinson's disease. Mov Disord 4: 586–594

Schingnitz G, Mireau J (1991) Postsynaptic dopamine agonistic effect of the autoreceptor agonist pramipexole. Biol Psychiatry 29: 609S

UK Bromocriptine Research Group (1982) Bromocriptine in Parkinson's disease: a double blind study comparing "low-slow" and "high-fast" introductory dosage regimens in de novo patients. J Neurol Neurosurg Psychiatry 52: 77–82

Vidailhet MJ, Bonnet AM, Belal S, Dubois B, Marle C, Agid Y (1990) Ropinirole without levodopa in Parkinson's disease (letter). Lancet 336: 316–317

Wachtel H, Dorow R, Sauer G (1984) Novel 8-aplha-ergolines with inhibitory and stimulatory effects on prolactin secretion in rats. Life Sci 35: 1859–1867

Weill E (1884) De l'apomorphine dans certains troubles nerveux. Lyon Med 40: 411–419

Zierz S, Gueldenberg V, Boeke-Kuhn K, Herschel M (1992) Talipexole: effects, safety and tolerability during long-term treatment in an open follow-up trial in advanced Parkinson's disease. Mov Disord 7 [Suppl 1]: 99

Authors' address: Dr. F. Piccoli, Institute of Neuropsychiatry, University of Palermo, Via G. La Loggia 1, I-90124 Palermo, Italy.

J Neural Transm (1995) [Suppl] 45: 197–202
© Springer-Verlag 1995

The response of "de novo" Parkinson's disease patients to Bromocriptine in a "low and slow" regimen is predictive for prognosis

C. Sampaio[1], **T. Coelho**[2], **A. Castro-Caldas**[3], **A. Bastos-Lima**[2], and **A. Levy**[3]

[1] Instituto de Farmacologia e Terapêutica Geral, Lisbon Faculty of Medicine, Lisbon,
[2] Department of Neurology, Hospital de St° António, Porto, and [3] Centro de Estudos Egas Moniz, Lisbon Faculty of Medicine, Lisbon, Portugal

Summary. It is possible that Bromocriptine only determines a complete antiparkinson effect in a subset of P.D. patients that have a good dopaminergic reserve. Our study intent to demonstrate that a good short-term response to Bromocriptine used in a "low and slow" regimen is a marker of long term good prognosis. We studied a series of 36 sequencial "de novo" P.D. patients treated with Bromocriptine in a "low and slow" regimen. The principal end-point was the introduction of Levodopa. "Good prognosis" was definied as no need of Levodopa until five years of follow-up. An improvement greater than 33% in the Columbia rating scale, at the 6th month of treatment, was the cut-off point to decide that a patient had a good short term response to Bromocriptine. Nine patients fulfilled the criteria for beeing good short term responders. Multiple regression analysis showed that this outcome could not be predicted by the clinical characteristics of the patients at admission. The sensitivity and the specificity of the short term response to Bromocriptine to predict a good prognosis were 70% and 90.5% respectively. We conclude that Bromocriptine in monotherapy is an efficient antiparkinson agent in 1/3 of "de novo" P.D. patients and good short term response to Bromocriptine is an acceptable marker for a good prognosis. Therefore it is possible that the response to Bromo criptine is a discriminator for a subset of P.D. patients in the early phases of the disease.

Introduction

The role of dopamine agonists in monotherapy or in early association with Levodopa/Dopa decarboxylase inhibitor (LD/DDI) for "de novo" Parkinson's disease (P.D.) patients is still a matter of controversy (Factor and Weiner, 1993; Rinne, 1993). One factor that contributes for the difficulties on analysing the data from trials is the heterogeneity of P.D. patients in what concerns progression of the disease. Other important point is the possibility that some drugs work better in a yet unidentified subgroup of patients. It is possible that a full antiparkinson effect is only achieved when at least D1 and D2 dopamine receptors are activated (Robertson, 1992). Bromocriptine is a selective agonist for D2 receptors therefore the presence of endogenous dopamine is necessary to fulfill the requirement of D1 activation (Goldstein et al., 1985; Robertson and Robertson, 1987). It is legitimate to presume that those patients that get a major antiparkinson effect with Bromocriptine are those that have a good dopaminergic reserve. This study intents to demonstrate that a good short term response to Bromocriptine used in a "low and slow" regimen is a marker for a good long term prognosis.

Patients and methods

Trial design

This was an open, non-comparative trial. The patients were sequentially admitted. The protocol was approved by the Ethical committee of the Lisbon Faculty of Medicine/ Hospital Santa Maria.

Subjects

Thirty-six patients were included (15 female and 21 male). The decision for inclusion was based on the following criteria: An unequivocal diagnosis of idiopathic Parkinson's disease according with a careful clinical examination and a complete questionnaire concerning potential iatrogenic drugs; No previous use of any antiparkinsonian drugs except for anticholinergics if they were withdrawn one month before enrollment; Staging I or II Hoehn and Yahr scale. Patients were excluded if they suffered from an additional disorder which would interfere with the clinical ratings, with the adherence to the protocol or with the expected survival.

Informed consent was obtained.

Evaluations

The tools used were the Columbia rating scale, the Hoehn and Yahr staging and questionnaires for side-effects, motor fluctuations and dyskinesias. These evaluations were timed at: 0 (baseline); 15th day, 1st month, 3rd month, 6th month, 1st year and yearly thereafter.

Drug titration

The starting dose of Bromocriptine was 3.75 mg achieved during the first 15 days with increments of 1.25/day. Until the end of the 1st month the dose was 7.5 mg. After this the dosage could be slowly increased (increments of 1.25 mg) until a maximum of 30 mg/day.

End-points

The primary end-point was the level of disability that implied the need for Levodopa. This decision was based on a clinical judgement. A "good prognosis" was defined as no need of Levodopa in the first 5 years of treatment. "Short-term good responders to Bromocriptine" were those patients that showed a decrease greater than 33% in the score of the Columbia rating scale, at the 6th month of treatment UK Bromocriptine research group (1989).

Statistical methods

The "survival curve" for the need of Levodopa was calculated. The patients included in the trial were stratified in two groups according to their short-term response to Bromocriptine ("good" or "not good") and according to the existence of a "good prognosis". The ability for the "short term response to Bromocriptine" to predict a "good prognosis" was measure calculating the sensibility and the specificity. In this circumstances the "short term response to Bromocriptine" was taken as a screening test for the outcome "good prognosis". Multiple regression analysis was used to identify any factors associated with the classification as a "good short-term responder".

Results

1. Characteristics of the population

Table 1 shows the characteristics of the population admitted, in what concerns: Age, mean duration of the disease before admission, the total and partial scores of the Columbia rating scale at baseline and the Hoehn and Yahr stage.

From the 36 patients admitted we had 4 drop-outs: Three were lost for follow-up because the patient did not return to the outpatient clinic. The other abandoned the use of Bromocriptine due to the appearance of dyskinesias of the left foot and shoulder at the first month of treatment with the drug.

2. Timing for the introduction of Levodopa

The figure represents the "survival curve" based on the time elapsed between the initiation of the treatment with Bromocriptine and the decision to use Levodopa. The cumulative probability for the need of Levodopa before the 2nd year is 48.4 ± 17.6%. The mean follow-up of the patients were 6.56 ± 1.2 years.

3. Response to Bromocriptine

At the 6th month of treatment 9 (36%) patients showed an improvement greater than a 33% decrease in the Columbia rating scale; Twenty-five (64%)

Table 1

	Mean	St. deviation	Range
Age (years)	58.4	8.9	40–70
Duration of the disease (months)	17.5	15.8	3–72
Stage (H&Y)	1.6	0.55	0–2
Total score	17.3	7.1	6–33
Tremor score	2.6	1.8	0–8
Rigidty score	4.3	3.3	0–10
Akinesia score	8.3	3.8	3–16

(N = 36; 15 female, 21 male)

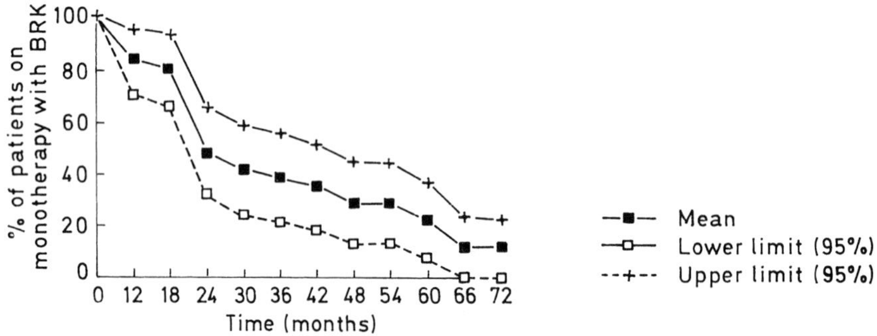

patients did not reached a decrease of 33%. From these, 12 (48%) patients had an improvement between 0 and 33% and 13 (52%) patients did not improve. Multiple regression analysis showed that the outcome — improvement greater than 33% — cannot be predicted by the clinical characteristics of the patients at admission.

Table 2 condenses the stratification of the patients according to the "short-term response to Bromocriptine" and with the quality of the prognosis ("good" or "not good"). The "short term response to Bromocriptine" as a screening test for "good prognosis" has a Sensitivity = 70%, Specificity = 90.5%, a Positive predictive value = 77.7% and a Negative predictive value = 90.4%.

4. Side-effects

There were 12 events (Nausea and Vomiting = 9; Epigastric distress = 1; Ortostatic Hypotension = 1; Hallucinations = 1) classified as side-effects of Bromocriptine. These events occurred in 9 patients. All side-effects were transient and could be controlled either by reducing Bromocriptine dosage or adding Domperidone until a maximum dosage of 30 mg/day. After introduction of Levodopa 10 patients developed motor fluctuations (wearing-off); 5 patients developed peak-dose dyskinesias, 3 patients suffered psychosis and 1 patient developed end-of-dose dystonia.

Table 2. Short-term response to bromocriptine (6th month)
versus long-term prognosis

	Good short-term response	No good short-term response
Good long-term prognosis	7	2
No good long-term prognosis	3	19

Discussion

Our data showed that Bromocriptine in monotherapy is an efficient antiparkinson agent in 1/3 of a population of "de novo" P.D. patients in the early phase of the disease. This is a well-known figure since several other authors (Lees and Stern, 1981; Teychenne et al., 1982; Grimes and Delgado 1985; Tolosa et al., 1987) found similar percentages in their series. The development of unequivocal dyskinesias in a patient under recent use of Bromocriptine is an extraordinary finding in P.D. patients (UK Bromocriptine research group, 1989). Leiguarda et al. (1993) had found dystonia in aphasic patients treated with Bromocriptine, but the dosage used in their case was higher than ours.

The use of Bromocriptine proved to be able to postpone about two years the use of Levodopa in ~42% of patients. This can be an interesting asset if the delay of introducing Levodopa proves to be useful on clinical grounds (Duvoisin, 1987).

The results also demonstrate that the patients who got an important antiparkinson effect with Bromocriptine were those who had have a good prognosis. This was found even when a very conservative definition of good prognosis is used (no need of Levodopa at 5 years of follow-up). The dosage reached is an important factor to take in consideration because UK Bromocriptine research group (1989) found that a "high and fast" regime can obtain a greater number of good short term responders than a "low and slow" regimen. It is suspected that the "low and slow" and the "high and fast" regimens had different pharmacodynamic profiles. Therefore it is impossible to known from our data if a good response to a "high and fast" regimen has the same impact in terms of prognosis.

We were unable to identify any clinical variable that could predict the improvement at the 6th month of treatment. One possible reason is the lack of statistical power due to a small sample size. However other series greater than ours (Rascol et al., 1979; Lees and Stern, 1981; UK Bromocriptine research group, 1989) found similar negative results. It is plausible to admit that if there is some predictive effect of a clinical variable this is a small one or it is confounded.

The existence of a subset of P.D. patients characterised for having a good therapeutic effect with Bromocriptine and a good long-term prognosis is of crucial importance for future comparative clinical trials. It is obvious that if this subset of patients is preferentially enrolled in one arm of a study, the results will be biased. Care should be taken to randomly distributed those patients.

References

Duvoisin RC (1987) To treat early or to treat late? Ann Neurol 21: 2–3

Factor SA, Weiner WJ (1993) Early combination therapy with bromocriptine and levodopa in Parkinson's disease. Mov Disord 8: 257–262

Goldstein M, Lieberman A, Meller E (1985) A possible molecular mechanism for the antiparkinsonian action of Bromocriptine in combination with levodopa. TIPS 6: 436–437

Grimes JD, Delgado MR (1985) Bromocriptine: problems with low-dose de novo therapy in Parkinson's disease. Clin Neuropharmacol 8: 73–77

Lees AJ, Stern GM (1981) Sustained bromocriptine therapy in previously untreated patients with Parkinson's disease. J Neurol Neurosurg Psychiatry 44: 1020–1023

Leiguarda R, Merello M, Sabe L, Starkstein S (1993) Bromocriptine-induced dystonia in patients with aphasia and hemiparesis. Neurology 43: 2319–2322

Rascol A, Guirand B, Montastruc JL, David J, Clanet M (1979) Long-term treatment of Parkinson's disease with bromocriptine. J Neurol Neurosurg Psychiatry 42: 143–150

Rinne UK (1993) Strategies in the treatment of early Parkinson's disease. Acta Neurol Scand 87 [Suppl 146]: 50–53

Robertson GS, Robertson HA (1987) D1 and D2 dopamine agonist synergism: separate sites of action? TIPS 8: 295–299

Robertson HA (1992) Synergistic interactions of D1- and D2-delective agonists in animal models for Parkinson's disease: sites of action and implications for the pathogenesis of dyskinesias. Can J Neurol Sci 19 [Suppl 1]: 147–52

Teychenne PF, Bergsrud MN, Racy A (1982) Bromocriptine: low-dosage in Parkinson's disease. Neurology 32: 577–83

Tolosa E, Blesa R, Bayes A (1987) Low-dose Bromocriptine in the early phases of Parkinson's disease. Clin Neuropharmacol 10: 169–174

UK Bromocriptine research group (1989) Bromocriptine in Parkinson's disease: a double-blind study comparing "low-slow" and "high-fast" introductory dosage regimens in de novo patients. J Neurol Neurosurg Psychiatry 52: 77–82

Authors' address: C. Sampaio, M.D., Instituto de Farmacologia e Terapêutica Geral, Faculdade de Medicina de Lisboa, Hospital de Santa Maria, P-1600 Lisboa, Portugal.

J Neural Transm (1995) [Suppl] 45: 203–212

Pergolide mesylate in Parkinson's disease treatment

G. Pezzoli, M. Canesi, A. Pesenti, and **C. B. Mariani**

Ospedale Maggiore Policlinico, Institute of Neurology, University of Milan,
Milan, Italy

Summary. In the past 15 years, clinical data of over 1,500 patients treated with pergolide mesylate have been published. Pergolide is a dopamine agonist with a potent stimulating effect on D2 and also on D1 receptors. This pharmacodynamic characteristic seems the most effective in increasing the motility in Parkinson's disease. Pergolide has been used almost exclusively as an adjunct to levodopa treatment. Its positive effects seems to be related to its long plasma half life, about 27 hours, and 5–6 hours of clinical activity; it has shown to be effective on all parkinsonian symptoms except for the reduction of postural reflexes, it reduces off periods and, compared to bromocriptine, it considerably improves the activities of daily living.

Adverse reactions are, for the most part, mild and reversible, they mostly include nausea and gastroenteric disturbances.

Introduction

Parkinson's disease is a neurodegenerative disorder, predominantly involving the dopaminergic neurons of the Substantia Nigra and the noradrenergic neurons of the Locus Coeruleus. Vast studies have been done, in the last decades, on the disease's anatomical, biochemical and functional damage (Oertel and Kupsch, 1993). In recent years the therapeutical advances have been among the most successful in the field of neurology. The substitutive therapy with levodopa, available since the end of the 60's, at first seemed to have completely resolved the problems related to this disease. In the years that followed it has been observed that the use of levodopa alone, or associated with decarboxylase inhibitors (DCI), resulted, after a few years of treatment, in "typical" side effects, mainly dyskinesias and dystonias that are called "long-term levodopa syndrome" (Poewe, 1994). PD patients present a polymorphic symptomatology according to the age of the onset of the disease and the therapy used. We have now arrived at the point where diagnostic and therapeutical algorithms are often available therefore facilitating the decisions the neurologist must make (Koller et al., 1994).

Dopamine agonists

During different periods of the disease dopamine agonists are suggested (Koller et al., 1994). Bromocriptine, lisuride, pergolide and apomorphine are the principal dopamine agonists available on the European market to-day (Montastruc et al., 1993). The advantages of dopamine agonists over levodopa (which is still the most effective drug in the treatment of Parkinson's disease) is linked to a precise neuropathological event. From the onset of Parkinson's disease, the dopaminergic nigrostriatal terminals are diminished and tend to progressively degenerate. As the disease progresses levodopa can not be transformed inside the dopaminergic terminals and is probably meta-bolised into dopamine in other brain cells such as the astroglial and endothelial cells. The non physiological compartmentalization of the dopam-ine could be one of the reasons for the "unpredictable on-off fluctuations" present in the advanced stages of the disease (Sage and Mark, 1994). The dopamine agonists are directly active on the dopaminergic receptor, independently from the presence of intact nigrostriatal terminals.

In the last twenty years, the pharmacological characteristics of these com-pounds have encouraged several pharmaceutical companies to continue basic and clinical research in this area; however to date molecules as effective as levodopa have not been found. A large number of clinical studies have shown the efficacy of these drugs in both monotherapy and as adjunct to levodopa therapy.

Most of the recent studies have shown that the combination of levodopa and dopamine agonists is better than levodopa by itself (Rinne, 1993).

In other research, not yet confirmed in humans, a neuroprotective effect of certain dopamine agonists has been shown on the nigrostriatal neurons (Glover et al., 1993).

Pergolide

Pergolide mesylate, a semisynthetic ergoline derivative, has a chemical struc-ture that is not so different from the other dopamine agonists (being more similar to lisuride than bromocriptine, Fig. 1), (Langtry and Clissold, 1990). Pergolide stimulates the receptors D1 and D2; this particular charac-teristic makes it different from bromocriptine which stimulates the D2 dopaminergic receptors and partially inhibits the D1 presynaptic receptors (Montastruc et al., 1993). It is believed that the "antiparkinson motor effect" is primarily due to the stimulation of the D2 receptors, but it is probably necessary to also have a D1 receptor stimulation for the optimal motor activity. These data has also been experimentally confirmed by using drugs that block the formation of dopamine in the presynaptic area: this treatment reduces the activity of bromocriptine but not that of pergolide (Lataste et al., 1989).

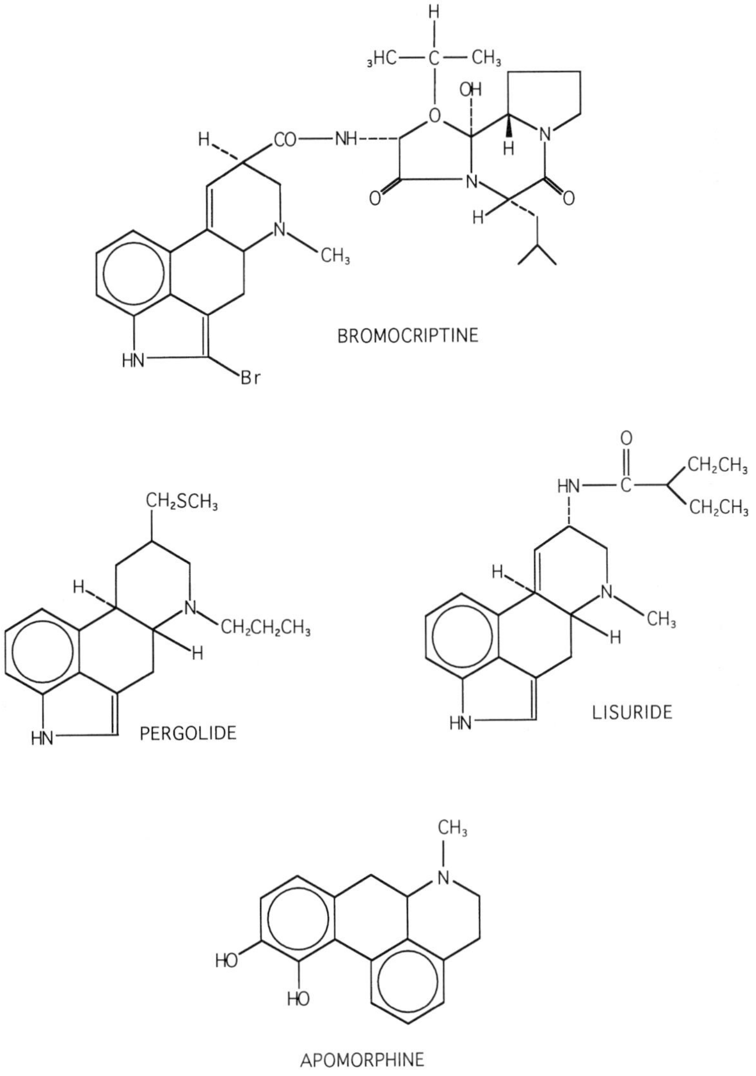

Fig. 1

Pergolide is rapidly absorbed in the gastrointestinal tract, beginning in the stomach and reaching its maximum plasmatic concentration at around 80 minutes: the effects last for about 5 hours. The radiolabelled compound is eliminated from the body in about 5 days. The half-life of the drug is about 27 hours, which is much longer than that of levodopa, allowing a sub-continuous stimulation of the dopaminergic receptors. Ninety per cent of pergolide binds to the plasmatic proteins (albumin and glycoprotein fractions). It is primarily eliminated in the urine (about 55%), in the faeces (about 50%) and through respiration (about 5%) (Rubin et al., 1981).

Table 1. Principal clinical studies on Pergolide from 1979 to 1994

Year	Reference	No. pt	Age PD	HY onset	Study design	No. week	Drug	Ldopa mean mg	Ldopa+pe	% Reduction	pe mean mg	% PD improvement
1979	Lieberman A	13			o	6	pe+Ld				2.4	40
1981	Lieberman A	13	11.9	3.6	o − db	2–10	pe+Ld − pe+Ld vs pl+Ld	965	680	29.5	2.4	14.6
1982	Tanner CM	23	13.0	3.0	o	24	pe + Ld				2.8	49.7
1982	Lang AE	26	7.5		o − db	20–38	pe+Ld − pe+Ld vs pl+Ld	1.100		30		
1982	Lieberman A	40	12.4		o − db cr	1–24	pe+Ld − pe+Ld vs pl+Ld	975			2.4	
1982	Lieberman A	56	12.8		o	56	pe+Ld	1,000		50	2.5	44
1983	Lieberman A	40	12.7	3.4	o − co	92	pe+Ld vs br+Ld	975			2.1	40 (on)
1983	LeWitt PA	24	11.0		db two period cr	7–10	pe+Ld vs br+Ld	792			3.3	
1983	Goetz CG	22	13.6	3.0	o	52	pe+Ld				2.85	32.3
1983	Ilson J	11	14.4		o − db cr − o	6	pe+Ld − pe+Ld cr pl+Ld − p	(2.35 g)*		50	2.9	
1983	Jankovic J	22	9.2		o − db − o	43	pe+Ld − pe+Ld vs pl+Ld	705	226	68	2.5	
1983	Klawans HL	16	12.6	3.0	o	24	pe+Ld					46.5
1984	Diamond SG	8	14.1	2.0	o	52	pe+Ld	(1.29 g)*	(1.10 g)*	14.7	2.1	30
1984	Mear JY	16	8.5	2.75	o	0	pe − pe+Ld	660			6.3	73
1984	Jeanty P	18	9.0		o	3–106	pe+Ld	843	283	66	3.8	24
1984	ibidem	8	2.5		o		pe	0			2.8	31
1984	Lieberman A	17	14	3.2	o	120	pe+Ld				2.2	20
1985	Sage JI	17			db	26	pe vs pl					
1985	Diamond SG	20	9.9	3.0	pa db	2 + 24	pe+Ld vs pl+Ld	941	677	28	3.14	
1985	Gonce M	9	8.6	3.7	o		pe+Ld	597.2	330.5	44.6	2.0	s.i.
1985	Goetz CG	10	12.2	3.0	o	260	pe+Ld after br	(4.8 g)*	(2.7 g)*	43.7	3.8	21.5
1985	Jankovic J	18			o	120	pe+Ld	694	468	32.5	3.2	36.7
1985	Kurlan R	9	16.9	4.0	o	172	pe+Ld	1,115			2.2	0
1986	Wright A	10 + 7	0.25	2.3	o	27.8	pe; mes	0	0	0	3.7	0
1986	Jankovic J	20	11.4	3.3	pa db	24	pe+Ld vs pl+Ld			46.4	4.6	
1986	Jankovic J	22	9.2	3.2	o − db	10	pe+Ld − pe+Ld vs pl+Ld	705	226	68	2.5	65
1986	ibidem	18	11	3.2	o	112	pe+Ld		232.6	33	3.2	42
1986	Sage JI	35			o no co	200	pe					
1986	Tanner CM	17	12	3.0	o no co	208	pe+Ld	(3.4 g)*			3.25	
1986	Markham CH	24	10	3.0	db ra	24	pe+Ld vs pl+Ld	941	677	28		
1987	Olanow CW	46	10.1	3.2	pa db	2 + 24	pe+Ld vs pl+Ld	910.7	596.4	35	2.5	43.7
1988	Factor SA	63	12.5	3.5	o re	4–148	pe+Ld					
1988	Ahlskog JE	39	12.2	3.0	o	130–156	pe+Ld					
1988	Ahlskog JE	49		3.0	db	2 + 24	pe+Ld vs pl+Ld	1,052	635	40	4.0	
1991	Zimmerman T	14	13.3	2.7	o re l	252	pe+Ld vs Ld	1,067	952	10.8	3.5	
1991	ibidem	12	9.7	2.7	o re ll	8.5	pe+Ld vs Ld	1,210				
1991	Pezzoli G	19	9	3.18	o no co	12	pe+Ld	680	540	21	1.63	
1994	Olanow CW	376	10.9	3.0	db	2 + 24	pe+Ld vs pl+Ld	891.4	656.1	26.4	2.94	25–50
1994	Pezzoli G	57	6.6	3.15	sb cr	2 + 24	pe+Ld vs br+Ld	658.3	635.1	3.5	2.3	

br bromocriptine; *co* comparative; *cr* crossover; *db* double blind; *HY* Hoehn Yahr stage at the onset of the treatment; *Ld* levo-dopa; *mes* mesulergine; *o* open; *pa* parallel; *pe* pergolide; *pl* placebo; *pt* patient; *ra* random; *re* retrospective; *red* reduction; *sb* single blind; *s.i.* significant improvement; * levo-dopa without DCI

Clinical studies

Pergolide has been studied in various pharmacological trials: comparative and non comparative studies of short and long duration, alone or associated with levodopa and levodopa plus decarboxylase inhibitors (Sinemet®, Madopar®). The comparative studies were done with placebo or dopamine agonists. More than 40 studies involving about 1,500 patients have been published over the past 15 years, most of them are listed in Table 1.

Non comparative studies

Most of the trials on pergolide, involving more than 850 cases, were non comparative (Lieberman et al., 1979, 1982, 1984; Lang et al., 1982; Tanner et al., 1982; Ilson et al., 1983; Mear et al., 1984; Gonce et al., 1985; Goetz et al., 1983; Klawans et al., 1983; Diamond and Markham, 1984; Jeanty et al., 1984; Jankovic, 1985; Kurlan et al., 1985; Sage and Duvoisin, 1986; Tanner et al., 1986; Factor et al., 1988; Ahlskog and Muenter, 1988; Pezzoli et al., 1991). The duration of these studies ranged from "single dose" to several years. In many of these trials it has been demonstrated that pergolide is effective in most PD patients. Pergolide is particularly effective in reducing the "off" time and most of the symptoms of PD. Due to the non rigorous design of these studies only limited conclusions can be drown. Most of the results of these trials, however, are in agreement with those of the comparative ones.

Monotherapy studies

No rigorously controlled trials have been performed on "de novo" patients (Mear et al., 1984). Very few non blind non parallel studies tend to demonstrate that pergolide is effective on the majority of PD symptoms however it is not as effective as levodopa. Only 25% of the patients in the third year of the disease had benefits from the monotherapy treatment (Rinne, 1986).

Controlled studies versus placebo

Eight controlled trials versus placebo with a total of 545 patients have been studied (Jankovic, 1983; Diamond et al., 1985; Sage and Duvoisin, 1985; Jankovic and Orman, 1986; Markham and Diamond, 1986; Olanow and Alberts, 1987; Ahlskog and Muenter, 1988; Olanow et al., 1994). Pergolide was given in doses ranging from 2.5 mg to 4.6 mg (mean daily dosage: about 3 mg). In pergolide treated patients levodopa dosage was reduced to about 35% (mean daily dose: 950 mg). Levodopa plus pergolide significantly reduced the "off" time from 26% to 76% (more than 35% mean reduction). The activity of daily living improved the mean score from 29% to 65% (35% mean improvement) and the severity of the disease, measured with various rating scales, was reduced from 22% to 58% (about 35% mean reduction). Over all the studies showed a great reduction of all principal PD symptoms (tremor, bradykinesia, rigidity), whereas no significant changes in balance were reported.

Controlled studies versus bromocriptine and lisuride

Two studies in double (Le Witt et al., 1983) and single blind crossover (Pezzoli et al., 1994) were conducted on 81 patients (24 and 57 respectively). Both studies had a similar experimental design and they are partially comparable. The initial levodopa dosage was 792 mg in the first study and 658 mg in the second; 3.3 and 2.3 mg of pergolide and 42.7 mg and 24.2 mg of bromocriptine were added, respectively. After the introduction of the dopamine agonist 22 patients out of 24 had benefits in the first study; 46 out of 57 in the second one.

At the end of the first study 11 patients preferred pergolide, 7 bromocriptine while 4 had no preferences. In the second study 29 patients preferred pergolide, 7 bromocriptine, 22 had no preferences. In the first study clinical evaluations showed no significant differences between the 2 drugs. In the second study pergolide proved to be superior to bromocriptine and particularly the activities of daily living improved considerably more in patients on pergolide compared to those on bromocriptine.

Table 2

	Incidence (%)	
Adverse effect	Pergolide (n = 189)	Placebo (n = 187)
Dyskinesia	62.4	24.6
Nausea	24.3	12.8
Dizziness	19.1	13.9
Hallucinations	13.8	3.2
Rhinitis	12.2	5.4
Dystonia	11.6	8.0
Confusion	11.1	9.6
Constipation	10.6	5.9
Somnolence	10.1	3.7
Postural hypotension	9.0	7.0
Insomnia	7.9	3.2
Pain	7.0	2.1
Diarrhoea	6.4	2.7
Dyspepsia	6.4	2.1
Anxiety	6.4	4.3
Abdominal pain	5.8	2.1
Injury, accident	5.8	7.0
Abnormal vision	5.8	5.4
Headache	5.3	6.4
Anorexia	4.8	2.7

From Olanow et al. (1994)

Table 3

	Incidence (%)	
Adverse effect	Pergolide (n = 68)	Bromocriptine (n = 68)
Nausea	5.8	8.8
Dyspepsia/heartburn	0	4.4
Abdominal pain	1.4	1.4
Postural hypotension	1.4	5.8
Syncope	1.4	0
Fatigue	0	2.9
Muscle cramps	1.4	0
Constipation	2.9	0
Diarrhoea	1.4	0
Intestinal obstruction*	1.4	0
Epistaxis*	1.4	0
Prostatitis*	1.4	0
Rectal cancer*	1.4	0

From Pezzoli et al. (1994). *Stated by the investigator as not drug-related

Few non rigorous studies of long duration showed that pergolide is more effective in reducing "off" time than both bromocriptine and lisuride (Lees and Stern, 1981). This may depend both on the pharmacokinetics and pharmacodynamics of pergolide. In fact, pergolide has a longer plasma half-life and a longer duration of action especially compared to lisuride. Pergolide, compared to bromocriptine, seems more effective on those patients with a poor preservation of presynaptic receptors.

Side effects

We here report the adverse events that are registered in the Eli Lilly file and that occurred in the double blind versus placebo study (Olanow et al., 1994), involving 376 patients (Table 2), and in the cross-over controlled study, pergolide versus bromocriptine (Pezzoli et al., 1994) involving 68 patients (Table 3). In Table 3, those side effects that are already rated in the motor scale are not listed.

Conclusions

It is apparently clear from this review that pergolide for its clinical activity is probably the most effective dopamine agonist in the treatment of PD, especially if complicated by on-off phenomena.

The fact remains, however, that the pharmacological treatment of parkinsonian patients must be empirically formulated and that a negative response to pergolide does not necessarily predict a negative response to other dopamine agonists.

References

Ahlskog JE, Muenter MD (1988) Treatment of Parkinson's disease with pergolide: a double-blind study. Mayo Clin Proc 63: 969–978

Ahlskog JE, Muenter MD (1988) Pergolide: long-term use in Parkinson's disease. Mayo Clin Proc 63: 979–987

Diamond SG, Markham CH (1984) One-year trial of pergolide as an adjunct to Sinemet in treatment of Parkinson's disease. Adv Neurol 40: 537–539

Diamond SG, Markham CH, Treciokas LJ (1985) Double-blind trial of pergolide for Parkinson's disease. Neurology 35: 291–295

Factor SA, Sanchez-Ramos JR, Weiner WJ (1988) Parkinson's disease: an open label trial of pergolide in patients failing bromocriptine therapy. J Neurol Neurosurg Psychiatry 51: 529–533

Glover V, Clow A, Sandler M (1993) Effects of dopaminergic drugs on superoxide dismutase: implications for senescence. J Neural Transm [Suppl] 40: 37–45

Goetz CG, Tanner CM, Glantz R, Klawans HL (1983) Pergolide in Parkinson's disease. Arch Neurol 40: 785–787

Goetz CG, Tanner CM, Glantz RH, Klawans HL (1985) Chronic agonist therapy for Parkinson's disease: a 5-year study of bromocriptine and pergolide. Neurology 35: 749–751

Gonce M, Delwaide PJ (1985) Etude clinique du pergolide dans la maladie de Parkinson. Presse Med 14: 1409–1411

Ilson J, Fahn S, Mayeux R, Cote LJ, Snider SR (1983) Pergolide treatment in parkinsonism. Adv Neurol 37: 85–94

Jankovic J (1983) Controlled trial of pergolide mesylate in Parkinson's disease and progressive supranuclear palsy. Neurology 33: 500–507

Jankovic J (1985) Long-term study of pergolide in Parkinson's disease. Neurology 35: 296–299

Jankovic J (1986) Pergolide: short-term and long-term experience in Parkinson's disease. In: Fahn S, et al (eds) Recent development in Parkinson's disease. Raven Press, New York, pp 339–345

Jankovic J, Orman J (1986) Parallel double-blind study of pergolide in Parkinson's disease. Adv Neurol 45: 551–554

Jeanty P, Van den Kerchove M, Lowenthal A, De Bruyne H (1984) Pergolide therapy in Parkinson's disease. J Neurol 231: 148–152

Klawans HL, Tanner CM, Glatt S, Goetz CG (1983) A 6-month trial of pergolide mesylate in the treatment of idiopathic Parkinson's disease. Adv Neurol 37: 75–83

Koller WC, Silver DE, Lieberman A (1994) An algorithm for the management of Parkinson's disease. Neurology 44 [Suppl 12]: 5–7

Kurlan R, Miller C, Levy R, Macik B, Hamill R, Shoulson I (1985) Long-term experience with pergolide therapy of advanced parkinsonism. Neurology 35: 738–742

Lang AE, Quinn N, Brincat S, Marsden CD, Parkes JD (1982) Pergolide in late-stage Parkinson disease. Ann Neurol 12: 243–247

Langtry HD, Clissold SP (1990) Pergolide. A review of its pharmacological properties and therapeutic potential in Parkinson's disease. Drugs 39: 491–506

Lataste X, Markstein R, Jaton AL (1989) Dopamine agonist: an update on the mode of action. In: Lieberman AN, Lataste X (eds) Parkinson's disease: the role of dopamine agonists. New trend in clinical neurology. Parthenon Publishing Group, Carnforth UK, pp 13–28

Lees AJ, Stern GM (1981) Pergolide and lisuride for levodopa-induced oscillation. Lancet ii: 577

LeWitt PA, Ward CD, Larsen TA, Raphaelson MI, Newman RP, Foster N, Dambrosia JM, Calne DB (1983) Comparison of pergolide and bromocriptine therapy in parkinsonism. Neurology 33: 1009–1014

Lieberman AN, Leibowitz M, Neophytides A, Kupersmith M, Mehl S, Kleinberg D, Serby M, Goldstein M (1979) Pergolide and lisuride for Parkinson's disease. Lancet ii: 1129–1130

Lieberman A, Goldstein M, Leibowitz M, Neophytides A, Kupersmith M, Pact V, Kleinberg D (1981) Treatment of advanced Parkinson disease with pergolide. Neurology 31: 675–682

Lieberman AN, Goldstein M, Neophytides A, Leibowitz M, Gopinathan G, Walker R, Pact V (1982) The use of pergolide, a potent dopamine agonist, in Parkinson's disease. Clin Pharmacol Ther 32: 70–75

Lieberman AN, Neophytides A, Leibowitz M, Gopinathan G, Pact V, Walker R, Goodgold A, Goldstein M (1983) Comparative efficacy of pergolide and bromocriptine in patients with advanced Parkinson's disease. Adv Neurol 37: 95–108

Lieberman AN, Goldstein M, Leibowitz M, Gopinathan G, Neophytides A, Hiesiger E, Nelson J, Walker R (1984) Long-term treatment with pergolide: decreased efficacy with time. Neurology 34: 223–226

Markham CH, Diamond SG (1986) Pergolide: a double-blind trial as adjunct therapy in Parkinson's disease. In: Fahn S, et al (eds) Recent development in Parkinson's disease. Raven Press, New York, pp 331–337

Mear JY, Barroche G, de Smet Y, Weber M, Lhermitte F, Agid Y (1984) Pergolide in the treatment of Parkinson's disease. Neurology 34: 983–986

Montastruc JL, Rascol O, Senard JM (1993) Current status of dopamine agonists in Parkinson's disease management. Drugs 46: 384–393

Oertel WH, Kupsch A (1993) Pathogenesis and animal studies of Parkinson's disease. Curr Opin Neurol Neurosurg 6: 323–332

Olanow CW, Alberts MJ (1987) Double-blind controlled study of pergolide mesylate in the treatment of Parkinson's disease. Clin Neuropharmacol 10: 178–185

Olanow CW, Fahn S, Muenter M, Klawans H, Hurtig H, Stern M, Shoulson I, Kurlan R, Grimes JD, Jankovic J, Hoehn M, Markham CH, Duvoisin R, Reinmuth O, Leonard HA, Ahlskog E, Feldman R, Hershey L, Yahr MD (1994) A multicenter double-blind placebo-controlled trial of pergolide as an adjunct to Sinemet in Parkinson's disease. Mov Disord 9: 40–47

Pezzoli G, Zecchinelli A, Mariani C, Reganati P, Scarlato G (1991) La pergolide mesilato nella terapia del morbo di Parkinson resistente ad altri trattamenti. Una prima esperienza italiana. Clin Ter 136(1): 39–45

Pezzoli G, Martignoni E, Pacchetti C, Angeleri VA, Lamberti P, Muratorio A, Bonuccelli U, De Mari M, Foschi N, Cossutta E, Nicoletti F, Giammona F, Canesi M, Scarlato G, Caraceni T, Moscarelli E (1994) Pergolide compared with bromocriptine in Parkinson's disease: a multicenter, crossover, controlled study. Mov Disord 9: 431–436

Poewe WH (1994) Clinical aspects of motor fluctuations in Parkinson's disease. Neurology 44 [Suppl 6]: 6–9

Rinne UK (1986) Dopamine agonist in the treatment of early Parkinson's disease. Adv Neurol 45: 519–523

Rinne UK (1993) Strategies in the treatment of early Parkinson's disease. Acta Neurol Scand [Suppl 1] 146: 50–53

Rubin A, Lemberger L, Dhahir P (1981) Physiologic disposition of pergolide. Clin Pharmacol Ther 30: 258–262

Sage JI, Duvoision RC (1985) Pergolide therapy in Parkinson's disease: a double-blind, placebo-controlled study. Clin Neuropharmacol 8: 260–265

Sage JI, Duvoisin RC (1986) Long-term efficacy of pergolide in patients with Parkinson's disease. Clin Neuropharmacol 9: 160–164
Sage JI, Mark MH (1994) Basic mechanisms of motor fluctuations. Neurology 44 [Suppl 6]: S10–S14
Tanner CM, Goetz CG, Glantz RH, Glatt SL, Klawans HL (1982) Pergolide mesylate and idiopathic Parkinson's disease. Neurology 32: 1175–1179
Tanner CM, Goetz CG, Glantz RH, Klawans HL (1986) Pergolide mesylate: four years experience in Parkinson's disease. Adv Neurol 45: 547–549
Wright A, Lees AJ, Stern GM (1987) Mesulergine and pergolide in previously untreated Parkinson's disease. J Neurol Neurosurg Psychiatry 50: 482–484
Zimmerman T, Sage JI (1991) Comparison of combination pergolide and levodopa to levodopa alone after 63 months of treatment. Clin Neuropharmacol 14: 165–169

Authors' address: G. Pezzoli, Ospedale Maggiore Policlinico, Pad. Ponti, Via F.Sforza 35, I-20122 Milan, Italy.

J Neural Transm (1995) [Suppl] 45: 213–224

Second generation of dopamine agonists: pros and cons

J. M. Rabey

Department of Neurology, Asaf Harofe Hospital, Zrifin, Iszael

Summary.   Dopamine agonists (DAGs) were first used in patients with moderate or advanced Parkinson's disease (PD). At that time, it was thought that DAGs could replace levodopa (LD) with fewer side effects. However, it soon became clear that while they could not replace LD, they did allow reduction of the dose of LD and diminished its side effects. Since the use of DAGs reduces response fluctuations as well as dyskinesias, there is a tendency to introduce them in the first stages of the disease, trying to delay motor fluctuations.

   While many DAGs have been developed, only four have been marketed and are used extensively for the treatment of Parkinson's disease: apomorphine, bromocriptine, lisuride and pergolide. In the present chapter, following a review of the "old" DAGs, the experience with three new promising DAGs is reported: cabergoline, ropinirole and pramipexole.

Introduction

Levodopa (LD), combined with a decarboxylase inhibitor, is the most effective treatment for Parkinson's disease (PD). However, chronic therapy can be associated with adverse effects such as dyskinesias and motor fluctuations (Marsden and Parkes, 1976; Fahn, 1980). Furthermore, a decline of LD efficacy often occurs as the disease progresses. While this may be due in part to the continuing loss of nigrostriatal neurons, other reasons may also play a role. LD may be unable to reverse parkinsonism because of impaired conversion to dopamine, or due to the limited capacity for dopamine storage and release by dopaminergic neurons. Another possibility for declining efficacy may be due to degeneration of the striatal dopamine receptors (Reisine et al., 1977). However, while some studies show a reduction in the number of those receptors (Reisine et al., 1977), others do not (O'Boyle and Waddington, 1987; Farde et al., 1988).

   Dopamine agonists (DAGs) have certain advantages over LD. DAGs, unlike LD, have not to be converted to dopamine by the failing nigrostriatal system. DAGs have been designed with both an increased potency and a greater selectivity, compared to LD, the natural neurotransmitter. Some

DAGs (i.e., apomorphine and lisuride) may also be administered by alternative routes of administration. Moreover, because DAGs decrease the requirements for LD, there is less accumulation of dopamine which is available to undergo auto-oxidation and generate cytotoxic free radicals. The generation of fewer cytotoxic free radicals and less oxidative stress may enhance the survival of the remaining dopamine neurons (Jenner, 1989). Another important point is the concept that pergolide (and possibly some other DAGs) exerts a protective effect on nigral cell cultures (Felton et al., 1992; Clow et al., 1992). This property may support the use of DAG early in the course of the disease as part of a "LD sparing" strategy (Olanow, 1992).

Historically, DAGs were first used in patients with moderate or advanced PD, who had been on high doses of LD and were experiencing a combination of decreased efficacy with response fluctuation and dyskinesias. At that time, it was thought that DAG could replace LD and provide an antiparkinsonian effect with fewer side effects (Vardi et al., 1977; Calne et al., 1978; Lieberman and Goldstein, 1985). It soon became apparent that DAG could not replace LD, but by reducing the dose of LD, many of the adverse effects could be ameliorated. This led to the use of DAGs in the first stages of the disease, before patients developed response fluctuations (Rascol et al., 1984; Rinne, 1987, 1989a).

Although it could be concluded that DAGs are superior to LD, there are also specific disadvantages inherent in this therapy. First, DAGs are clinically less effective than LD in reducing symptoms; some of them (bromocriptine) also require dopamine in the system in order to be effective; they show tachyphylaxis after prolonged use (bromocriptine, pergolide) which may be due to down regulation of dopamine receptor, progressive striatal cell loss or decoupling of the second messenger in the striatum (Riederer et al., 1978; Shibuya, 1979). The use of DAGs may produce more severe side effects than LD (nausea, vomiting, orthostatic hypotension, confusion and psychosis). Another important disadvantage of DAGs is their higher cost which makes them inaccessible to patients with low income without adequate medical insurance coverage.

While many DAGs have been developed, only four are extensively used in the treatment of PD: apomorphine, bromocriptine, lisuride and pergolide, the latter three of them ergoline derivatives. Three other drugs (cabergoline, ropinirole and pramipexole) are under intensive clinical investigations and should be available soon. Some of their pharmacological characteristics are summarized in Table 1.

Dopamine agonists as monotherapy

There have been several studies using DAGs as monotherapy. In five reports (Alberts et al., 1980; Nakamishi et al., 1989; Hely et al., 1989; Libman et al., 1989; Montrastuc et al., 1989), bromocriptine (415 patients) was compared to LD (325 patients). Because different PD evaluation scales were used

Table 1. Pharmacological profile of DA agonists

Drug	D1	D2	Other characteristics
Bromocriptine	antagonist	agonist	
Lisuride	antagonist	agonist	Serotonin receptors interaction; water soluble
Pergolide	agonist	agonist	Long T 1/2
Apomorphine	agonist	agonist	Short T 1/2; water soluble
Ropinirole		agonist	
Cabergoline		agonist	Long T 1/2
Pramipexole		agonist	

Table 2. Bromocriptine monotherapy in mild PD

Study	Pts	BC (mg)	BC (y)	Improved	Worsened	Fluctuations	Dyskinesia
Nakamishi et al. (1989)	286	10	2.0	125 (44%)	71 (25%)	3 (1%)	0
Hely et al. (1989)	66	18	3.0	15 (22%)	15 (22%)	0	0
Libman et al. (1989)	25	24	0.9	8 (31%)	0	0	0
Alberts et al. (1987)	23	17	1.4	7 (30%)	5 (22%)	0	1 (4%)
Montastruc et al. (1989)	15	50	2.7	13 (87%)	4 (31%)	0	0
Total	415	14 (mean)	2.1 (mean)	168 (40%)	95 (23%)	3 (0.7%)	1 (0.2%)
Range	—	(10–50)	(0.9–3.0)	(22–87%)	(0–31%)	(0–1%)	(0–1%)

(Webster, Parkinson's Disease Rating Scale, Unified Parkinson's Disease Rating Scale), change is reported as the percentage of patients in the study who improved or worsened compared to the baseline values. In these studies, the rescue drug in patients who deteriorated below baseline was LD (Tables 2, 3).

A significantly higher percentage of patients improved on LD compared to bromocriptine (68% va 40%). A similar percentage of patients worsened on LD compared to bromocriptine (24% vs 23%). The most significant difference was that the response fluctuation was higher in patients on LD than that on bromocriptine (9% vs 0.7%).

Dyskinesias were also significantly higher in patients on LD than in those on bromocriptine (13% vs 0.2%). The main reason for withdrawal of therapy on bromocriptine monotherapy was insufficient therapeutic response. Other reasons were nausea and vomiting, hallucinations, confusion, postural hypotension and pleurisy (Rinne, 1987, 1989a,b). All adverse effects were

J. M. Rabey

Table 3. Levodopa monotherapy in mild PD

Study	Pts	LD (mg)	LD (y)	Improved	Worsened	Fluctuations	Dyskinesia
Nakamishi et al. (1989)	200	368	2.0	145 (73%)	55 (27%)	20 (10%)	16 (9%)
Hely et al. (1989)	63	380	3.0	46 (73%)	21 (32%)	7 (11%)	14 (22%)
Libman et al. (1989)	25	252	0.9	8 (32%)	0	0	0
Alberts et al. (1987)	24	383	1.4	10 (25%)	2 (0.9%)	1 (0.4%)	9 (38%)
Montastruc et al. (1989)	135	442	2.7	13 (100%)	0	0	0
Total	325	365 (mean)	2.1 (mean)	222 (68%)	28 (9%)	28 (9%)	43 (13%)
Range	(252–442)	(0.9–3.0)	(252–100%)	(0–11%)	(0–11%)	(0–38%)	

reversible upon discontinuation of bromocriptine. A recently published study (Montastruc et al., 1993) of a 3-year follow-up utilizing bromocriptine monotherapy with a later addition of LD (26 patients) versus LD monotherapy (29 patients) confirmed that bromocriptine monotherapy was secondarily associated to delayed LD motor complications.

The results of monotherapy with lisuride (45 patients) (Giovannini et al., 1988) and MK458, a sustained-release formulation of napthoxazine (94 patients) (Koller et al., 1991) were similar to those reported with bromocriptine as monotherapy. Also, Rinne (1989), who used bromocriptine, lisuride and pergolide as monotherapy for PD, could not show any substantial difference among the various DAGs utilized (Table 4).

As can be seen from the literature, DAGs have been used successfully as monotherapy in newly diagnosed PD. In this aspect, although a smaller percentage of patients responded to DAGs monotherapy than to LD, a significantly smaller percentage of them developed response fluctuations with time. This concept, however, has been challenged recently by Weiner et al. (1993), who presented data pointing out that early bromocriptine use (as monotherapy or in addition to LD) does not prevent motor fluctuations in PD. On the contrary, this group even presented data suggesting that PD patients on bromocriptine monotherapy presented 83% of freezing episodes compared with 22% of patients treated with LD monotherapy. The only limitation of this well-designed study is the relatively small amount of patients studied (6 patients on bromocriptine, 9 patients on LD and 7 on combined therapy).

Bromocriptine, when used as monotherapy, delays the need for LD over 2 years, a delay similar to that seen with selegiline as monotherapy in de novo PD patients (Tetrud and Langston, 1989; The Parkinson's Study Group, 1989). Recent evidence showing that DAGs might have a protective as well as a symptomatic effect (Felton et al., 1992) suggests that the use of these drugs may preserve dopaminergic nigral neurons, and, in this way, explain why fewer response fluctuations are detected in long-term treatment.

Use of dopamine agonists in addition to LD

Our group (Vardi et al., 1977) among others (Calne et al., 1974; Parkes et al., 1976) reported that the beneficial effect of bromocriptine added to LD in advanced PD was even better than the use of LD in higher doses alone.

Bromocriptine was added to LD either in low dosages (less than 25 mg/day) (Caraceni et al., 1977; Fahn et al., 1979; Hoehn and Elton, 1985) or high dosages (26-mg–100 mg/day) (Glantz et al., 1981; Lees et al., 1978).

Several hypotheses have been proposed to explain the pharmacodynamic interaction at the striatal level between bromocriptine and LD (Goldstein et al., 1985). However, none has considered the possibility that LD may modify the kinetics of bromocriptine in the periphery and vice versa. We have shown that LD administered orally together with bromocriptine significantly reduces the plasma bromocriptine levels in PD-treated patients (Rabey et al., 1989). Moreover, we found that the addition of bromocriptine in patients with parkinsonism modifies plasma levels of LD (Rabey et al., 1990). In this last study, we showed that, in PD patients with diminished therapeutic response and severe akinesia, bromocriptine administered simultaneously with LD produced a reduced level of LD in the periphery. Contrarily, PD patients with an increased amount of dyskinesias showed that the addition of bromocriptine significantly elevated LD levels. We therefore postulated that PD patients with motor fluctuations under combined treatment should be monitored for plasma levels of LD if they showed marked akinesia or severe dyskinesia which could be related to the amount of LD available for conversion to dopamine in the striatum.

Lisuride is 10–20 times more potent on a milligram basis than bromo-criptine. The duration of its activity is shorter than that of bromocriptine, and its effectiveness appears to be independent of either dopamine storage or synthesis. In a 4-year study (Rabey et al., 1990), we compared the effect of lisuride in combination with a fixed dose of LD (24 patients) vs increased doses of LD (20 patients) in the treatment of advanced PD with motor fluctuations. After 4 years, 15 patients from the lisuride group were available for comparison with 13 from the LD groups. Analysis of the two groups revealed that lisuride was as effective as LD in controlling bradykinesia, rigidity and gait, but was statistically more effective in treating "off" episodes and dyskinesias (Figs. 1, 2). By the end of the fourth year, the mean daily dose of lisuride was just over 1 mg daily, which is about one-half of the daily dose taken by the same patients at the end of the first 6 months of the study. At low doses, lisuride was still a potent DA agonist after a long-term follow-up, suggesting the possible potentiation of its effect after chronic administration, as was also found in animal studies. This consistent dopaminergic effect observed with lisuride contrasts with the tolerance reported with bromocriptine (Lieberman et al., 1982) and pergolide (Lieberman et al., 1984).

An interesting observation reported by our (Rabey et al., 1990) and another group (Le Witt et al., 1982) is the weight gain in about 25% of our lisuride-treated PD patients. Lisuride is a central serotonin agonist, and we

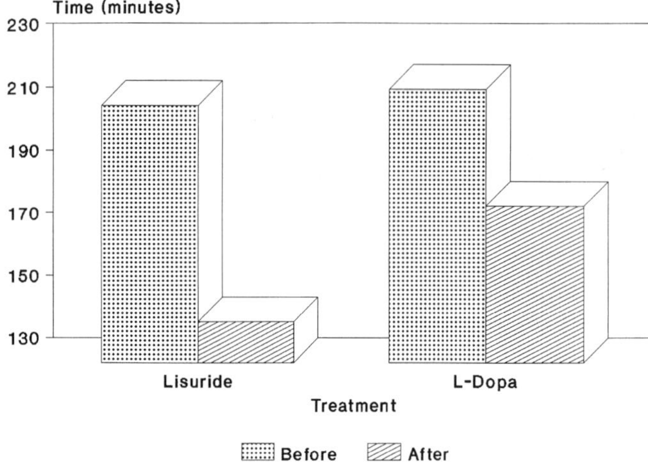

Fig. 1. Comparison of "off" episodes (mean of the daily group in minutes) in patients treated with lisuride (11 of 15) vs levodopa (9 of 13) before and after 4 years

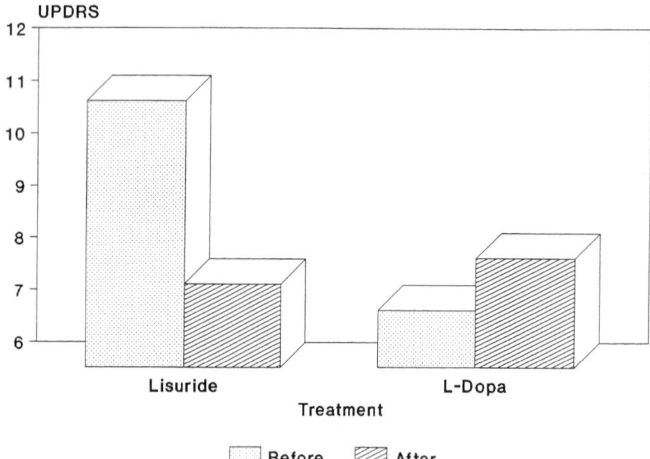

Fig. 2. Comparison of dyskinesia (daily mean of the group) in patients treated with lisuride (10 of 15) vs levodopa (11 of 13) before and after 4 years

hypothesized it may thus affect eating behavior (increased food ingestion), an important feature since many PD patients lose weight with progression of the disease (Vardi et al., 1976).

Apomorphine (as well as lisuride) is water soluble, and has been administered parenterally in severe cases of PD, where oral medication no longer controlled motor symptoms and fluctuations. Its 100% first-pass effect prevents oral administration. Different groups (Frenkel et al., 1990; Stocchi et al., 1991) have confirmed its beneficial effect in chronic PD patients with motor fluctuations. Despite the promising benefit of chronic parenteral administration of DAGs, it is important to mention that the main limiting factors are the production of skin nodules and infections at the site of the injections.

Pergolide mesylate is a semisynthetic ergoline derivative which had been developed in the hope that it would have a longer and stronger potency than other known agonists (Goldstein et al., 1980; Rabey et al., 1981). Several studies (Lees and Stern, 1981; Lieberman et al., 1981) have shown that pergolide added to LD reduces motor fluctuations by substantially decreasing "off" time and increasing "on" time in PD patients. Although pergolide suppresses prolactin release longer than bromocriptine or lisuride, the duration of its clinical effect on motor performance of parkinsonian patients seems to be similar to the other available ergots.

The beneficial effect of adding pergolide to LD was confirmed recently in an American multicenter double-blind placebo-controlled trial of pergolide as an adjunct to Sinemet (LD with carbidopa) performed in 376 subjects (Olanow et al., 1994). In that study, an addition of a mean dose of 2.94 mg/day of pergolide to LD achieved a statistically significant improvement in activities of daily life and motor performance with less "off" episodes. At the same time, a diminution of 25% of LD was obtained.

New dopamine agonists

Although several drugs have been tested during the last 5 years, there is some doubt whether they will be introduced into the market. Among them, one of the most promising DAGs is cabergoline, which is a new ergoline derivative with potent and long-lasting dopamine activity. Its long plasma half-life (65 hours) allows a single daily dose administration (Lera et al., 1990). We recently published (Rabey et al., 1994) a 1-year follow-up of 17 PD patients with motor fluctuations in whom cabergoline (5 mg daily) was added to levodopa. Eight patients completed the first year follow-up, showing significant improvement in their motor performance and in the proportion of "off" hours spent during waking time.

Ropinirole and pramipexole which are two "pure" dopamine type 2 receptor agonists are presently under intensive study in Europe and in the United States, and both drugs may become available within the next few years.

Forty-seven PD patients were randomized (1:1) to ropinirole or placebo added to an optimized LD dose over a 3-month study duration (Rascol et al., 1993). Seventy-five percent of ropinirole and 29% of placebo patients responded with >30% reduction in awake "off" periods (p = 0.006). UPDRS and finger tapping were also more improved by ropinirole than by placebo. The usual pharmacological classic side effects were observed in the ropinirole group.

In another multicenter study (Korczyn et al., 1993), 63 PD patients with motor fluctuations treated with LD were administered ropinirole (46 patients) or placebo (22 patients). During the initial incremental dose titrations of ropinirole, LD had to be maintained on a constant level. Over a second 6-week period, LD could be reduced. Responsiveness criteria required at least 20% reduction in LD from baseline, without deteriorations of the clinical state. Overall, 62.9% of patients on ropinirole and 29% in the placebo group (0.01) responded to treatment. Side effects were minimal.

Pramipexole was used in a single-blind, placebo-controlled, randomized prospective trial in patients with advanced PD (Molho et al., 1993). Twenty-three patients were enrolled (12 active, 11 placebo). The study lasted 14 weeks, with 7 weeks of dose escalations, 3 weeks of maintenance and a 1-week dose reduction. Patients treated with pramipexole showed significant improvement of "off" periods, of the activities of daily living score and a significant reduction in LD dose; no significant improvement was observed in the placebo group. Seventy-five percent (8/12) of the active patients had reductions of "off" time, compared with 45% (3/11) of placebo patients. The severity of dyskinesia increased in 50% (6/12) of active patients despite significant reduction in LD doses. There were no serious adverse side events.

One of the main subjects which remains unclear is what clinical differences may be obtained from a pure dopamine D2 receptor agonist compared with drugs which are mixed D1 and D2 agonists (see Table 1).

Comparison between different DAGs in chronic PD

One of the crucial questions which neurologists currently ask themselves is whether there is a difference in the clinical response of PD patients exposed to the different available DAGs. Another point is whether a declining efficacy of one DAG observed in some PD patients might not imply a negative response to another. According to the available current data, the response (or lack of response) of a PD patient to one drug does not predict what will be the response to another DAG. In an attempt to answer questions of this nature, we just completed a long-term study using two combined DAGs added together to the optimized amount of LD for the management of motor fluctuations in 8 PD patients (Rabey and Orlov, in preparation). Those patients were treated with LD (mean dose 750 mg/day, 8 patients), and bromocriptine (mean dose 22 mg, 5 patients) or lisuride (mean dose 1.5 mg, 3 patients) during the last few years and showed diminished response (in 6) or complained of increased dyskinesia (2 patients). Pergolide (mean dose 0.9 mg in 6 patients) and lisuride (mean dose 1.5 mg in 2 patients) were added. A modified Webster score and a Global and Physician Impression Scale were assessed before and after every 3 months. Long-term follow-up (20–30) months showed an improved gait with less "offs", freezings and falling episodes. However, no change in dyskinesias were observed. In our view, combined DAGs may be a good approach for the treatment of the axial features frequently observed in PD.

Concerning the comparison of different DAGs, our group has just finished the analysis of a double blind cabergoline versus bromocriptine trial in PD patients with motor fluctuations (Inzelberg et al., in preparation) as part of an extensive European multicenter study. A one-year analysis of our patients receiving cabergoline (up to 4 mg, 25 patients) vs bromocriptine (up to 40 mg, 19 patients) showed that both drugs were mainly effective in alleviating bradykinesia, rigidity and the amount of awake hours spent during "off" periods. In patients who received a low DA dose before the study, bradykinesia scores and the percentage of "off" hours decreased significantly with cabergoline but did not change with bromocriptine. Both drugs were equally effective when pre-study doses of LD had been higher. Adverse effects included hallucinations, dyskinesia, erythromelalgia, orthostatic hypotension, nausea, headache and insomnia. These side effects and dyskinesias were similar for both drugs. We have concluded, after using cabergoline in our center for 5 years, that a once daily dose of cabergoline is safe and at least as effective as bromocriptine in PD patients with motor fluctuations.

Le Witt et al. (1982) compared lisuride (mean dose 4.5 mg) to bromocriptine (mean dose 56.5 mg) in 28 patients enrolled in a double-blind crossover study (7 to 10 weeks of each drug titrated to an optimal dosage). According to their data, the effect of both drugs on parkinsonian symptomatology was quite similar and comparable. Le Witt et al. (1983) also compared bromocriptine (mean dose 51.7 mg) and pergolide (mean dose 3.1 mg) in a crossover study of 13 patients over a period of 10 weeks. Both drugs were similarly effective.

Lieberman et al. (1983, 1985) compared lisuride in an open study with bromocriptine and pergolide, and confirmed that lisuride (in dosages up to 5 mg daily or until side-effects prevented further increases) caused a significant improvement in PD symptomatology similar or even slightly superior to bromocriptine. Pergolide had a similar effect, possibly related to its long half-life, resulted in a greater improvement in the "on" hours than lisuride (175% vs 115%). Factor et al. (1988) classified 63 patients in whom bromocriptine therapy failed into several groups: loss of efficacy, lack of efficacy plus adverse events and only adverse effects. Pergolide was of benefit in 46% of these patients, and this benefit appeared in all the groups examined.

The only study which compared the addition of bromocriptine, lisuride and pergolide to LD in the same patients was published by Le Witt and Calne (1983). According to their data (open trial, 13 patients, mean dose of lisuride 3.6 mg, pergolide 3 mg and bromocriptine 51.7 mg), the addition of the different DAGs produced similar clinical responses. Most of the patients also reported no differences in the duration of response with the three drugs.

The hope in the future for fluctuating PD patients will be the development of more effective DAGs.

The ideal DAG should be one which produces complete amelioration of parkinsonian symptomatology without showing undesirable side effects. It should also exert clinical efficacy similar to LD, considered the "gold standard" medication for PD. Considering the efforts being invested in the last decade, we feel that this goal may finally be achieved.

References

Alberts MJ, Stajich JU, Olanow CW (1980) A randomized blinded study of low dose bromocriptine versus low dose carbidopa-levodopa in untreated Parkinson's patients. In: Fahn S, Marsden CD (eds) Recent developments in Parkinson's disease. Macmillan, New York, pp 201–208

Calne DB, Teychenne PE, Claveria LE, Eastman R, Greenacre JK, Petrie A (1974) Bromocriptine in Parkinsonism. Br Med J 4: 442–444

Calne DB, Williams AC, Neophytides A (1978) Long-term treatment of Parkinsonism with bromocriptine. Lancet i: 735–738

Caraceni TA, Celano I, Parati E, Girotti F (1977) Bromocriptine alone or associated with l-dopa plus benserazide in Parkinson's disease. J Neurol Neurosurg Psychiatry 40: 1142–1146

Clow A, Hussain T, Glover V, Sandler M, Walker M, Dexter D (1992) Pergolide can induce soluble superoxide dismutase in rat striata. J Neural Transm 90: 27–31

Factor SA, Sanchez-Ramos JR, Weiner WJ (1988) Parkinson's disease: an open label trial of pergolide in patients failing bromocriptine therapy. J Neurol Neurosurg Psychiatry 51: 529–533

Fahn S (1980) "On off" phenomenon with levodopa therapy in Parkinsonism. Neurology 24: 431–441

Fahn S, Cote LJ, Snider SR, Barrett RE, Isgreen WP (1979) The role of bromocriptine in the treatment of Parkinsonism. Neurology 29: 1077–1083

Farde L, Wiesel FA, Norstrom AL, Sedvall G (1988) PET examination of human D1 and D2 characteristics. Psychopharmacology (Berl) 96 [Suppl]: 79

Felten DL, Felten SY, Fuller RW, Romano TD, Smalstig EB, Wong DT, Clemens JA (1992) Chronic dietary pergolide preserves nigrostriatal neuronal integrity in aged Fisher 344 rats. Neurobiol Aging 13: 339–351

Frenkel JP, Lees AJ, Kempster PA, Stern GM (1990) Subcutaneous apomorphine in the treatment of Parkinson's disease. J Neurol Neurosurg Psychiatry 53: 96–101

Giovannini P, Scigliano G, Piccolo I, Soliveri P, Suchy I, Caraceni T (1988) Lisuride in Parkinson's disease: four year follow-up. Clin Neuropharmacol 11: 201–211

Glantz R, Goetz CG, Nausieda A, Weiner WJ, Klawans HL (1981) The effect of bromocriptine on the on-off phenomenon. J Neural Transm 52: 41–47

Goldstein M, Lieberman A, Lew J, Asano J, Rosenfeld M, Matwan M (1980) Interaction of pergolide with central dopaminergic receptors. Neurobiology 77: 3725–3728

Goldstein M, Lieberman A, Meller E (1985) A possible molecular mechanism for the antiparkinsonian action of bromocriptine in combination with levodopa. Trends Pharmacol Sci 6: 436–437

Hely MA, Morris J, Rail D (1989) The Sydney Multicentre Study of Parkinson's disease: a report on the first 3 years. J Neurol Neurosurg Psychiatry 52: 324–328

Hoehn MM, Elton RL (1985) Is low dose bromocriptine effective in Parkinsonism? Neurology 35: 199–206

Inzelberg R, Nissipeanu P, Rabey JM, Katz T, Orlov E, Kipervasser S, Schechtman E, Korczyn AD (1995) Comparison of cabergoline and bromocriptine in Parkinson's disease patients with motor fluctuations (in preparation)

Jenner P (1989) Clues to the mechanism underlying dopamine cell deth in Parkinson's disease. J Neurol Neurosurg Psychiatry 52 [Suppl]: 228

Koller WC, Block GA, Ahlskog JE, Cederbaum JM, Cyhan G, Goetz C, Le Witt PA (1991) Effect of MK-458 (HPMC) in Parkinson's disease previously untreated with dopaminergic drugs. Clin Neuropharmacol 14: 322–329

Korczyn AD, Abbot RJ, Playfer JR, Foster J, Wells TJ, Brooks DJ, Spokes G, Sagar H, Aharon J (1993) Ropinirole, a placebo controlled study of efficacy as adjunct therapy in Parkinsonian patients not optimally controlled on LD. New Trends Clin Neuropharmacol [Suppl] VII: 131

Lees AJ, Stern GM (1981) Pergolide and lisuride for levodopa induced oscillations. Lancet ii: 577

Lees AJ, Haddad S, Shaw KM, Kohut LJ, Stern GM (1978) Bromocriptine in Parkinsonism: a long-term study. Arch Neurol 35: 503–505

Le Witt PA, Calne DB (1983) Experience with dopamine agonists in Parkinson's disease and related disorders. In: Calne DB, Horowski R, Mc Donald RJM, Wuttke (eds) Lisuride and other dopamine agonists. Raven, New York, pp 474–480

Le Witt PA, Gopinathan G, Sanes JN, Dambrosia JM, Durso R, Calne DB (1982) Lisuride versus bromocriptine in Parkinson's disease: a double — blind study. Neurology 32: 69–72

Le Witt PA, Ward CD, Larsen TA, Raphaelson MI, Newman RP, Foster N, Dambrosia JM, Calne DB (1983) Comparison of pergolide and bromocriptine therapy in Parkinsonism. Neurology 33: 1009–1014

Lera G, Vaamonde J, Muruzabal J, Obeso JA (1990) Cabergoline: a long-acting dopamine agonist in Parkinson's disease. Ann Neurol 28: 593–594

Libman I, Gawel M, Riopelle R (1989) A comparison of bromocriptine (Parlodel) and levodopa-carbidopa (Sinemet) for treatment of "de novo" Parkinson's disease patients. Can J Neurol Sci 14: 576–580

Lieberman A, Goldstein M (1985) Bromocriptine in Parkinson's disease. Pharmacol Rev 37: 217–227

Lieberman A, Goldstein M, Leibowitz M, Neophytides A, Kupersmith M, Pact V, Kleinberg M (1981) Treatment of advanced Parkinson's disease with pergolide. Neurology 12: 243–247

Lieberman A, Kupersmith M, Neophytides A (1982) Bromocriptine in Parkinson's disease: report on 108 patients treated for up to 5 years. In: Goldstein M (ed) Ergot compounds and brain function: neuroendocrine and neuropsychiatric aspects. Plenum, New York, pp 45–53

Lieberman A, Goldstein M, Gopinathan G, Neophytides A, Leibowitz M, Walker R, Heisiger E (1983) Lisuride in Parkinson's disease and related disorders. In: Calne DB, Horowski R, McDonald RJ, Wittke W (eds) Lisuride and other dopamine agonists. Raven, New York, pp 419–429

Lieberman A, Kupersmith M, Neophytides A (1984) A long-term treatment with pergolide: decreased efficacy with time. Neurology 34: 223–226

Lieberman A, Leibowitz, Gopinathan G, Walker R, Heisiger E, Nelson J, Goldstein M (1985) The use of pergolide and lisuride, two experimental dopamine agonists, in patients with advanced Parkinson's disease. Am J Med Sci 290: 102–106

Marsden CD, Parkes JD (1977) Success and problems of long-term levodopa therapy in Parkinson's disease. Lancet i: 345–349

Molho ES, Factor SA, Weiner WJ, Sanchez-Ramos JR, Singer C, Shulman L (1993) The use of Pramipexole, a novel dopamine (DA) agonist, in advanced Parkinson's disease (1993). Neurology 43 [Suppl]: A384

Montastruc JL, Rascol O, Rascol A (1989) A comparison of bromocriptine versus levodopa in previously untreated parkinsonian patients: a three year follow-up. J Neurol Neurosurg Psychiatry 52: 773–775

Montastruc JL, Rascol O, Senard JM, Rascol A (1993) Does initial bromocriptine treatment delay L-Dopa-induced motor complications in Parkinson's disease? A prospective randomized controlled study. Neurology 43 [Suppl]: A348

Nakamishi T, Iwata M, Goto I (1989) Second interim report of the nation-wide collaborative study on the long term effects of bromocriptine in the treatment of Parkinsonian patients. Eur Neurol 29 [Suppl I]: 3–8

O'Boyle KM, Waddington JL (1987) New substituted 1-phenyl-3-benzapine analogues of SKF-38393 and N-methyl thienopyridine analogues of dihydroxynomifensine with selective affinity for the D1 receptor in human postmortem brain. Neuropharmacology 256: 1807–1810

Olanow CW (1992) An introduction to the free radical hypothesis in Parkinson's disease. Ann Neurol 32 [Suppl]: S2–S9

Olanow CW, Fahn S, Muenter M, Klawans H, Hurtig H, Stern M, Shoulson I, Kurlan R, Grimes JD, Jankovic J, Hoehn M, Markham CH, Duvoisin R, Reinmuth O, Leonard HA, Ahlskog E, Feldman R, Hershey L, Yahr MD (1994) A multicenter double-blind placebo-controlled trial of pergolide as an adjunct to Sinemet in Parkinson's disease. Mov Disord 9: 40–47

Parkes JD, Debono AG, Marsden CD (1976) Bromocriptine in Parkinsonism: long term treatment dose response and comparison with levodopa. J Neurol Neurosurg Psychiatry 39: 1101–1108

Rabey JM, Orlov E (1995) Long-term evaluation of two combined dopamine agonists for the management of motor fluctuations in Parkinson's disease (in preparation)

Rabey JM, Passeltiner P, Markey K, Asano T, Goldstein M (1981) Stimulation of pre- and post-synaptic dopamine receptors by an ergoline and by a partial ergoline. Brain Res 225: 347–356

Rabey JM, Oberman Z, Scharf M, Isakov A, Bar M, Graff E (1989) The influence of levodopa in the pharmacokinetics of bromocriptine in Parkinson's disease. Clin Neuropharmacol 12: 440–447

Rabey JM, Schwartz M, Graff E, Harsat A, Vered Y (1990) The influence of bromocriptine on the pharmacokinetics of levodopa in Parkinson's disease. Clin Neuropharmacol 14: 514–522

Rabey JM, Streifler M, Treves T, Korczyn AD (1990) The beneficial effect of chronic lisuride administration compared with levodopa in Parkinson's disease. In: Streifler M, Korczyn AD, Melamed E, Youdim MBH (eds) Advances in neurology, vol 53. Parkinson's disease: anatomy, pathology and therapy. Raven, New York, pp 451–455

Rabey JM, Nissipeanu P, Inzelberg R, Korczyn AD (1994) Beneficial effect of cabergoline: a new long lasting D2 agonist in the treatment of Parkinson's disease. Clin Neuropharmacol 17: 286–293

Rascol O, Lees AJ, Senard JM, Pirtosek D, Murray G (1993) Ropinirole: a double-blind placebo controlled study of efficacy and safety as adjunct therapy in Parkinsonian patients with "on/off" fluctuations. Neurology 43 [Suppl]: A348

Rascol A, Montastruc JL, Rascol O (1984) Should dopamine agonists be given early in the treatment of Parkinson's disease? J Neurol Sci [Suppl]: 229–238

Reisine TD, Fields JZ, Yamamura HJ (1977) Neurotransmitter receptor alterations in Parkinson's disease. Life Sci 21: 335–344

Riederer P, Rausch WD, Birkmayer W, Jellinger K, Danielczyk W (1978) Dopamine sensitive adenylate cyclase activity in the caudate nucleus and adrenal medulla in Parkinson's disease and in liver cirrhosis. J Neural Transm 14 [Suppl]: 153

Rinne UK (1987) Early combination of bromocriptine and levodopa in the treatment of Parkinson's disease: a five-year follow-up. Neurology 37: 826–828

Rinne UK (1989a) Dopamine agonist treatment in early Parkinson's disease. In: Przuntek H, Riederer P (eds) Early diagnosis and preventive therapy in Parkinson's disease. Springer, Wien New York, pp 343–348

Rinne UK (1989b) Lisuride, a dopamine agonist in the treatment of early Parkinson's disease. Neurology 39: 336–339

Shibuya M (1979) Dopamine-sensitive adenylate cyclase activity in the striatum in Parkinson's disease. J Neural Transm 44: 287–295

Stocchi F, Ruggieri S, Bramante L, Monge A, Viselli F, Lucarelli C, Agnoli A (1991) Subcutaneous continuous infusion in fluctuating patients with Parkinson's disease: apomorphine and lisuride. In: Rinne UK, Nagatsu T, Horowski R (eds) From basic research and early diagnosis to long-term treatment. Medicom, Asten, pp 296–306

Tetrud JW, Langston JW (1989) The effect of deprenyl (selegiline) on the natural history of Parkinson's disease. Science 41: 519–522

The Parkinson Study Group (1989) Effect of deprenyl on the progression of disability in early Parkinson's disease. N Engl J Med 321: 1364–1371

Vardi J, Oberman Z, Streifler M, Rabey JM (1976) Weight loss in elderly Parkinsonian patients on long-term levodopa therapy. J Neurol Sci 30: 33–40

Vardi J, Rabey JM, Streifler M (1977) Bromocriptine combined with levodopa plus a decarboxylase inhibitor in advanced Parkinsonism. Harefuah 93: 129–133

Weiner WJ, Factor SA, Sanchez-Ramos JR, Singer C, Sheldon RN, Cornelius L, Ingenito A (1993) Early combination therapy (bromocriptine and levodopa) does not prevent motor fluctuations in Parkinson's disease. Neurology 43: 21–27

Author's address: Prof. J. M. Rabey, Department of Neurology, Asaf Harofe Hospital, Zrifin , 70300 Israel.

J Neural Transm (1995) [Suppl] 45: 225–230
© Springer-Verlag 1995

The use of pramipexole, a novel dopamine (DA) agonist, in advanced Parkinson's disease

E. S. Molho[1], S. A. Factor[1], W. J. Weiner[2], J. R. Sanchez-Ramos[2], C. Singer[2], L. Shulman[2], D. Brown[1], and C. Sheldon[2]

[1] Albany Medical College, Department of Neurology Albany, New York, and
[2] University of Miami School of Medicine, Department of Neurology, Miami, Florida, U.S.A.

Summary. We evaluated the efficacy, safety and tolerability of a new dopamine D-2 receptor agonist, pramipexole [(S)-2-amino-4,5,6,7-tetrahydro-6-propylamino-benzathiazol-dihydrochloride], as adjunctive therapy in patients with advanced Parkinson's disease (PD). Twenty-four PD patients with motor fluctuations were treated in an 11 week prospective, single-blind parallel-group, placebo-controlled trial. The pramipexole treated group experienced a significant improvement in "off" time functioning as measured by the activities of daily living portion of the United Parkinson's Disease Rating Scale. In addition, the active treatment group was able to reduce total levodopa dose by 30% ($p < 0.05$). Pramipexole was well tolerated and the side effects reported were typical of other dopamine agonists. We conclude that pramipexole has antiparkinsonian effects which make it potentially useful in the treatment of motor fluctuations in PD.

Introduction

For more than 20 years, levodopa in combination with a dopa decarboxylase inhibitor (carbidopa or benserazide) (L/D) has been the cornerstone of therapy in Parkinson's disease (PD). Despite its dramatic initial benefit in relieving PD symptoms, long-term treatment is often complicated by progressive disability, motor fluctuations and dyskinesias (Marsden and Parkes, 1977; Rinne, 1983). Dopamine (DA) receptor agonists have been widely employed in patients with these complications and their beneficial effects are well documented. They can be particularly useful for stabilizing fluctuations in motor response to L/D and in improving "off" period disability and discomfort (Hoehn, 1985; Lieberman et al., 1987). However, therapy with DA agonists is associated with its own limitations, including hallucinations, delusions, dyskinesias, loss of efficacy and individual variations in therapeutic response (Lieberman et al., 1987). Given these problems, new DA agonists have been sought which might be better tolerated and more effective in treating advanced PD.

Pramipexole (Prx) is a new synthetic benzothiazole derivative [(S)-2-amino-4,5,6,7-tetrahydro-6-propylamino-benzathiazol-dihydrochloride] which has selective D-2 DA receptor agonist activity. In rats with unilateral 6-hydroxydopamine lesions or monkeys exposed to neuroleptics or MPTP, Prx has potent direct post-synaptic D-2 DA receptor agonist activity (Mierau and Schingnitz, 1992). In a single dose response study in patients it has shown significant anti-PD effects (Albani et al., 1992). The purpose of this preliminary trial is to evaluate the tolerability, safety and efficacy of Prx in PD patients experiencing motor fluctuations on L/D therapy.

Material and methods

Twenty four PD patients (16 men and eight women) gave consent and were enrolled. All patients had stage II-IV PD on the Hoehn and Yahr scale (Hoehn and Yahr, 1967) and were experiencing motor fluctuations while being treated with L/D. Motor fluctuations included "wearing-off" response, early morning akinesia, random "on-off" oscillations and L/D-induced dyskinesia. The mean age of the patients was 66.5 years (range, 49 to 81) and the mean duration of illness was 11.9 years (range, four to 21). Patients with atypical or secondary parkinsonism, dementia, hallucinations or epilepsy and patients with clinically significant cardiac, hepatic, or renal disease were excluded. Any patient with a supine systolic blood pressure (BP) <100 mm Hg, standing diastolic BP <50 mm Hg or an orthostatic drop in systolic BP of 20 mm Hg or greater was also excluded. Standard preparations of L/D, anticholinergic medications and amantadine were allowed during the trial, but other DA agonists, selegiline, and sustained release L/D had to be discontinued at least one month prior to administration of the study medication. If necessary, restricted medications were replaced by standard L/D prior to initiation of the study.

We evaluated all patients in a prospective, single-blind, parallel group, randomized, placebo-controlled manner. The study coordinators at each site had access to patient treatment group assignments, but all patients and all investigators were blinded to this information. The study design included a three week screening period during which L/D dose was optimized and an 11 week active treatment phase. The L/D dose was stable for at least one week prior to baseline evaluations. Patients were randomized (12 placebo and 12 Prx) at the start of the treatment phase. The ascending dose interval lasted up to seven weeks (dose levels 1 to 7) followed by a three week maintenance phase and a one week dose reduction. The dose of Prx was 0.1 mg t.i.d. at dose level 1, 0.25 mg t.i.d. at level 2, 0.5 mg t.i.d. at level 3, 0.75 mg t.i.d. at level 4, 1.0 mg t.i.d. at level 5, 1.25 mg t.i.d. at level 6 and 1.5 mg t.i.d. at level 7. During dose escalation, L/D dose could be decreased but not increased beyond the dose utilized at baseline. If dose-limiting side effects occurred beyond dose level 3, patients were allowed to enter the maintenance phase early. Patients were evaluated in hospital for dose levels 1 to 4 (16 days) for close BP monitoring and as outpatients for the remainder of the study.

We evaluated patients weekly with the following: the Unified Parkinson's Disease Rating Scale (UPDRS) (Fahn et al., 1987); modified Schwab and England disability scale (S-E) for "on" and "off" periods (Fahn et al., 1987; Schwab and England, 1969); modified Hoehn and Yahr scale (Hoehn and Yahr, 1967; Fahn et al., 1987) and a Parkinson's dyskinesia scale (graded assessment of dyskinesia intensity for the head, trunk and each limb, on a 0 to 4 scale with 0 = normal and 4 = incapacitating). Adverse experiences were monitored at each visit. The motor portion of the UPDRS and the dyskinesia scale were performed only when the patients were "on", approximately one to two hours after a dose of L/D. The activities of daily living (ADL) portion was utilized for "on" and "off" periods. Patients kept daily, hour by hour, diaries and mean hours "off", "on", and "on" with dyskinesia were calculated at each dose level (or weekly). An electrocardiogram was performed at each visit. In addition, blood chemistries, a complete blood count and an

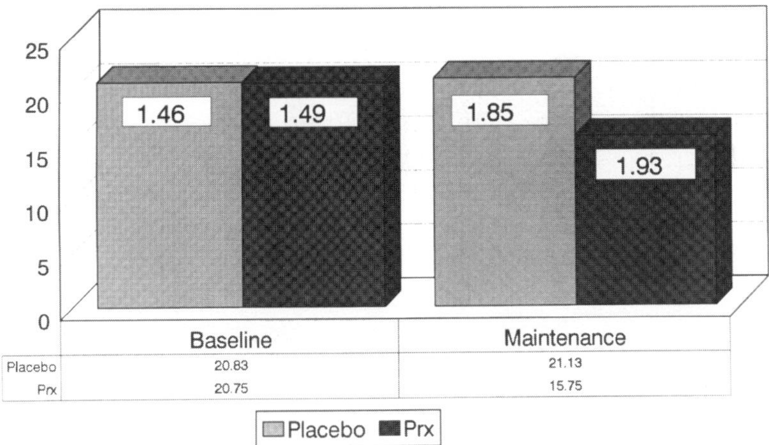

Fig. 1. ADL-"off" scores at baseline and at maintenance. The ADL score of the Prx group was significantly improved at maintenance compared to baseline (p < 0.05). Bar insert shows the standard error of the mean

urinalysis was performed at regular intervals. Supine and standing BP measurements were taken prior to, and at hourly intervals for four hours after, all doses while in the hospital and after the first dose of study medication at each new dose level as an outpatient.

The primary efficacy endpoints of this study were the ADL portion of the UPDRS and the diary results, particularly mean hours "off". All other clinical assessments were considered secondary efficacy endpoints. Statistical analysis included a direct comparison of Prx patients and placebo patients at baseline and at maintenance using a Student's t-test. The maintenance score was the mean of the three maintenance visit scores. The efficacy of Prx and placebo were also evaluated by comparing the baseline and maintenance scores for each treatment group using a paired t-test. Subsection scores examined included the ADL-"on", ADL-"off", and motor examination portions of the UPDRS. The data reported and analyzed here represent a portion of a larger multi-center trial.

Results

The Prx and placebo groups did not differ with regard to any of their disability scores at baseline. Patients treated with Prx showed a statistically significant improvement in their ADL-"off" score when compared to baseline (Fig. 1; paired t-test; p < 0.05). The overall score of the Prx treated group dropped from a mean of 20.75 pretreatment to a mean of 15.75 at maintenance. The placebo group showed no significant improvement in their ADL-"off" score. The ADL-"on" score was not significantly improved in either group.

The Prx group had a decrease in the UPDRS motor examination score at maintenance when compared to baseline of 12%. This change was not statistically significant. The total daily "off" time at maintenance was not significantly improved when compared to baseline for either group. However, 5 of 12 patients in the Prx treated group experienced a dramatic reduction in "off" time. The average reduction was 5.2 hours (56%) in these patients.

The placebo group experienced a 26% reduction in UPDRS motor examination score at maintenance when compared to baseline (p < 0.05). Four of 12

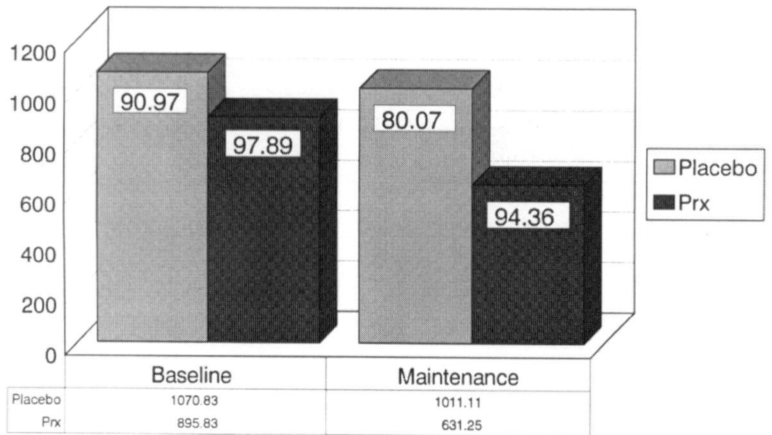

Fig. 2. Total daily levodopa dose (mg) at baseline and at maintenance. The levodopa dose of the Prx group is significantly decreased at maintenance compared to baseline (p = 0.004). Bar insert shows the standard error of the mean

Table 1. Clinical adverse experiences

	Prx (n = 12)	Placebo (n = 12)
Increased Dyskinesia	6	2
Confusion	3	1
Hallucinations	3	2
Insomnia	3	4
Dizziness	2	1
Nausea	2	1
Anxiety	2	1
Leg Pain	2	4
Symptomatic Hypotension	1	0
Depression	1	1
Headache	1	0
Blurred Vision	1	0

patients experienced a 40% or greater improvement. However, when the Prx group was compared directly to the placebo group at maintenance the difference did not reach significance (p = 0.06).

Levodopa dose decreased significantly in the Prx group (Fig. 2; paired t-test; p = 0.004) from a pretreatment mean of 895.8 mg to a mean at maintenance of 631.2 mg (30%). The mean Prx dose achieved at maintenance was 3.53 mg. This decrease in L/D dose was not accompanied by any significant worsening on UPDRS ADL scale, UPDRS motor scale, modified S-E disability scale or diary assessments of "on"/"off" time. The placebo group had no significant change in their L/D dose.

No serious adverse events occurred and all 24 patients that were enrolled completed the study. Clinical adverse events are listed in Table 1. Worsening of dyskinesia was reported by six of 12 patients in the Prx group during the dose escalation phase of the study (UPDRS Part IV "Complications of Therapy"). Five of these six patients required reduction of their L/D dose. Only two of 12 placebo patients reported worsening of dyskinesia. However, at maintenance there was no statistically significant change in the Parkinson's dyskinesia scale score of either group. Other adverse experiences were those typically observed with DA receptor agonists.

Discussion

The results of this preliminary, controlled clinical trial indicate that Prx: [1] has obvious dopaminergic activity when utilized in patients with advanced PD, and [2] has some efficacy in improving motor fluctuations when used as an adjunct to L/D. The Prx treated group was able to reduce their mean dose of L/D by 30% at a mean maintenance Prx dose of 3.53 mg. This reduction of L/D was not associated with a worsening of any measure of disability or parkinsonian signs. On the contrary, the active treatment group experienced a significant improvement in "off" time functioning as measured by the ADL portion of the UPDRS, a primary efficacy endpoint. There was also an increase in dyskinesia in the Prx group during dose escalation. Despite these findings, there was no significant improvement in diary measurements of "on" or "off" time. There was also no significant improvement in any secondary endpoint measures. This would suggest that Prx provides only a modest improvement in advanced PD.

The relatively small patient population and the study design may, in part, contribute to these modest results. Motor examinations were only performed when patients were near peak performance after a dose of L/D. The results indicate that the addition of Prx as an adjunct to L/D did not improve peak performance significantly. However, since Prx seems to improve "off" time functioning it may have been useful to look at "off" period motor examinations as well and this should be considered when studying other DA agonists. The reason for the improvement in the motor examination score of the placebo group is unclear but, it may be due to the effects of weekly monitoring and increased medication compliance. This "placebo" effect has been seen in other clinical trials (Olanow et al., 1994) and was likely magnified by the small patient population studied.

Prx is safe and well tolerated in doses ranging from 0.1 mg t.i.d. to 1.5 mg t.i.d. in this patient population. Side effects typical of other DA agonists such as worsening of dyskinesia, confusion and hallucinations occurred but, were generally controlled by lowering the dose of L/D.

Although Prx was not efficacious in all patients, there appears to be a select group of PD patients who respond favorably to this agent. This individual variation in response is typical of other DA agonists and an individual patient's response or lack of one to a particular agent may not be useful in predicting their response to others (Factor et al., 1988). Therefore, the development of effective new agonists can only add to the clinician's ability to treat advanced PD.

Acknowledgements

This work was supported by a grant from Boehringer Ingelheim Pharmaceuticals, Inc., the Albany Medical College Parkinson Research Fund and the National Parkinson Foundation.

References

Albani C, Popescu R, Lacher R, Boke-Kuhn K (1992) Single dose response to pramipexole in patients with Parkinson's disease [Abstract]. Mov Disord 7 [Suppl 1]: 98

Factor SA, Sanchez-Ramos JR, Weiner WJ (1988) Parkinson's disease: an open label trial of pergolide in patients failing bromocriptine therapy. J Neurol Neurosurg Psychiatry 51: 529–533

Fahn S, Elton RL, members of the UPDRS committee (1987) In: Fahn S, Marsden CD, Calne DB, Goldstein M (eds) Recent developments in Parkinson's disease, vol 2. McMillan Health Care Information, Florham Park NJ, pp 153–163, 293–304

Hoehn MM (1985) The result of chronic levodopa therapy and its modification by bromocriptine in Parkinson's disease. Acta Neurol Scand 71: 97–106

Hoehn MM, Yahr MD (1967) Parkinsonism: onset, progression, and mortality. Neurology 17: 427–442

Lieberman A, Goldstein M, Gopinathan G, Neophytides A (1987) D-1 and D-2 agonists in Parkinson's disease. Can J Neurol Sci 14: 466–473

Marsden CD, Parkes JD (1977) Success and problems of long-term levodopa therapy in Parkinson's disease. Lancet ii: 345–349

Mierau J, Schingnitz G (1992) Biochemical and pharmacological studies on pramipexole, a potent and selective D-2 receptor agonist. Eur J Pharmacol 215: 161–170

Olanow CW, Fahn S, Muenter M, Klawans H, Hurtig H, Stern M, Shoulson I, Kurlan R, Grimes JD, Jankovic J, Hoehn M, Markham CH, Duvoisin R, Reinmuth O, Leonard HA, Ahlskog E, Feldman R, Hershey L, Yahr MD (1994) A multicenter double-blind placebo-controlled trial of pergolide as an adjunct to Sinemet in Parkinson's disease. Mov Disord 9: 40–47

Rinne UK (1983) Problems associated with long-term levodopa treatment of Parkinson's disease. Acta Neurol Scand 68 [Suppl 95]: 19–26

Schwab RS, England AC (1969) Projection technique for evaluating surgery in Parkinson's disease. In: Gillingham FJ, Donaldson IM (eds) Third symposium on Parkinson's disease. Livingstone, Edinburgh, pp 152–157

Authors' address: S. A. Factor, D.O., Albany Medical College, Department of Neurology (A70), Albany, New York 12208, U.S.A.

J Neural Transm (1995) [Suppl] 45: 231–238
© Springer-Verlag 1995

Ropinirole in the symptomatic treatment of Parkinson's disease

D. J. Brooks, N. Torjanski, and **D. J. Burn**

MRC Cyclotron Unit, Hammersmith Hospital, London, United Kingdom

Summary.   Ropinirole is a novel, non-ergoline dopamine agonist chemical name with a very high specificity for dopamine D_2-like receptors, currently being investigated for the symptomatic treatment of Parkinson's disease. The efficacy of ropinirole has been investigated in three placebo-controlled studies: one using ropinirole as monotherapy in early Parkinson's disease and two using it as an adjunct to L-dopa in patients who are experiencing fluctuations in motor response. Ropinirole therapy for 12 weeks was an effective symptomatic therapy in both patient groups, as measured by either a significant improvement in the motor score of the UPDRS, reduction of awake time spent "off" or a reduction in the dose of L-dopa. Ropinirole therapy was generally well tolerated, the most frequent adverse events being nausea and vomiting which are typical of all dopamine agonists, but unlike other dopamine agonists, CNS side-effects were of the same magnitude as found patients receiving placebo.

Introduction

Dopamine agonists provide an important addition to the armamentarium of drugs used in the symptomatic treatment of Parkinson's disease. Patients receiving a dopamine agonist, such as bromocriptine, as an adjunct to L-dopa experience fewer fluctuations in motor response, and for the majority of patients it may also be possible to reduce the dose of L-dopa (Goetz, 1990; Montastruc et al., 1993). However, the use of those dopamine agonists that are commercially available may be limited by their association with CNS side-effects, which may necessitate either a reduction in dosage or withdrawal of the drug (Goetz, 1990; Montastruc, 1993).

Ropinirole (4-[2-(dipropylamino) ethyl]-1,3 dihydro-2-H-indol-2-one monohydrochlatide) name is a novel, non-ergoline, specific dopamine agonist that binds specificaly to dopamine D_2-like receptors (Eden et al., 1991). The selectivity of ropinirole for these receptors is similar to that of dopamine (Fears et al., 1993). Early clinical studies have suggested that ropinirole is effective in the symptomatic treatment of Parkinson's disease, and that therapy is well tolerated (Kapoor et al., 1989; Vidailhet et al., 1990). It is thought that, like other dopamine agonists, ropinirole may be able to reduce the incidence of motor fluctuations commonly associated with L-dopa treatment, while its non-ergoline structure may produce fewer dose-limiting side-effects.

Current research with ropinirole is concentrating on two aspects of treatment:

a) The use of ropinirole as monotherapy in patients in the early stages of Parkinson's disease who have had little or no prior exposure to L-dopa or dopamine agonists. The objectives of ropinirole treatment in these patients are to provide an effective symptomatic treatment for the early stages of Parkinson's disease.

b) The use of ropinirole as adjunct therapy in patients in the later stages of Parkinson's disease who are also receiving L-dopa. The objective of ropinirole treatment in these patients is either to reduce the incidence and severity of fluctuations in the motor response to L-dopa or to reduce the dose of L-dopa.

This review focuses on three Phase II clinical studies which have recently been presented at international meetings (Lees et al., 1994; Rascol, 1994; Sagar, 1994) and which examined the efficacy and safety of ropinirole either as early monotherapy or as adjunct therapy with L-dopa in the later stages of Parkinson's disease. The analysis is limited to preliminary results with respect to the primary efficacy variable, patient withdrawal and adverse events.

Patients and methods

Early monotherapy

The efficacy and safety of ropinirole as monotherapy in the treatment of the early stages of Parkinson's disease was evaluated in an international, double-blind study involving patients at Hoehn and Yahr stages I-IV of Parkinson's disease. Patients had received dopamine therapy for less than 6 months, and this was stopped 2 weeks prior to a 7-day screening period. After the screening period, patients were randomized to receive either ropinirole (n = 41) or placebo (n = 22) for 12 weeks. The mean age of patients was 59.2 years in the ropinirole group (range 38–74) and 56.5 years in the placebo group (range 36–72). Patients in the ropinirole group received an initial dose of 0.5 mg twice daily, titrated to a maximum dosage of 5 mg twice daily. Assessments of motor function were made using the Unified Parkinson's Disease Rating Scale (UPDRS). The primary endpoint was an improvement of at least 30% in the motor score of UPDRS. Efficacy was also measured by a finger tap test and a clinician's global evaluation. The safety of treatment was assessed by a full physical examination, vital signs, laboratory data, ECG, adverse event reports and the dyskinesias score section of the UPDRS. Statistical analyses were performed using analysis of variance (ANOVA), the Mantel-Haenszel procedure, the Mann-Whitney test and chi-squared or Fisher's exact tests.

Adjunct therapy

Two double-blind, Phase II studies have been carried out to assess the efficacy and safety of ropinirole as adjunct therapy in patients not optimally controlled on L-dopa and exhibiting mild to moderate "on/off" fluctuations. In both studies, patients who had been treated with L-dopa for more than 3 years were randomized to receive either ropinirole or placebo as an adjunct to L-dopa for 12 weeks.

Study A

In the first study, 46 patients at Hoehn and Yahr stages I-IV of Parkinson's disease were randomized to either the ropinirole treatment group or the placebo group (23 patients in each group) after a 7-day period to establish baseline status. Patients in the ropinirole group received a dose of 0.5 mg ropinirole twice daily, increasing to 4 mg twice daily. The patients were aged between 44 and 78 years with a mean age of 61.5 years and 63 years in the ropinirole and placebo groups, respectively. The dose of L-dopa was kept constant throughout the study. The primary efficacy parameter was a reduction in the duration of "off" periods, as determined from patients' daily diary cards, with response defined as a reduction from baseline of 30% or more. Parkinsonian symptoms were also assessed by means of a clinicians global evaluation, the Unified Parkinson's Disease Rating Scale (UPDRS) and finger tap tests. The safety of treatment was evaluated using vital signs, laboratory data and adverse events monitoring. Statistical analyses were performed using ANOVA, the Mantel-Haenszel procedure, the Mann-Whitney test and chi-squared or Fisher's exact tests.

Study B

In this study, 41 patients at Hoehn and Yahr stages II to IV of Parkinson's disese received ropinirole and 22 received placebo. Patients in the ropinirole group received a dose of 0.5 mg ropinirole twice daily, increasing to 5 mg twice daily. The mean age of the patients was 62.3 years (range 36–78) in the ropinirole group and 63.7 years (range 41–78) in the placebo group. The dose of L-dopa was held stable for the first 6 weeks of the study and then reduced if an improvement in Parkinsonian symptoms was observed. The primary measure of efficacy was a 20% or greater reduction in the dose of L-dopa while maintaining symptom control. Efficacy was also measured by the motor component of the UPDRS. The duration of "on/off" periods was determined from daily diary cards. The safety of treatment was determined by physical examination, laboratory data and adverse event reports. Statistical analyses were performed using ANOVA, the Mantel-Haenszel procedure, the Mann-Whitney test and chi-squared or Fisher's exact tests.

Results

Early monotherapy

In total, 36 patients (87.8%) in the ropinirole group and 19 (86.4%) patients in the placebo group completed the study. Of the 5 patients in the ropinirole group who withdrew from the study, three did so because of adverse events and two for other reasons. One patient in the placebo group withdrew because of adverse events and two withdrew because of insufficient therapeutic effect.

According to the clinicians global evaluation, a significantly higher proportion of patients in the ropinirole group showed an overall improvement in their parkinsonian symptoms at the endpoint of the study (last observation carried forward) compared with patients in the placebo group. For the inten-

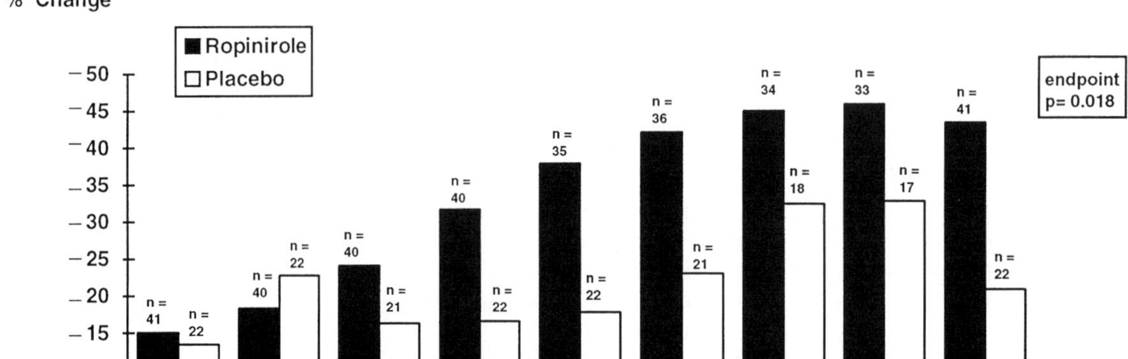

Fig. 1. The mean percentage change from baseline in total UPDRS motor score in the intention to treat population during treatment of early PD with ropinirole

tion to treat population, an improvement of at least 30% in the motor score of the UPDRS was achieved by 70.7% of the patients treated with ropinirole compared with 40.9% of the patients treated with placebo (p = 0.021). The percentage mean change in UPDRS score from baseline to endpoint was also significantly greater in the ropinirole group (Fig. 1). A greater improvement in the results of the finger tap test was observed in patients treated with ropinirole compared with patients treated with placebo, though this difference was not statistically significant. In the ropinirole group, 85.4% of patients experienced one or more adverse events, compared with 68.2% of patients in the placebo group. This difference was not statistically significant. In the ropinirole group, nausea, dizziness, somnolence and vomiting were experienced by 10% or more of patients. No single adverse event was experienced by 10% or more of patients the placebo group.

Adjunct therapy

Study A

Treatment with ropinirole as adjunct therapy with L-dopa was more effective than placebo in patients with Parkinson's disease not optimally controlled by L-dopa alone (Table 1). In the intention to treat population at endpoint, 65% of patients in the ropinirole group had a 30% reduction in awake time spent "off", compared with 39% of patients in the placebo group (p = 0.077). The clinicians global evaluation indicated that there was an improvement in 78% of patients treated with ropinirole compared with 35% of patients who received placebo (p = 0.04).

Table 1. Treatment with ropinirole compared with placebo as adjunct therapy to L-dopa

	Ropinirole group	Placebo group	p
Primary efficacy variable (percentage of patients with ≥30% improvement in 'on/off' periods)	65 (15/23)	39 (9/23)	<0.077
Proportion of awake time spent 'off' (%)	−44.3	−24.0	<0.085
% patients improved in clinicians global evaluation	78.3	34.8	<0.01

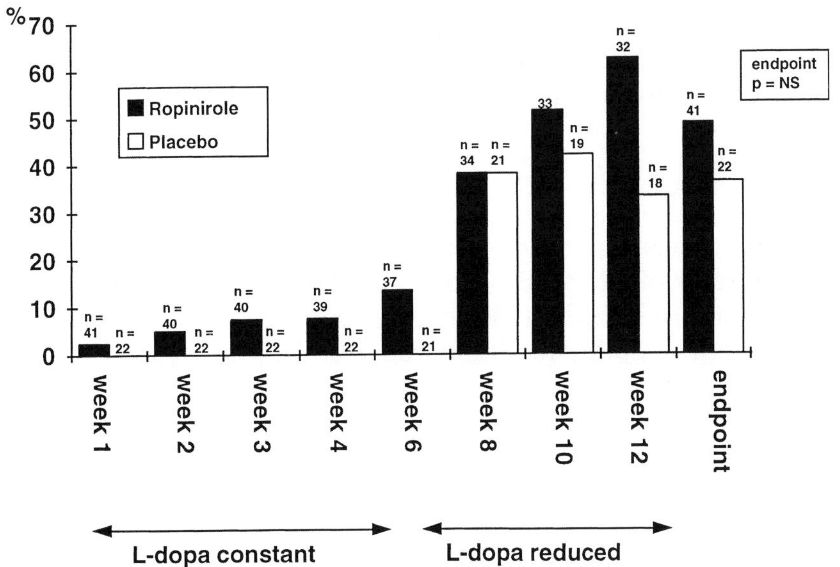

Fig. 2. The mean percentage change from baseline in total daily dose of L-dopa in the intention to treat population during treatment with ropinirole (% patients with >20% reduction in L-dopa)

In the placebo group, significantly more patients withdrew from the study; more patients withdrew because of adverse events or insufficient therapeutic effect than in the ropinirole group. One or more adverse events were experienced by 91.3% of patients in the ropinirole group and 78.3% of patients in the placebo group, but this difference was not statistically significant. The most commonly reported adverse events were asthenia, dizziness, dyskinesia, headache, nausea and somnolence, but there was no significant difference between treatment groups in the frequency of any individual adverse event.

Study B

The proportion of patients in the intention to treat population who had a reduction in their dose of L-dopa of at least 20% at endpoint, while maintaining control of parkinsonian symptoms, was 49% in the ropinirole group and 36% in the placebo group. This difference was not significant (Fig. 2).

Table 2. The most frequently reported adverse events in patients receiving ropinirole or placebo for up to 12 weeks

Non-dopaminergic	Ropinirole (n = 215)	Placebo (n = 67)	
Dyskinesia	16 (7.4%)	7 (10.4%)	
Headache	27 (12.6%)	7 (10.4%)	
Parkinsonism aggravated	6 (2.8%)	6 (6.0%)	
Somnolence	39 (18.1%)	4 (6.0%)	
Dopaminergic	Ropinirole: adjunct (n = 129)	Ropinirole: early (n = 52)	Placebo (n = 67)
Dizziness	44 (34.1%)	16 (30.8%)	13 (19.4%)
Nausea	50 (38.8%)	37 (71.2%)	12 (17.9%)
Vomiting	15 (11.6%)	8 (15.4%)	3 (4.5%)

Although the aim of the study was to keep symptoms constant, 66.7% of patients in the ropinirole-treated group had an improvement in the clinicians global evaluation at endpoint, compared with 54.6% in the placebo-treated group.

The proportion of patients withdrawing because of adverse events was similar in both treatment groups; 17% in the ropinirole group, 14% in the placebo group. One or more adverse events were experienced by 76% of the patients treated with ropinirole and 73% of the patients who received placebo. The most commonly reported adverse events in the ropinirole group were dizziness, dyskinesia, headache, nausea and somnolence. In the placebo group, postural hypotension, dizziness, headache and nausea were the most common adverse events. The percentage of patients withdrawing from the study was higher in the ropinirole group than in the placebo group, though the difference was not statistically significant.

Overall tolerability

In the course of the ropinirole programme to date, a total of 215 patients have been exposed to treatment with ropinirole for up to 12 weeks, while 67 patients received placebo. Overall, the treatment was well tolerated. The most frequently reported non-dopaminergic adverse events in the ropinirole-treated patients were headache and somnolence, while higher percentages of patients in the placebo-treated group reported dyskinesias and an aggravation of their parkinsonism (Table 2). The dopaminergic adverse events that were reported most frequently by both groups of patients were nausea, vomiting and dizziness, although all three were more common in ropinirole-treated patients (Table 2). In this database, hallucinations have been reported by only 2.3% of patients receiving ropinirole, compared with 1.5% of placebo-treated patients.

Discussion

Ropinirole was shown to be significantly more effective than placebo in the treatment of patients in the early stages of Parkinson's disease, as determined by the analysis of improvement in the motor score of the UPDRS.

Although dopamine agonists have usually been used as an adjunct to L-dopa as Parkinson's disease progresses and fluctuations in motor response develop, there has also been some interest in the use of dopamine agonists as early monotherapy for Parkinson's disease. A recent open study in the UK has compared bromocriptine with L-dopa and L-dopa plus selegiline as symptomatic treatment for the early stages of Parkinson's disease (Parkinson's Disease Research Group of the United Kingdom, 1993). All three treatments provided improvement in symptoms after 12 months of treatment but both L-dopa and L-dopa plus selegiline were significantly more effective than bromocriptine after three years. However, the patients who did receive treatment with bromocriptine for three years had a lower incidence of treatment-induced dyskinesias and "on/off" fluctuations in response compared with patients in the other two groups (Parkinson's Disease Research Group of the United Kingdom, 1993). The results of the present study with ropinirole, which showed that it provides an effective symptomatic treatment for the early stages of Parkinson's disease while being associated with fewer dyskinesias and on-off fluctuations than are experienced in patients receiving L-dopa alone, are in agreement with those of the UK study, although further study is needed to discover whether this efficacy is maintained. This is being investigated in an extension to the existing trial and in an ongoing programme.

The studies described here have also shown that ropinirole has good efficacy compared with placebo as an adjunct to L-dopa in the later stages of Parkinson's disease. This is not unexpected as there is already a wealth of evidence supporting the benefits of dopamine agonists in this indication; both well-established agents such as bromocriptine, pergolide and lisuride (Goetz, 1990; Montastruc et al., 1993) and newer compounds, including cabergoline (Lera et al., 1993; Lieberman et al., 1993) and the lisuride derivative, terguride (Pacchetti et al., 1993).

Overall, ropinirole was well-tolerated, both as monotherapy in patients in the early stages of Parkinson's disease, and also in patients in the later stages of the disease whose symptoms were not adequately controlled by L-dopa alone. The principal side-effects of nausea, vomiting and dizziness were typical of all dopamine agonists (Goetz, 1990; Montastruc et al., 1993; Lera et al., 1993) but were mostly tolerated with continued therapy. Of the 215 patients who received ropinirole, only 25 withdrew from the studies because of adverse events.

A feature of the side-effects profile of ropinirole in these studies was the low incidence of any neuropsychiatric effects, such as hallucinations, which can be a complication of treatment with the ergoline dopamine agonists, especially in patients in the later stages of Parkinson's disease (Goetz, 1990; Montastruc et al., 1993). The low incidence of such effects with non-ergoline dopamine agonists has already been reported for apomorphine (Lees, 1993), and this may prove to be a significant advantage for ropinirole in the treatment of Parkinson's disease. This, along with further studies of its efficacy, will be investigated in the ongoing clinical research programme.

References

Eden RJ, Costall B, Domeney AM, Gerrard PA, Harvey CA, Kelly ME, Naylor RJ, Owen DAA, Wright A (1991) Preclinical pharmacology of ropinirole (SK&F 101468-A) a novel dopamine D_2 agonist. Pharmacol Biochem Behav 38: 147–154

Fahn S, Calne DB (1978) Considerations in the management of Parkinsonism. Neurology 28: 5–7

Fears R, Bowen WP, Brown F, Coldwell MC, Riley GJ (1993) The novel dopaminergic agent ropinirole selectively binds to cloned dopamine D_3 receptors. Can J Neurol Sci 20 [Suppl 4]: S68

Goetz CG (1990) Dopaminergic agonists in the treatment of Parkinson's disease. Neurology 40 [Suppl 3]: 50–54

Kapoor R, Pirtosek Z, Frankel JP, Stern GM, Lees AJ, Bottomley JM, Sree Haran N (1989) Treatment of Parkinson's disease with novel dopamine D_2 agonist SK&F 101468. Lancet i: 1445–1446

Lees AJ (1993) Dopamine agonists in Parkinson's disease: a look at apomorphine. Fundam Clin Pharmacol 7: 121–128

Lees AJ, Pirtosek D, Rascol O (1994) Anti-Parkinson efficacy of ropinirole vs placebo as adjunct therapy in Parkinsonian patients not optimally controlled on L-dopa. 11th International Symposium on Parkinson's disease. Rome, Italy

Lera G, Vaamonde J, Rodriguez M, Obeso JA (1993) Cabergoline in Parkinson's disease: long-term follow-up. Neurology 43: 2587–2590

Lieberman A, Imke S, Muenter M, Wheeler K, Ahlskog JE, Matsumoto JY, Maraganore DM, Wright KF, Schoenfelder J (1993) Multicenter study of cabergoline, a long-acting dopamine receptor agonist, in Parkinson's disease patients with fluctuating responses to levodopa/carbidopa. Neurology 43: 1981–1984

Montastruc JL, Rascol O, Senard JM (1993) Current status of dopamine agonists in Parkinson's disease management. Drugs 46: 384–393

Pacchetti C, Martignoni P, Bruggi P, Godi L, Aufdembrinke B, Miltenburger C, Voet B, Nappi G (1993) Terguride in fluctuating parkinsonian patients: a double-blind study versus placebo. Mov Disord 8: 463–465

Parkinson's Disease Research Group in the United Kingdom (1993) Comparisons of therapeutic effects of levodopa, levodopa and selegiline, and bromocriptine in patients with early, mild Parkinson's disease: three year interim report. BMJ 307: 469–472

Rascol O, on behalf of the Ropinirole Early PD Study Group (1994) Anti-Parkinson efficacy of ropinirole vs placebo as early therapy in Parkinson's disease. 11th International Symposium on Parkinson's disease. Rome, Italy, p 279

Sagar H (1994) Anti-Parkinson efficacy (L-dopa sparing effect) of ropinirole vs placebo as adjunct therapy in Parkinsonian patients not optimally controlled on L-dopa. 11th International Symposium on Parkinson's disease. Rome, Italy, p 321

Vidailhet MJ, Bonnet AM, Belal S, Dubois B, Marle C, Agid Y (1990) Ropinirole without levodopa in Parkinson's disease. Lancet 336: 316–317

Authors' address: Dr. D. J. Brooks, MRC Cyclotron Unit, Hammersmith Hospital, Du Cane Road, London W12 0NN, United Kingdom.

J Neural Transm (1995) [Suppl] 45: 239–245
© Springer-Verlag 1995

Dihydroergocryptine in the treatment of Parkinson's disease

U. Bonuccelli, P. D'Antonio, C. D'Avino, P. Piccini, and **A. Muratorio**

Institute of Clinical Neurology, University of Pisa, Italy

Summary. In the last 20 years dopamine agonists have been considered more and more helpful as primary therapy for Parkinson's disease (PD). Recently the neuroprotective activity and the therapeutic efficacy of a new ergot derivative, α-dihydroergocryptine (DHEC), has been highlighted.

In the present work we resume the experimental and clinical data reported about this drug.

The rationale for dopamine (DA) agonists as primary therapy for Parkinson's disease (PD) is based on the possibility to delay the onset of long term l-dopa syndrome (LTS) (King, 1992); moreover DA agonists seem to exert a neuroprotective effect on substantia nigra neurons. In fact, they stimulate DA receptors bypassing the degenerating nigrostriatal neurons and their metabolic machinery (Lieberman, 1992; Olanow, 1992); more recently, some studies have shown that these drugs have a direct protective effect too (Felten et al., 1992; Yoshikawa et al., 1994). In this minireview we resume the data reported about neuroprotective activity and therapeutic efficacy of a new ergot derivative, α-dihydroergocryptine (DHEC).

Neuroprotective activity

In animal models, DHEC has shown a protective activity against total cerebral ischemia $MgCl_2$-induced, histocytic anoxia by NaCN, and intracerebroventricular glutamate- and NMDA-induced convulsions (Maggioni et al., 1992). Some investigators have demonstrated that DHEC is able to prevent striatal dopamine loss induced by MPTP in mice (Coppi, 1993) and in monkeys (Marzatico et al., 1993; Bernocchi et al., 1990); moreover, DHEC is able to reduce the formation of intraneuronal peroxides by exposure to glutamate (Canonico and Favit, 1993). The molecular mechanisms underlying the neuroprotective action of DHEC probably consist in modifying some cerebral antioxidant enzyme activities (i.e. superoxide dismutase, glutathione reductase or oxidase) (Benzi et al., 1988; Villa et al., 1992; Marzatico et al., 1993), and in increasing the forebrain content of reduced glutathione (Benzi et al., 1991). The neuroprotective activity of DHEC is supported also by clinical studies on neurodegenerative diseases; for example, in trials vs placebo DHEC has proved to be effective in senile psycho-organic syndrome (Scarzella et al., 1992).

Pharmacodynamics

As for the symptomatic effectiveness of DHEC in PD, it depends on its potent D_2 receptor agonist activity, demonstrated by studies on receptorial binding in striatum (Canonico et al., 1988; Groppetti et al., 1989). On the contrary, the activity on D_1-receptors is still controversial (Markstein, 1983; Canonico et al., 1988). As far as the other cathecholaminergic systems are concerned, DHEC seems to have no serotoninergic activity and a very slight interaction with α-adrenergic receptors: this might explain the low incidence of cardiovascular side effects reported for this drug (Mailland, 1989; Martucci et al., 1989; Piolti et al., 1989).

Symptomatic activity

Some preliminary studies demonstrated that DHEC has a symptomatic effect in PD patients if added to l-dopa (Martucci et al., 1989; Battistin et al., 1991; Martignoni et al., 1991) (Table 1). In "de novo" PD patients DHEC shows a similar efficacy than BCR, when compared to this drug (Bergamasco et al., 1989; Piolti et al., 1989; Rodriguez et al., 1990) (Table 2).

Table 1. Clinical studies: DHEC in l-dopa treated patients

	Martucci et al. (1989)	Battistin et al. (1991)	Martignoni et al. (1991)
Patients			
No.	20	68	20
Age (years)	60.2 ± 4.6	64.7 ± 8.6	60.30 ± 6.18
H & Y	I–II–III	I–II–III–IV–V	II–III
Methods			
Design	double-blind vs BCR	double-blind vs LIS	double-blind vs PLA
Duration	1.5 months	2 months	6 months
DHEC			
max daily dosage (mg)	73 ± 29	60	56.6 ± 5
Results			
Efficacy	DHEC > BCR	DHEC = LIS	DHEC > PLA
Tolerability	DHEC > BCR	DHEC > LIS	DHEC < PLA

BCR Bromocriptine, *DHEC* α-Dihydroergocriptine, *LIS* Lisuride, *PLA* Placebo

Table 2. Clinical studies: DHEC in de novo patients

	Piolti et al. (1989)	Scarzella and Bergamasco (1989)	Rodriguez et al. (1990)	Bonuccelli et al. (1994)
Patients				
No.	28	13	20	14
Age (years)	61–74	54–68	<75	48–70
H & Y	I–II–III	I–II–III	I–II	I–II
Methods				
Design	double-blind vs BCR	open	double-blind vs BCR	double-blind cross-over vs BCR
Duration	6 months	24 months	2 months	6 months
DHEC max daily dosage (mg)	100	30.8 ± 12.6	120	60
Results				
Efficacy	DHEC = BCR	good therapeutic activity	DHEC = BCR	DHEC > BCR
Tolerability	DHEC > BCR	DHEC > BCR	DHEC > BCR	DHEC > BCR

BCR Bromocriptine, *DHEC* α-Dihydroergocriptine

Tolerability

Both in de novo patients and in patients treated with l-dopa, DHEC shows slight side effects (Table 3).

Our study

Recently in a double-blind cross-over studie with DHEC vs BCR we compared the effectiveness and tolerability of DHEC and BCR in the treatment of "de novo" patients affected by PD (Table 1) (Bonuccelli et al., 1994).

Our data indicate that at low doses DHEC can be a useful drug in the early treatment of PD, with an even greater efficacy and tolerability than BCR at low dosage.

Slight side effects were observed after DHEC administration, in agreement with the AA who used similar dosages (Martignoni et al., 1989, 1991; Battistin et al., 1991); when DHEC and BCR were administered at higher dosages, side effects were more numerous and more severe (Piolti et al., 1989; Rodriguez et al., 1990). The low incidence of cardiovascular side effects

                    U. Bonuccelli et al.

Table 3. DHEC side effects in clinical studies

	Martucci et al. (1989)	Piolti et al. (1989)	Scarzella and Bergamasco (1989)	Rodriguez et al. (1990)	Battistin et al. (1991)	Martignoni et al. (1991)	Bonuccelli et al. (1994)
No. of patients	10	13	22	10	32	10	14
Anorexia				1			
Anxiety	1			1	3		
Confusion					1		
Constipation	1	2		1			
Depression				4			
Dermatological disorders		1			1		
Diskynesias		1					
Dizziness		1		8	1	1	
Dry mouth				2			
Gastric pain		5	6	4			1
Hallucination					1		
Headache			2			5	
Hypotension	3		5	1	3		
Legs edema		2					
Myalgia				1			
Nausea	2	2		6		6	
Palpitation			1	2			
Paresthesia				1			
Sleep disorders				2	1		
Tremor					1		
Vomiting		1		2		1	
Weakness				8			

observed with DHEC may be due to its little interaction with α-adrenoreceptors (Mailland, 1989).

The peculiar design of our study (double-blind cross-over with a short wash-out period) allows us to make some additional observations. In fact we observed a different response to DHEC and BCR depending on the administration sequence. When DHEC was administered first, a significant improvement in motor performances was obtained, whereas no improvement could be seen both when DHEC was administered after BCR (and one-week wash-out period) and when BCR was administered after DHEC. This different response could be explained by a mutual interference between the two drugs. Similar results have been observed in studies in which BCR was alternate to pergolide (Goetz et al., 1985, 1989). The discrepancies in these results could be due to pharmacodynamic differences, in particular because of their different behaviour on D_1 receptors; in fact, while all DA agonists considered have a D_2 agonist activity, BCR has a D_1 antagonist activity, whereas pergolide acts as a D_1 agonist, and DHEC is a partial D_1 agonist (Markstein, 1983). The sinergy between D_1 agonist and D_2 agonist activity has been considered very important for the best treatment of PD (Robertson, 1992). Recently experimental studies have shown that D_1 agonist activity could be involved in long-term neuronal alterations, such as the synthesis of substance P and dinorphine, co-transmitters in the striatonigral GABAergic neurons (Gerfen et al., 1990; Robertson, 1992), receptorial changes and neuronal plasticity (Goelet et al., 1986; Robertson and Dragunow, 1990), via the increase of the expression of c-fos gene, involved in the regulation of gene transcription processes (Young et al., 1991).

On these bases, we suggest that, when a DA agonist is replaced by another, receptorial changes induced by the first might led to an altered response to the other.

Conclusions

DHEC, as well as the other DA agonists, can be considered a helpful drug in the treatment of PD de novo patients either because its symptomatic and its protective activity.

In particular, the main peculiarity of DHEC consists in its greater tolerability, associated with a similar therapeutic efficacy, in comparison with the other DA agonists.

References

Battistin L, Bardin PG, Ferro-Milone F, Ravenna C, Toso V (1991) Diidroergocriptina e morbo di Parkinson: studio multicentrico in doppio cieco vs lisuride. In: Agnoli A, Fabbrini G, Stocchi F (eds) Proceedings of "1st European Conference on Parkinson's disease and Extrapyramidal disorders", Rome 1990. John Libbey CIC, Rome, pp 31–50

Benzi G, Pastoris O, Villa RF (1988) Changes induced by aging and drug treatment on cerebral enzymatic system. Neurochem Res 13: 467–478

Benzi G, Pastoris O, Gorini A, Marzatico F, Villa RF, Curti D (1991) Influence of aging on the acute depletion of reduced glutathione induced by electrophilic agents. Neurobiol Aging 12: 227–231

Bergamasco B, Scarzella L, Cantello R, Delsedine M, Gilli M, Pinessi L, Riccio A (1989) La diidroergocriptina nel Morbo di Parkinson: risultati preliminari. Giorn Neuropsicofarmacol 4 [Suppl]: 22–26

Bernocchi G, Gerzeli G, Scherini E, Vignola C (1990) Neuroprotective effects of α-dihydroergocriptine against damages in the substantia nigra caused by severe treatment with 1-methyl-4-phenyl-1,2,3,6-tetrahydropyridine. Acta Neuropathol [Berl] 85: 404–413

Bonuccelli U, D'Antonio P, D'Avino C, Muratorio A (1994) α-dihydroergocriptine in Parkinson's disease: a double-blind cross-over study. In: Korczyn AD (ed) Dementia in Parkinson's disease. International symposium, Jerusalem, 1994. Monduzzi Editore, Bologna, pp 137–141

Canonico PL, Favit A (1993) Molecular mechanism underlying the neuroprotective action of dihydroergocryptine. New Trends Clin Neuropharmacol 7: 80

Canonico PL, Mailland F, Scapagnini U (1988) Diidroergocriptina e recettori dopaminergici a livello ipofisario e striatale. In: Agnoli A, Battistin L (eds) Morbo di Parkinson e demenze: metodologie diagnostiche. Atti Congresso LIMPE, Alba 1987. Don Guanella, Roma, pp 413–427

Coppi G (1993) Neuroprotective activity of α-dihydroergocryptine in animal models. New Trends Clin Neuropharmacol 7: 79–80

Felten DL, Felten SY, Fuller RW, Romano TD, Smalstig EB, Wong DT, Clemens JA (1992) Chronic dietary pergolide preserves nigrostriatal neuronal integrity in aged-Fisher-344 rats. Neurobiol Aging 13: 339–351

Gerfen CR, Engber TM, Mahan LC, Susel Z, Chase TN, Monsma FJ Jr, Sibley DR (1990) D_1 and D_2 dopamine receptor-regulated gene expression of striatonigral and striatopallidal neurons. Science 250: 1429–1432

Goelet P, Castellucci VF, Schacher S, Kandel ER (1986) The long and the short of long-term memory-a molecular framework. Nature 322: 419–422

Goetz CG, Tanner CM, Glantz RH, Klawans HL (1985) Chronic agonist therapy for Parkinson's disease: a 5-year study of bromocriptine and pergolide. Neurology 35: 749–751

Goetz CG, Shannon KM, Tanner CM, Carroll VS, Klawans HL (1989) Agonist substitution in advanced Parkinson's disease. Neurology 39: 1121–1122

Groppetti A, Ceresoli G, Del Monaco S, Parenti M (1989) Diidroergocriptina: studio degli effetti sui recettori dopaminergici striatali. Giornale di Neuropsicofarmacologia 4: 10–15

King DB (1992) The place of the dopaminergic agonists in the treatment of Parkinson's disease: the view from the trenches. Can J Neurol Sci 19: 156–159

Lieberman A (1992) Dopamine agonists used as monotherapy in de novo PD patients: comparisons with selegiline. Neurology 42 [Suppl 4]: 37–40

Maggioni A, Falcone A, Coppi G (1992) Activity of α-dihydroergocriptine in some animal models of cerebral anoxia and ischemia. Pharmacol Res 26 [Suppl 1]: 69

Mailland F (1989) Pharmacology of dihydroergokyptine and its role in the management of Parkinson's disease. In: Nappi G, Caraceni T (eds) Parkinsonism: diagnosis and treatment. Laurel House Publishing Company, London, pp 173–181

Markstein R (1983) Dopamine receptor profile of co-dergocrine (Hydergine) and its components. Eur J Pharmacol 86: 145–155

Martignoni E, Pacchetti C, Sibilla L, Bruggi P, Pedevilla M, Nappi G (1989) Studio clinico in doppio cieco vs placebo della diidroergocriptina nel Morbo di Parkinson. Giorn Neuropsicol 4 [Suppl]: 32–36

Martignoni E, Pacchetti C, Sibilla L, Bruggi P, Pedevilla M, Nappi G (1991) Dihydroergokryptine in the treatment of Parkinson's disease: a six months' double-blinde clinical trial. Clin Neuropharmacol 14: 78–83

Martucci N, Fabbrini G, Levi Minzi A, Pedevilla M (1989) La diidroergocriptina nella terapia del Morbo di Parkinson. Giorn Neuropsicol 4 [Suppl]: 37–39

Marzatico F, Café C, Taborelli M, Benzi G (1993) Experimental Parkinson's Disease in monkeys. Effect of ergot alkaloid derivative on lipid peroxidation in different brain areas. Neurochem Res 18: 1101–1106

Olanow CW (1992) A rationale for dopamine agonists as primary therapy for Parkinson's disease. Can J Neurol Sci 19: 108–112

Piolti R, Bergamaco B, Scarzella L, Scarzella R, Rivoira M, Apollonio I, Frattola L (1989) Diidroergocriptina versus bromocriptina nella terapia dei pazienti parkinsoniani "de novo". Giorn Neuropsicofarmacol 4: 27–31

Robertson HA (1992) Dopamine receptor interactions: some implications for the treatment of Parkinson's disease. Trends Neurosci 15: 201–206

Robertson HA, Dragunow M (1990) From synapse to genome: the role of immediate-early genes in permanent alterations in the central nervous system. Curr Aspects Neuro-Sciences 2: 143–157

Rodriguez M, Mailland F, Obeso JA, Martinez-Lage JM (1990) Diidroergocriptina nella malattia di Parkinson: studio doppio cieco vs bromocriptina. Poli symposium. Proceedings Atti, European Conference on Parkinson's disease and Extrapyramidal disorders, Rome 1990, pp 19–30

Scarzella L, Bono G, Bergamasco B (1992) Dihydroergocryptine in the management of senile psycho-organic syndrome. Int J Clin Pharm Res 12: 37–46

Villa RF, Arnaboldi R, Ghigini B, Gorini A (1992) Mitochondrial factors involved in Parkinson's disease by MPTP toxicity in Macaca fascicularis and drug effect. Neurochem Res 17: 1147–1154

Yoshikawa T, Minamiyama Y, Naito Y, Kondo M (1994) Antioxidant properties of bromocriptine, a dopamine agonist. J Neurochem 62: 1034–1038
Young ST, Porrino LJ, Iadarola MJ (1991) Cocaine induces striatal c-fos immunoreactive proteins via dopaminergic D1 receptors. Proc Natl Acad Sci USA 88: 1291–1295

Authors' address: Prof. U. Bonuccelli, Institute of Clinical Neurology, University of Pisa, Via Roma 67, I-56100 Pisa, Italy.

J Neural Transm (1995) [Suppl] 45: 247–257
© Springer-Verlag 1995

Lack of pharmacokinetic interaction between the selective dopamine agonist cabergoline and the MAO-B inhibitor selegiline

P. Dostert[1], M. Strolin Benedetti[1], S. Persiani[1], R. La Croix[1], M. Bosc[1], F. Fiorentini[1], D. Deffond[2], D. Vernay[2], and G. Dordain[2]

[1] Pharmacia, Department of Pharmacokinetics and Metabolism, Milan, Italy
[2] Hôpital Nord-Cebazat, Neurology Service, Clermont-Ferrand, France

Summary. The addition of a dopamine agonist and of a monoamine oxidase type B inhibitor to l-dopa has been suggested in the therapy of Parkinson's disease. The plasma pharmacokinetics of both cabergoline and l-dopa have previously been shown to remain unaffected when the two drugs are given concomitantly. This study aimed at examining whether the plasma pharmacokinetic parameters of cabergoline and selegiline are modified when given in combination. Selegiline is hardly detectable in plasma. Therefore, the plasma levels of its metabolites amphetamine, methamphetamine and desmetylselegiline were used to assess the effect of cabergoline co-administration. Plasma levels of the selegiline metabolites were determined first after selegiline administration (10 mg/day) for 8 days, and then after administration of both drugs for 22 additional days (day 30). Cabergoline plasma levels were measured on day 30, and then after administration of cabergoline (1 mg/day) alone for further 22 days. No statistical difference was found between the $C_{max,ss}$, $t_{max,ss}$, $AUC_{0-24h,ss}$, $C_{0h,ss}$, $C_{24h,ss}$ values of cabergoline and of the selegiline metabolites when the two drugs were given alone or in combination, indicating the absence of pharmacokinetic interaction between cabergoline and selegiline.

Introduction

Cabergoline, 1-[(6-allylergolin-8β-yl)carbonyl]-1-[3(dimethylamino)propyl]-3-ethylurea (FCE 21336, Fig. 1) is a new ergoline derivative. Cabergoline was shown to be a potent and selective agonist of dopamine D_2 receptors (Carfagna et al., 1991), with a IC_{50} value of 1.5 nM for the inhibition of N-propylnorapomorphine binding to rat striatum dopamine receptors (Strolin Benedetti et al., 1990).

Cabergoline displays long-lasting inhibitory activity on basal secretion and pharmacological and physiological hypersecretion of prolactin in the rat (Di Salle et al., 1982, 1983). In healthy male volunteers, cabergoline has a potent

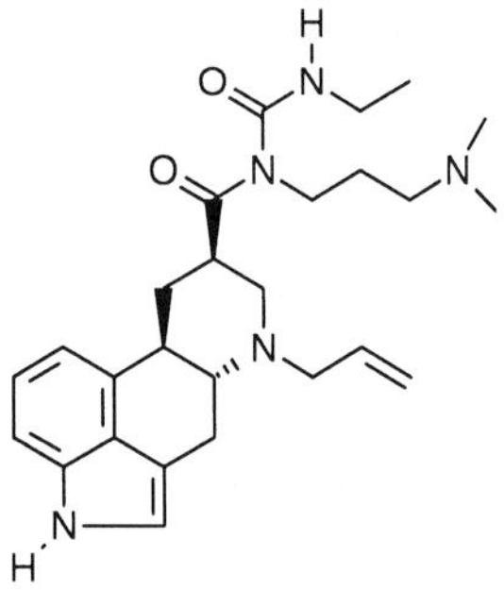

Fig. 1. Structure of cabergoline

prolactin lowering effect lasting up to 4 and 7 days after single oral doses of 0.2–0.3 mg and 0.6 mg, respectively (Pontiroli et al., 1987), while prolactin levels are decreased by 72–75% for at least 9 days in healthy female volunteers given a 1 mg dose of cabergoline as tablets or as a solution (Persiani et al., 1994). In hyperprolactinemic patients, a single oral dose of 0.3 mg cabergoline induced a marked and long-lasting fall in serum prolacting levels (Ferrari et al., 1986).

In MPTP-treated monkeys, a single subcutaneous dose of 0.5–1 mg/kg cabergoline completely restores locomotor activity for 24–70 h (Fariello et al., 1991), while a 0.25–0.5 mg/kg dose reduces L-dopa-induced dyskinesia (Grondin et al., 1994). In addition to its antiprolactin activity, cabergoline is undergoing clinical evaluation for the treatment of Parkinson's disease (Franceschi et al., 1988; Jori et al., 1990; Hutton et al., 1993; Lieberman et al., 1993). A global evaluation of the clinical data available at present suggests antiparkinson efficacy for cabergoline, as assessed by the use of specific rating scales and by patient self-assessment of daily fluctuations in motor performance.

Cabergoline concentrations in human plasma and urine were determined by HPLC with electrochemical detection with a limit of quantitation (LOQ) of 250 and 300 pg/ml, respectively (Pianezzola et al., 1992), and by radioimmunoassay with a LOQ of 12 and 120 pg/ml for plasma and urine, respectively (Persiani et al., 1992). In healthy female volunteers given a single oral dose of 1 mg cabergoline, the elimination half-life of the unchanged drug calculated from the data of the mean urinary excretion rate plotted on a semilogarithmic scale against the mid-point of the collection interval was 68 h, in good agreement with the long-lasting duration of prolactin decrease (Persiani et al., 1994). In healthy male volunteers given single oral doses of 0.5, 1, and 1.5 mg cabergoline, plasma C_{max} and AUC values and the percentage of urinary excretion indicated that the pharmacokinetics of cabergoline is dose-independent in the range of doses used (Pontiroli et al., 1993). The linearity of cabergoline pharmacokinetics was further evaluated in parkinsonian patients after repeated administration of single daily doses of 3, 5 and 7 mg. No significant differences were detected for C_{min}, C_{max} and AUC_{0-24h} values at steady-state after normalization to the dose, showing the linearity of cabergoline plasma pharmacokinetics, at least up to the dose of 7 mg (Strolin Benedetti et al., 1991). Moreover, the C_{max} and AUC_{0-24h} values at steady-state determined in another study (Del Dotto et al., 1994), in which parkinsonian patients received single oral daily doses of 2 mg cabergoline, were found to fit in well with the previous values.

In humans, after single oral administration of a 1 mg dose of ^{14}C-cabergoline, about 22% of the administered radioactivity was eliminated in urine within 20 days. Fecal excretion, about 57% dose during the same interval, was the main route of elimination of radioactivity (Battaglia et al., 1993). Cabergoline undergoes extensive metabolism, with unchanged drug amounting to about 1% of 0–24 h urinary radioactivity. The AUC_{0-8h} value of cabergoline was found to be about 6% of that of total plasma radioactivity (unpublished results). In the 0–24 h urine fraction, 8 metabolites were detected, 5 of which, accounting for 71% of urinary radioactivity, were identified. The main metabolite (41% urinary radioactivity) is the acid derivative resulting from the hydrolysis of the acylurea bond. The oxidative metabolism leading to the loss of the 3-dimethylaminopropyl group and to the dealkylation of the piperidine nitrogen is a minor pathway in humans.

The association of a dopamine D_2 agonist with L-dopa therapy is one of the treatments commonly used in patients with early Parkinson's disease, as well as in the management of fluctuations in mobility or dyskinesia which occur more frequently during long-term treatment (Calne, 1993). There is no compelling evidence for choosing one therapy or the other in the treatment of newly diagnosed Parkinson's disease, and the combination of a dopamine agonist, monoamine oxidase (MAO)-B inhibitor and l-dopa has been suggested among other approaches (Rinne, 1989). It has recently been established that l-dopa/carbidopa therapy does not influence cabergoline pharmacokinetics at steady-state (Del Dotto et al., 1994), and vice versa (Bonuccelli et al., 1993). The objective of this study was to examine whether

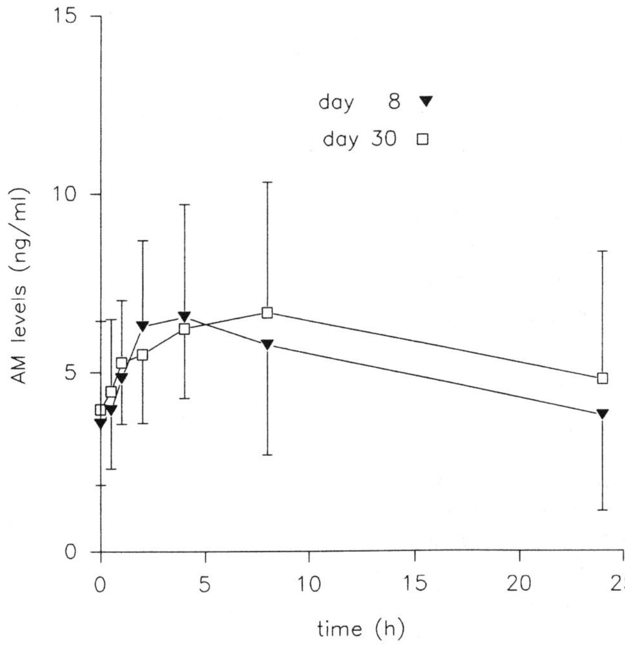

Fig. 2. Mean (± S.D.) plasma levels of amphetamine (AM) in parkinsonian patients after administration of selegiline (10 mg/kg) for 8 days and selegiline plus cabergoline (1 mg/kg) for further 22 days

the plasma pharmacokinetics of cabergoline and of the selective MAO-B inhibitor selegiline are modified when both drugs are given concomitantly. Amphetamine, methamphetamine and desmethylselegiline have been shown to be the main metabolites of selegiline in mammals including man (Reynolds et al., 1978, 1979; Philips, 1981; Yoshida, 1986) (Fig. 2), as a result of cytochrome P-450-dependent oxidative dealkylation of selegiline. It is worth noting that desmethylselegiline has been shown to be also a potent inhibitor of MAO-B in vivo (Borbe et al., 1990). Since selegiline is not easily detectable in human blood, likely as a consequence of its rapid metabolism (Lee et al., 1989), the plasma pharmacokinetics of selegiline was assessed by measuring the concentrations of its main metabolites.

Materials and methods

Subjects and study design

Five male de novo patients and one female patient, whose treatment with the dopamine agonist piribedil was discontinued 2 months before inclusion, completed the study. Another patient was excluded due to the appearance of aphasia during the second week of the study. In this patient, brain TC scan revealed the presence of a frontal meningioma which justified the transfer to the neurosurgery department. The evaluated patients were aged 57.5 ± 7.1 years (mean ± SD), had a Hoehn and Yahr score of 1–1.5, and a duration of the disease from 4 to 24 months (Table 1). Patients were fully informed of the nature of the study. Only subjects free of history or presence of psychiatric, severe cardiovascular and metabolic disorders, and with normal kidney and liver functions were enrolled. Patients received 10 mg selegiline once a day for 8 days, then concomitantly the same daily dose of selegiline plus cabergoline at the dose of 1 mg/day for 22 days followed by cabergoline alone (1 mg/day) for further 22 days.

Blood sampling and plasma preparation

Blood samples (8 ml) were collected in heparinized tubes. The times of blood sampling were: prior to any treatment (blank sample), and on days 8, 30 and 52: immediately before drug intake and at 0.5, 1, 2, 4, 8 and 24 h post-dosing.

Table 1. Characteristics of the evaluated patients

Patient No.	Sex	Age (y)	Weight (kg)	Height (cm)	Hoehn and Yahr grade	Duration of the disease (months)	Pretreatment with dopamine agonist
1	M	61	80	168	1.5	14	—
2	M	51	78	172	1	4	—
3	M	56	71	162	1	6	—
4	M	66	53	155	1	10	—
5	F	63	92	185	1	24	+*
6	M	48	76	170	1.5	7	—
mean ± SD		57.5 ± 7.1	75 ± 12.8	168.6 ± 10.1		10.8 ± 7.3	

*In this patient, treatment with the dopamine-agonist piribedil had been discontinued 2 months before study start

The blood samples were cooled in ice-water and immediately centrifuged, at 4°C, at 1.200 g for 10 min. The resulting plasma sample was divided into three tubes, which were stored at −20°C pending analysis. The whole procedure was carried out within 30 min from blood collection.

Plasma kinetics of selegiline metabolites were determined on days 8 and 30, while plasma kinetics of cabergoline were determined on days 30 and 52.

Analytical assays

The plasma concentrations of amphetamine, methamphetamine and desmethylselegiline were determined simultaneously using an HPLC method with fluorescence detection, after precolumn derivatisation with 9-fluorenylmethyl chloroformate (FMOC-Cl) (La Croix et al., 1994). Briefly, plasma samples were brought to pH 11 with 0.5 M borate buffer and extracted with diethyl ether. After back-extraction with 0.1 M HCl, the aqueous phase was subjected to derivatisation by reaction with FMOC-Cl in the presence of borate buffer (pH 8) and proline. Aliquots were injected directly into the HPLC system. This consisted of an Isochrom isocratic pump with a 200 μl loop, a FP 821 fluorescence detector, a SP 4270 integrator and a Winner 386 data acquisition system with "Labnet" software. All instruments were from Thermo Separation Products, except the detector, which was purchased from Jasco. The chromatographic conditions were: a Nova-Pak Phenyl column (150 × 3.9 mm I.D., particle size 4 μm) equipped with a precolumn filter, acetonitrile — 50 mM phosphate buffer pH 6.0 (50:50 v:v) as mobile phase, flow rate 1.0 ml/min. The fluorescence detector was set at 260 nm (excitation wavelength) and 315 nm (emission wavelength). The LOQ for the three derivatives was 0.5 ng/ml plasma.

Plasma concentrations of cabergoline were determined by radioimmunoassay using an antiserum raised in rabbits with an immunogen produced by conjugation of cabergoline to bovine serum albumine (Persiani et al., 1992). The LOQ was 12 pg/ml plasma, and the specificity with respect to structurally close analogues and other agents that could simultaneously be present in plasma of treated Parkinson's disease patients was excellent.

Pharmacokinetic analysis

Plasma pharmacokinetics of cabergoline and selegiline metabolites (amphetamine, methamphetamine and desmethylselegiline) were calculated by standard non-compartmental methods. For all pharmacokinetic parameters the actual sampling times were used. The area under the plasma concentration-time curve at steady-state ($AUC_{0-24h,ss}$) was calculated within the 24-h dosing interval using the linear trapezoidal rule. $C_{max,ss}$ and $t_{max,ss}$ were read as the coordinates of the highest concentration measured. $C_{0h,ss}$ and $C_{24h,ss}$ were taken as the concentration values determined prior to and 24 h after dosing on the day of treatment, respectively.

$AUC_{0-24h,ss}$, $C_{0h,ss}$, $C_{24h,ss}$ and $C_{max,ss}$, determined on days 8 and 30 for selegiline metabolites and on days 30 and 52 for cabergoline, were compared using Student's t-test for paired data. $T_{max,ss}$ values obtained on days 8 and 30 for selegiline metabolites and on days 30 and 52 for cabergoline were compared using the non-parametric Wilcoxon signed-rank test. Statistical analysis was performed at 0.05 significance level.

Results

Minor and well-tolerated adverse events were noted in two patients. Nightmares, insomnia and nausea occurred in patient 1 when this patient was under the association selegiline plus cabergoline. These effects disappeared on discontinuation of selegiline. Patient 3 suffered from mild nightmare episodes on the association of both drugs.

Mean plasma concentration profiles of amphetamine, methamphetamine, desmethylselegiline and cabergoline are shown in Figs. 2–5. Mean $AUC_{0-24h,ss}$, $C_{max,ss}$, $t_{max,ss}$, $C_{0h,ss}$ and $C_{24h,ss}$ values determined on days 8 and 30 for the selegiline metabolites and on days 30 and 52 for cabergoline are given in

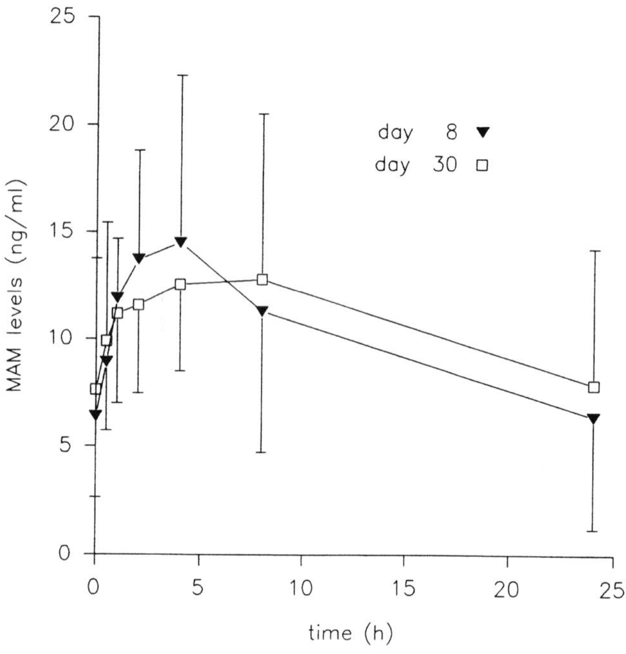

Fig. 3. Mean ($\pm$ S.D.) plasma levels of methamphetamine (MAM) in parkinsonian patients after selegiline (10 mg/kg) for 8 days and selegiline plus cabergoline (1 mg/kg) for further 22 days

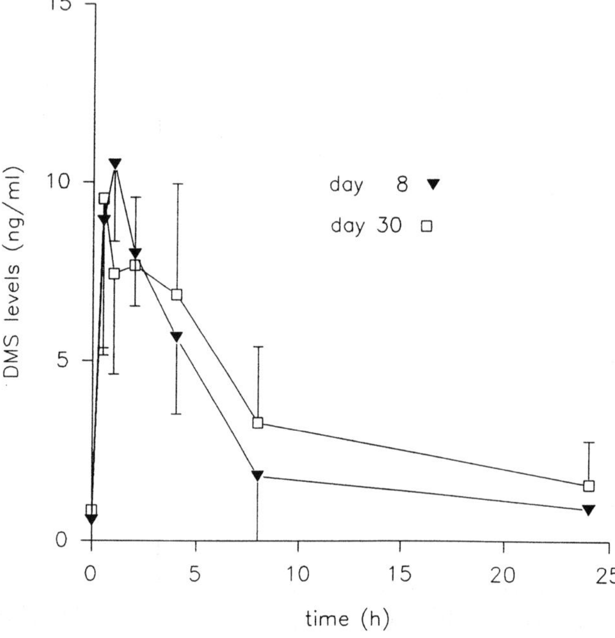

Fig. 4. Mean ($\pm$ S.D.) plasma levels of desmethylselegiline (DMS) in 6 parkinsonian patients after selegiline (10 mg/kg) for 8 days and selegiline plus cabergoline (1 mg/kg) for further 22 days

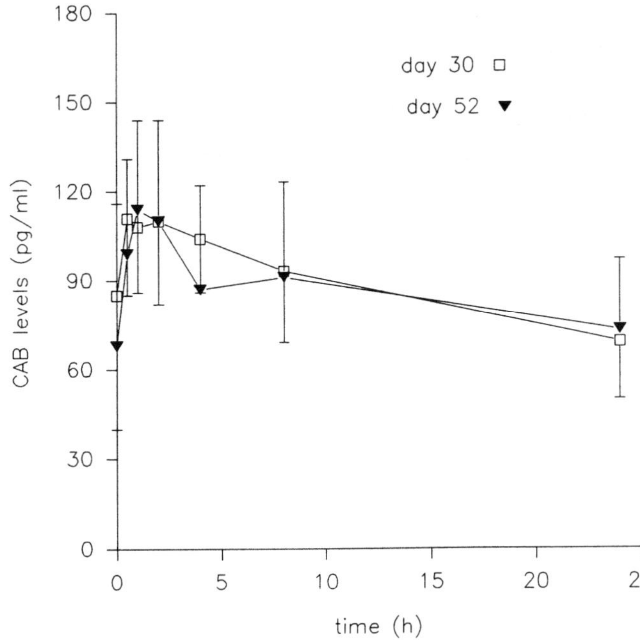

Fig. 5. Mean (± S.D.) plasma levels of cabergoline (CAB) in 6 parkinsonian patients after administration of selegiline (10 mg/kg) plus cabergoline (1 mg/kg) for 22 days and cabergoline alone for further 22 days

Table 2. Mean $AUC_{0-24h,ss}$, $C_{max,ss}$, $t_{max, ss}$, $C_{0h,ss}$ and $C_{24h,ss}$ values (±S.D.) of amphetamine (AM), methamphetamine (MAM), desmethylselegiline (DMS) and cabergoline (CAB) in 6 parkinsonian patients given selegiline (10 mg/day) and cabergoline (1 mg/day) alone or in combination

	AM		MAM		DMS		CAB	
	D_8	D_{30}	D_8	D_{30}	D_8	D_{30}	D_{30}	D_{52}
$AUC_{0-24h,ss}$ (ng.h/ml*)	123.3 (63.1)	139.9 (74.9)	243.5 (136.1)	263.4 (149.9)	58.2 (37.1)	83.2 (46.2)	2,087 (665)	2,138 (527)
$C_{max,ss}$ (ng/ml**)	6.98 (3.0)	7.21 (3.19)	15.66 (6.96)	15.05 (6.73)	11.03 (1.90)	11.01 (2.88)	122 (30)	121 (24)
$t_{max,ss}$ (h)	2.71 (1.0)	3.71 (2.61)	2.38 (1.34)	3.63 (2.72)	1.06 (0.55)	1.36 (1.48)	1.32 (0.62)	1.36 (1.49)
$C_{0h,ss}$ (ng/ml**)	3.56 (1.71)	3.97 (2.46)	6.41 (3.76)	7.63 (6.13)	0.56[a]	0.89[a]	68 (28)	85 (31)
$C_{24h,ss}$ (ng/ml**)	3.77 (2.66)	4.78 (3.56)	6.41 (5.22)	7.98 (6.35)	0.84[a]	1.56 (1.22)	73 (24)	69 (19)

[a] estimates based on the approximation that the values below the limit of quantitation are equal to zero; for cabergoline: *pg.h/ml, **pg/ml

Table 2. It is worth noting that, except for desmethylselegiline, the plasma concentrations of all the analytes were found to be always higher than the LOQ. For desmethylselegiline the plasma concentrations were sometimes, especially at t_0 and t_{24}, lower than the LOQ, which was set at 2 ng/ml for the analysis of real plasma samples due to the occurrence of interference problems. When the concentration was below the LOQ, the corresponding value was taken as zero, with consequent underestimate of the $AUC_{0-24h,ss}$ value.

For the three selegiline metabolites, the values of $C_{max,ss}$ $t_{max,ss}$, $AUC_{0-24h,ss}$, $C_{0h,ss}$ and C_{24h} obtained on day 8 after selegiline alone and on day 30 on coadministration with cabergoline resulted not significantly different. In the same way, no statistically significant difference was found for the pharmacokinetic parameters of cabergoline as determined on day 30 and day 52.

Discussion

The mean $AUC_{0-24h,ss}$, $C_{0h,ss}$, $C_{24h,ss}$, $C_{max,ss}$ and $t_{max,ss}$ values for cabergoline and the selegiline metabolites amphetamine, methamphetamine and desmetylselegiline were found not to be statistically different in the two sessions, on day 8 and day 30 for the selegiline metabolites and on day 30 and day 52 for cabergoline. These results show the absence of pharmacokinetic interaction when the two drugs are given concomitantly, as it could be expected considering their respective metabolism. Although selegiline is a weak inhibitor of cytochrome P-450 activities in rat liver microsome preparations (Dupont et al., 1987), and gives only weak type I interactions with microsomal cytochrome P-450$_s$ from rats either untreated or pretreated with classical inducers (D. Mansuy, personal communication), cytochrome P-450$_s$ are clearly involved in the dealkylation of selegiline (Yoshida et al., 1986). In addition, the binding of selegiline to liver cytochrome P-450$_s$ is not significantly affected by the presence of cabergoline. Also cabergoline was found to give very weak type I interactions with rat liver cytochrome P-450$_s$ (D. Mansuy, unpublished results). Since the main metabolic pathway of cabergoline is not cytochrome P-450-dependent and is essentially similar in the rat and the human (Battaglia et al., 1989), and since the repeated administration of cabergoline to rats causes marginal or moderate changes in the activity of only a few cytochrome P-450 families, with both weak inhibition and induction effects being found (F. Oesch, unpublished results), it is not surprising, therefore, that the plasma pharmacokinetics of either drug is not influenced when they are given concomitantly.

Selegiline was also found not to affect l-dopa plasma pharmacokinetics (Cedarbaum et al., 1990). Administration of l-dopa to bromocriptine-treated parkinsonian patients has been shown to decrease bromocriptine plasma levels (Rabey et al., 1989), while the effects of administration of bromocriptine on l-dopa plasma concentrations in l-dopa treated patients are not clear, with no change, increase or decrease being reported (Bentué-Ferrer et al., 1988; Rabey et al., 1990). In contrast, the plasma pharmacokinetic parameters of cabergoline and l-dopa remained virtually unaffected when the two drugs were administered concomitantly (Bonuccelli et al., 1993; Del Dotto et al., 1994).

In this study, a simple and sensitive HPLC method was developed for the determination of amphetamine, methamphetamine and desmethylselegiline concentrations in plasma (La Croix et al., 1994). The LOQ reached (0.5 ng/ml) is much lower than that reported by numerous authors (see references in Reimer et al., 1993). Using a more sophisticated gas chromatography/mass spectrometry method, Reimer et al. reported a LOQ of 0.1 ng/ml for amphetamine and methamphetamine and of 0.25 ng/ml for desmethylselegiline. As concerns cabergoline, it is worth nothing that the plasma levels at steady-state found in the present study conducted mainly in de novo parkinsonian patients fit in reasonably well with the plasma levels of cabergoline determined after administration of 3, 5 and 7 mg doses to older idiopathic Parkinson's disease patients suffering from l-dopa-associated motor fluctuations (Strolin Benedetti et al., 1991).

Tatton and Greenwood (1991) have suggested that selegiline exerts a neuroprotective action. This, in fact, should more appropriately be regarded as being a "neurorescue", in which selegiline would prevent the death and degeneration of neurons after damage that would otherwise be considered lethal has occurred. The mechanisms of such an activity of selegiline are unclear and may involve interactions with the normal mechanisms of programmed cell death (apoptosis). That cabergoline does not affect the plasma levels of selegiline metabolites is of potential interest since Tatton et al. (1994), using PC12 cells deprived of trophic proteins, have recently reported that selegiline would reduce the programmed cell death, whereas its metabolites amphetamine and methamphetamine would have the opposite effect.

Acknowledgement

The authors wish to warmly thank Ms. A. Zeni for the preparation of the manuscript.

References

Battaglia R, Strolin Benedetti M, Mantegani S, Castelli MG, Cocchiara G, Dostert P (1993) Disposition and urinary metabolic pattern of cabergoline, a potent dopaminergic agonist, in rat, monkey and man. Xenobiotica 23: 1377–1389

Bentué-Ferrer D, Allain H, Reymann JM, Sabouraud O, Van den Driessche J (1988) Lack of pharmacokinetic influence on levodopa by bromocriptine. Clin Neuropharmacol 11: 83–86

Bonuccelli U, Del Dotto P, Colzi A, Piccini P, Strolin Benedetti M, Dubini A, Fariello RG, Muratorio A (1993) Clinical and pharmacokinetic evaluation of levodopa and cabergoline co-treatment in Parkinson's disease. New Trends Clin Neuropharmacol 7: 120

Borbe HO, Niebch G, Nickel B (1990) Kinetic evaluation of MAO-B-activity following oral administration of selegiline and desmethylselegiline in the rat. J Neural Transm [Suppl] 32: 131–137

Calne DB (1993) Treatment of Parkinson's disease. N Engl J Med 329: 1021–1027

Carfagna N, Caccia C, Buonamici M, Cervini MA, Cavanus S, Fornaretto MG, Damiani D, Fariello RG (1991) Biochemical and pharmacological studies on cabergoline, a new putative antiparkinsonian drug. 21st Annual Meeting Society for Neuroscience, New Orleans, November 10–15. Soc Neurosci Abstr 17: 1075

Cedarbaum JM, Silvestri M, Clark M, Harts A, Kutt H (1990) L-deprenyl, levodopa pharmacokinetics and response fluctuations in Parkinson's disease. Clin Neuropharmacol 13: 29–35

Del Dotto P, Dostert P, Pardini C, Strolin Benedetti M, Persiani S, Fariello RG, Bonuccelli U (1994) Cabergoline pharmacokinetics in de novo PD: influence of L-Dopa. 11th International Symposium on Parkinson's disease, Rome, March 26–30 (Abstracts, p 293)

Di Salle E, Ornati G, Briatico G (1982) FCE 21336 a new ergoline derivative with a potent and long-lasting lowering effect on prolactin secretion in rats. J Endocrinol Invest 5 [Suppl 1]: 45

Di Salle E, Ornati G, Giudici D, Briatico G (1983) Prolactin lowering effect of a new ergoline derivative, FCE 21336, in the rat: a comparison with bromocriptine. Acta Endocrinol 103 [Suppl 256]: 265

Dupont H, Davies DS, Strolin Benedetti M (1987) Inhibition of cytochrome P-450-dependent oxidation reactions by MAO inhibitors in rat liver microsomes. Biochem Pharmacol 36: 1651–1657

Fariello RG, Carfagna N, Buonamici M, Dubini A (1991) Cabergoline a long acting D_2 agonist with antiparkinsonian properties. Preclinical studies. Ann Neurol 30: 258–259

Ferrari C, Barbieri C, Caldara R, Mucci M, Codecasa F, Paracchi A, Romano C, Boghen M, Dubini A (1986) Long-lasting prolactin lowering effect of cabergoline, a new dopamine agonist, in hyperprolactinemic patients. J Clin Endocrinol Metab 63: 941–945

Franceschi M, Bassi S, Calloni E, Camerlingo M, Frattola L, Giusti MC, Jori MC, Mamoli A, Piolti R, Canal N (1988) Evaluation of cabergoline, a new ergoline derivative, for the treatment of Parkinson's disease. J Neurol 235 [Suppl 1]: S53–S54

Grondin R, Blanchet PJ, Bédard PJ (1994) Cabergoline, a long-acting dopamine D-2 receptor agonist, reduces L-dopa-induced dyskinesia in MPTP monkeys. Can J Physiol Pharmacol [Suppl 1] 72: 385

Hutton JT, Morris JL, Brewer MA (1993) Controlled study of the antiparkinsonian activity and tolerability of cabergoline. Neurology 43: 613–616

Jori MC, Franceschi M, Giusti MC, Canal N, Piolti R, Frattola L, Bassi S, Calloni E, Mamoli A, Camerlingo M (1990) Clinical experience with cabergoline, a new ergoline derivative, in the treatment of Parkinson's disease. Adv Neurol 53: 539–543

La Croix R, Pianezzola E, Strolin Benedetti M (1994) Sensitive high-performance liquid chromatographic method for the determination of the three main metabolites of selegiline (L-deprenyl) in human plasma. J Chromatogr B 656: 251–258

Lee DH, Mendoza M, Dvorozniak MT, Chung E, van Woert MH, Yahr MD (1989) Platelet monoamine oxidase in Parkinson patients: effect of L-deprenyl therapy. J Neural Transm [P-D Sect] 1: 189–194

Lieberman A, Imke S, Muenter M, Wheeler K, Ahlskog JE, Matsumoto JY, Maraganore DM, Wright KF, Shoenfelder J (1993) Multicenter study of cabergoline, a long-acting dopamine receptor agonist, in Parkinson's disease patients with fluctuating responses to levodopa/carbidopa. Neurology 43: 1981–1984

Persiani S, Pianezzola E, Broutin F, Fonte G, Strolin Benedetti M (1992) Radioimmunoassay for the synthetic ergoline derivative cabergoline in biological fluids. J Immunoassay 13: 457–476

Persiani S, Sassolas G, Piscitelli G, Bizzolon A, Poggesi I, Pianezzola E, Edwards DMF, Strolin Benedetti M (1994) Pharmacodynamics and relative bioavailability of cabergoline tablets vs solution in healthy volunteers. J Pharm Sci 83: 1421–1424

Philips SR (1981) Amphetamine, p-hydroxyamphetamine and β-phenethylamine in mouse brain and urine after (−)- and (+)-deprenyl administration. J Pharm Pharmacol 33: 739–741

Pianezzola E, Bellotti V, La Croix R, Strolin Benedetti M (1992) Determination of cabergoline in plasma and urine by high-performance liquid chromatography with electrochemical detection. J Chromatogr 574: 170–174

Pontiroli AE, Viberti GC, Mangili R, Cammelli L, Dubini A (1987) Selective and extremely long inhibition of prolactin release in man by 1-ethyl-3-(3'-dimethylaminopropyl)-3-(6'-allylergoline-8'-β-carbonyl)-urea-diphosphate (FCE 21336). Br J Clin Pharmacol 23: 433–438

Pontiroli AE, Andreotti AC, Pianezzola E, Persiani S, Pacciarini MA, Strolin Benedetti
M (1993) Pharmacokinetics and prolactin lowering effect of cabergoline in healthy
men. 75th Annual meeting of the Endocrine Society, Las Vegas, June 9–12, 1993
(Abstracts, p 153)

Rabey JM, Oberman Z, Scharf M, Isakov A, Bar M, Graff E (1989) The influence of
levodopa on the pharmacokinetics of bromocriptine in Parkinson's disease. Clin
Neuropharmacol 12: 440–447

Rabey JM, Oberman Z, Harset A, Graff E, Vered Y (1990) Mutual interaction of
bromocriptine and levodopa in the periphery in Parkinson disease (PD). Mov Disord
[Suppl 1] 5: 50

Reimer MLJ, Mamer OA, Zavitsanos AP, Siddiqui AW, Dadgar D (1993) Determination
of amphetamine, methamphetamine and desmethyldeprenyl in human plasma by gas
chromatography/negative ion chemical ionization mass spectrometry. Biol Mass
Spectr 22: 235–242

Reynolds GP, Elsworth JD, Blau K, Sandler M, Lees AJ, Stern GM (1978) Deprenyl is
metabolized to methamphetamine and amphetamine in man. Br J Clin Pharmacol 6:
542–544

Reynolds GP, Riederer P, Sandler M (1979) 2-phenylethylamine and amphetamine in
human brain: effects of L-deprenyl in Parkinson's disease. Biochem Soc Trans 7: 143–
145

Rinne UK (1989) Combination of a dopamine agonist, MAO-B inhibitor and levodopa —
a new strategy in the treatment of early Parkinson's disease. Acta Neurol Scand 126:
165–169

Strolin Benedetti M, Dostert P, Barone D, Efthymiopoulos C, Peretti G, Roncucci R
(1990) In vivo interaction of cabergoline with rat brain dopamine receptors labelled
with [^{3}H]N-n-propylnorapomorphine. Eur J Pharmacol 187: 399–408

Strolin Benedetti M, Pianezzola E, Persiani S, Grimaldi R, Obeso JA (1991) Evaluation
of the linearity of cabergoline pharmacokinetics in parkinsonian patients. 10th International Symposium on Parkinson's Disease, Tokyo, October 27–30, 1991 (Abstracts,
p 240)

Tatton WG, Greenwood CE (1991) Rescue of dying neurons: a new action of deprenyl in
MPTP parkinsonism. J Neurosci Res 30: 666–672

Tatton W, Wadia J, Ju W, Holland D, Seniuk-Tatton N (1994) (−)-Deprenyl blocks
mitochondrial depolarization and programmed cell death in trophically-deprived
cells. Can J Physiol Pharmacol 72 [Suppl 1]: 36

Yoshida T, Yamada Y, Yamamoto Y, Kuroiwa Y (1986) Metabolism of deprenyl, a
selective monoamine oxidase (MAO) B inhibitor in rat: relationship of metabolism to
MAO-B inhibitory potency. Xenobiotica 16: 129–136

Authors' address: Dr. P. Dostert, Pharmacia, R&D/Pharmacokinetics & Metabolism
Department, Via Bisceglie, 104, I-20152 Milan, Italy.

J Neural Transm (1995) [Suppl] 45: 259–265
© Springer-Verlag 1995

Cabergoline improves motor disability without modifying L-DOPA plasma levels in fluctuating Parkinson's disease patients

P. Del Dotto[1], A. Colzi[1], C. Pardini[1], C. Lucetti[1], A. Dubini[2], R. Grimaldi[2], and U. Bonuccelli[1]

[1] Institute of Clinical Neurology, University of Pisa, and [2] Pharmacia, Milano, Italy

Summary. Studies on the influence of some dopamine agonists, particularly bromocriptine, on the pharmacokinetics of L-dopa have furnished contrasting results. Thus, any possible pharmacokinetic interaction should be taken into consideration when adding a new dopamine agonist to L-dopa treatment. In 12 Parkinson's disease (PD) patients with motor fluctuations, cabergoline was added in an 8-week study to their usual L-dopa/carbidopa therapy. Cabergoline was administered once a day at increasing doses of 0.5, 1, 2, and 3 mg/day for a period of one week per dose, and 4 mg/day for three weeks. Motor performance was assessed weekly evaluating the motor examination of the Unified Parkinson's Disease Rating Scale (UPDRS) and the patients' diaries of daily on-off time. Blood levels of both L-dopa and 3-O-methyldopa (3-OMD) were assayed by HPLC in two different days, over an 8-hour period, before initiating cabergoline and at the end of the study.

The results of this study confirm that cabergoline is effective in the management of PD motor fluctuations without modifying L-dopa and 3-OMD pharmacokinetics.

Introduction

L-dopa therapy is still the most effective drug for the treatment of Parkinson's disease (PD); however, in a high proportion of patients, its administration is accompanied by the development of motor fluctuations after few years of treatment. The use of dopamine agonists to control the wearing-off or on-off phenomena is well-established; the administration of lisuride and apomorphine by continuous subcutaneous infusion has been reported to be of particular benefit, probably by virtue of continuous stimulation of dopaminergic receptors (Obeso et al., 1987). Such an approach, however, is an impractical treatment strategy.

Cabergoline is a dopaminergic agonist specific for the D2 receptors, with an elimination half-life of approximately 65 hours. In PD patients with motor fluctuations cabergoline administered once daily has been proved to be effective and well-tolerated (Lera et al., 1990; Jori et al., 1990; Hutton et al., 1993;

Lieberman et al., 1993; Rabey et al., 1994). The long cabergoline half-life enables this drug to provide a hypothetical continuous stimulation of dopaminergic receptors; this might be the reason of its effectiveness in the treatment of parkinsonian motor fluctuations. However, we cannot rule out that this long-lasting effect may be due to an interaction with L-dopa pharmacokinetics and bioavailability.

Studies concerning the influence of some dopamine agonists, particularly bromocriptine, on the pharmacokinetics of L-dopa, have provided contrasting data. For instance, Rabey et al. (1991) found that the administration of bromocriptine plus L-dopa can produce an increase, a decrease or no effect on L-dopa plasma levels in different groups of parkinsonian patients. Sutton et al. (1990) observed that chronic bromocriptine co-therapy increases peak plasma concentration of L-dopa. Other Authors, in contrast, showed no influence on L-dopa pharmacokinetic parameters by oral bromocriptine (Bentuè-Ferrer et al., 1988; Contin et al., 1992).

Since co-administration of cabergoline and L-dopa is to be expected in the clinical practice for the treatment of parkinsonian patients suffering from motor fluctuations, it is interesting to investigate the possible pharmacokinetic interactions between the two compounds.

The present study focuses on the clinical efficacy of cabergoline as well as the pharmacokinetics of L-dopa before and after the adjunct of cabergoline according to an open, rising-dose study have been evaluated in a group of fluctuating PD patients.

Patients and methods

Subjects

Twelve PD patients (6 males, 6 females) under chronic L-dopa therapy completed the study; all patients showed motor fluctuations of the wearing-off type. The clinical characteristics of the study population are reported in Table 1.

All patients took L-dopa/carbidopa at a mean L-dopa daily dose of 760 ± 99 mg/day (ranging from 625 to 875 mg/day), divided in 3.8 ± 0.7 administrations per day.

Table 1. Clinical characteristics of the study population

No.	12
Sex(M/F)	6/6
Age (mean ± SD)	57.7 ± 6.9 yrs
Disease duration (mean ± SD)	8.4 ± 4.0 yrs
Hoehn-Yahr (mean ± SD)	2.9 ± 0.6
L-DOPA therapy	
duration(mean ± SD)	6.9 ± 2.3 yrs
dose (mean ± SD)	760 ± 99 mg/day

Protocol

The study, approved by the local Ethics Committee, was carried out under open conditions at the Institute of Clinical Neurology of Pisa (Italy).

Baseline visit was performed four weeks after the discontinuation of excluded medications, such as other dopamine agonists, anticholinergics, selegiline or amantadine (wash-out period). During weeks 3 to 4 of this period the L-dopa dose was optimized.

At the end of the wash-out period (day 0) the patients were admitted to the hospital after an overnight fast; baseline blood samples for the first kinetic session were drawn. Starting from the following day (day 1) cabergoline was added, as a single morning daily dose, to the L-dopa/carbidopa therapy at increasing doses of 0.5, 1, 2 and 3 mg/day for a period of one week per dose, and 4 mg/day for the following three weeks. At the end of this treatment period (day 49) the patients returned to the hospital for the second kinetic session, as well as for clinical evaluations.

During the study the L-dopa/carbidopa dose was maintained unchanged and no other antiparkinsonian drugs were started.

Clinical evaluation of parkinsonian disability was rated at baseline and after the adjunct of cabergoline (days 7, 14, 21, 28 and 49) by means of:

1) Unified Parkinson's Disease Rating Scale (UPDRS, motor examination) during on and off conditions;
2) on-off diary card of daily motor conditions;
3) Clinical Global Impression (CGI).

Pharmacokinetic sessions

Blood samples were collected in the morning (starting between 8 am-9 am) on day 0 and day 49 of the study before and 0.5, 1, 2, 3, 4, 5, 6, 7, 8 h after administration of 250/25 mg of L-dopa/carbidopa. On day 49 L-dopa/carbidopa was administered together with 4 mg of cabergoline.

A low protein breakfast and lunch were provided at 10 am and 1 pm, respectively.

The blood samples were collected in heparinized tubes and immediately centrifuged at 2500 g for 10 min at 4°C. After centrifugation, plasma was separated and stored at -70°C until analysis.

L-dopa and 3-O-methyldopa (3-OMD) were assayed by high-pressure liquid chromatography (HPLC) with coulometric detection according to the method described by Gerlach et al. (1986) with modifications. The maximum plasma concentration (C_{max}) and the time of maximum concentration (T_{max}) of L-dopa were determined by inspection of the data.

Areas under the curve (AUC) for L-dopa and 3-OMD were determined by the trapezoidal rule.

In seven randomized patients the minimal steady-state plasma concentrations ($C_{min,ss}$) of cabergoline were measured on days 46, 47, and 48 (after three weeks of receiving a stable dose of 4 mg/day) to evaluate the compliance of the patients and to check that steady state had in fact been reached. Blood samples were collected in heparinized tubes before the morning cabergoline dose; plasma was separated and stored at -70°C until assay by radioimmunoassay (Persiani et al., 1992) at the Department of Pharmacokinetics and Metabolism of Pharmacia (Milano, Italy).

Statistics

Statistical analysis was performed using ANOVA with repeated measures and multiple comparisons, the Student t test, and the Wilcoxon test as appropriate. Significant values were considered when $p < 0.05$.

Results

Clinical observations

A significant dose-dependent decrease of "off" hours and an improvement in UPDRS motor examination (evaluated during the "off" condition) was observed for the dose of 2, 3 and 4 mg/day of cabergoline (Figs. 1 and 2). No change in UPDRS was observed during the "on" periods. None of the patients experienced an increase in dyskinesia severity.

According to the Global Improvement score subitem of CGI evaluated at last visit, 1 patient was judged very much improved, 6 patients were judged much improved and 1 patient was judged minimally improved as compared to their baseline conditions; only in 4 patients parkinsonian symptoms were judged unmodified; no patient was judged to have deteriorated.

The results of the Patient Judgement score subitem of CGI were substantially superimposable on the ones given by the investigators (3 patients judged their own conditions very much improved, 4 as much improved and 1 as minimally improved as compared to baseline; 4 patients judged their own conditions as unmodified).

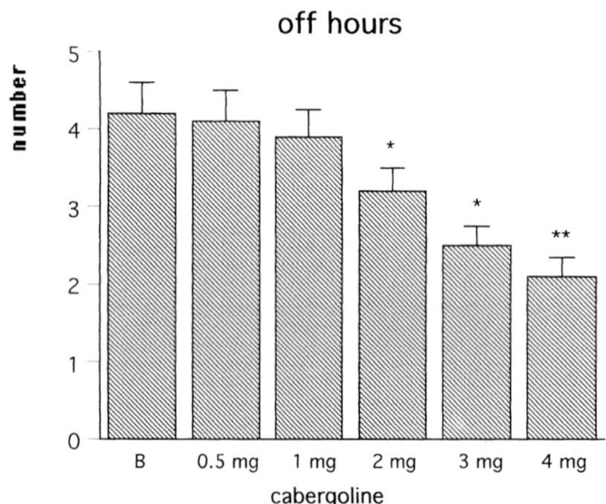

Fig. 1. Off hours at baseline (B) and after the adjunct of 0.5, 1, 2, 3, and 4 mg/day of cabergoline in 12 fluctuating PD patients. Values are expressed as mean ± SD. *p < 0.05 compared to baseline; **p < 0.02 compared to baseline

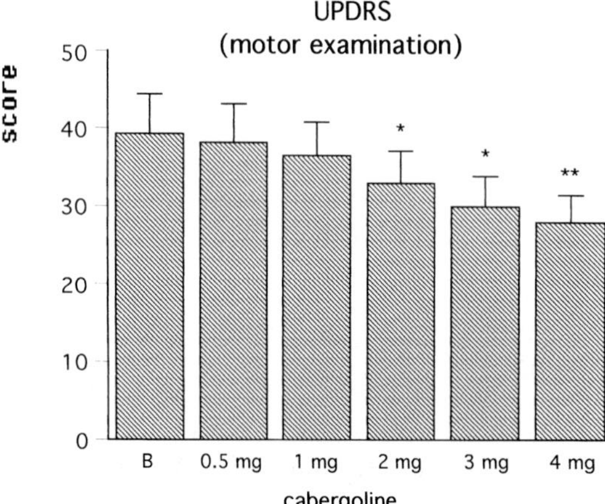

Fig. 2. UPDRS motor examination scores evaluated during off conditions at baseline (B) and after the adjunct of 0.5, 1, 2, 3, and 4 mg/day of cabergoline in 12 fluctuating PD patients. Values are expressed as mean ± SD. *p < 0.05 compared to baseline; **p < 0.02 compared to baseline

The following adverse effects were noted: 1 patient experienced orthostatic hypotension; 1 patient experienced dizziness; another patient complained of constipation. However, the severity of these side effects did not require the discontinuation of cabergoline in any patient.

A clinically significant increase in total bilirubin was reported in one patient; however, at baseline bilirubin levels were already above the normal range, an underlying hepatic problem was likely.

Pharmacokinetics

L-dopa pharmacokinetic parameters (C_{max}, T_{max} and $AUC_{(0-8h)}$) and $AUC_{(0-8h)}$ of 3-OMD are reported in Table 2 and Fig. 3. No statistically significant differences were observed before or after the addition of cabergoline.

The $C_{min,ss}$ of cabergoline measured in seven patients at the end of the study was $225.6 \pm 66.7\,pg/ml$.

Discussion

In spite of the short duration of the trial, our clinical data confirm that cabergoline is well tolerated and effective in the control of parkinsonian motor fluctuations.

Table 2. L-DOPA pharmacokinetic parameters (mean $\pm$ SD) without and with cabergoline therapy

	L-dopa/carbidopa alone (No. = 12 pts)	L-dopa/carbidopa + cabergoline (No. = 12 pts)	
Cmax (μg/ml)	1.17 ± 0.31	1.20 ± 0.37	NS
Tmax (min)	60.7 ± 24.5	57.7 ± 19.2	NS
AUC L-dopa (0–8 h) (μg/mlxh)	2.46 ± 1.43	2.29 ± 1.25	NS
AUC 30MD (0–8 h) (μg/mlxh)	13.95 ± 4.10	13.22 ± 4.19	NS

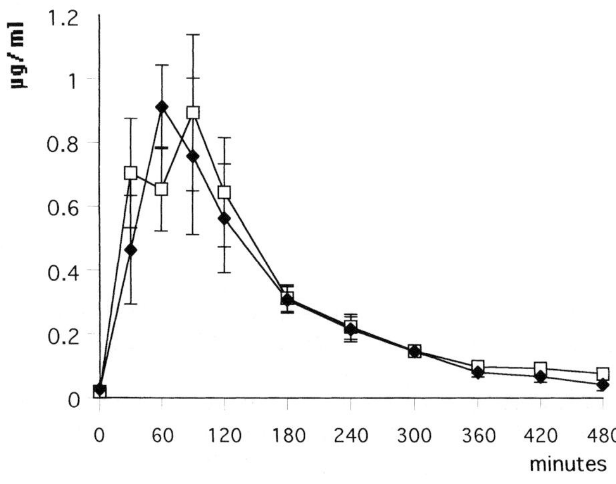

Fig. 3. Mean plasma levels (±SE) of L-dopa administered alone (250/25 mg L-dopa/carbidopa) (-□-) or with cabergoline (4 mg) (-◆-) in 12 fluctuating PD patients

The extent of such improvement (decrease of "off" hours, reduction in "off" disability scores) is similar to that reported by Hutton et al. (1993), Lieberman et al. (1993), Ahlskog et al. (1994), and appears to be dose-dependent. Even better results are reported in fluctuating PD patients by Lera et al. (1993) using higher doses of cabergoline (about 12 mg/day). The improvement seen in our unblinded, open-label trial is unlikely to be due to a placebo effect, as a clear-cut improvement did not occur for the lower doses of 0.5 and 1 mg/day of cabergoline.

The main goal of the present study was, however, to evaluate the possible effects of chronic cabergoline on L-dopa pharmacokinetics in parkinsonian patients; to our knowledge this is the first report concerning this matter. Our results demonstrate that L-dopa and 3-OMD pharmacokinetic parameters with and without cabergoline are not statistically different. Plasma concentrations of cabergoline measured in 7 patients at steady state fit reasonably well with the values observed by Strolin Benedetti et al. (1991) and Lera et al. (1993) in parkinsonian patients with motor fluctuations, providing evidence of a good patient compliance.

Some authors have studied the possible pharmacokinetic influence on plasma L-dopa of another dopamine agonist, bromocriptine, with the aim of explaining the beneficial effect of the addition of this drug on parkinsonian symptomatology, apart from its pharmacodynamic action. Bentuè-Ferrer et al. (1988) and Contin et al. (1992) did not find any significant effect of acute or chronic treatment with bromocriptine on oral L-dopa pharmacokinetics. On the other hand, Rabey et al. (1991) found some influence of bromocriptine on the L-dopa pharmacokinetics in parkinsonian patients; particularly, in a subgroup of fluctuating patients, L-dopa plasma levels were significantly lower; in some of these patients off hours were greater and dyskinesias less severe when the two drugs were given together; in another group L-dopa levels were higher and dyskinesias were at times more severe during co-administration, suggesting that bromocriptine may interfere with the peripheral pharmacokinetics of L-dopa and contribute to the fluctuations in the therapeutic response to L-dopa itself. Our pharmacokinetic results suggest that the long-lasting clinical effect of once-a-day cabergoline in parkinsonian patients with motor fluctuations is not due to an increase in L-dopa bioavailability; it might be attributable to the prolonged stimulation of dopaminergic receptors in keeping with the long cabergoline elimination half-life. In such patients cabergoline may represent a practical approach to providing easy continuous dopaminergic stimulation by the oral route even when taken only once a day.

References

Ahlskog JE, Muenter MD, Maraganore DM, Matsumoto JY, Lieberman A, Wright KF, Wheeler K (1994) Fluctuating Parkinson's disease. Treatment with the long-acting dopamine agonist cabergoline. Arch Neurol 51: 1236–1241

Bentuè-Ferrer D, Allain H, Reymann JM, Sabouraud O, Van der Driessche J (1988) Lack of pharmacokinetics influence on L-dopa by bromocriptine. Clin Neuropharmacol 11: 83–86

Contin M, Riva R, Martinelli P, Albani F, Baruzzi A (1992) No effect of chronic bromocriptine therapy on L-dopa pharmacokinetics in patients with Parkinson's disease. Clin Neuropharmacol 15: 505–508

Gerlach M, Klaunzer N, Przuntek H (1986) Determination of L-dopa and 3-O-methyldopa in human plasma by extraction using C18 cartridges followed by high-performance liquid chromatographic analysis with electrochemical detection. J Chromatogr 180: 378–385

Hutton TJ, Jerry LM, Brewer MA (1993) Controlled study of the antiparkinsonian activity and tolerability of cabergoline. Neurology 43: 613–616

Jori MC, Franceschi M, Giusti MC, Canal N, Piolti R, Frattola L, Bassi S, Calloni E, Mamoli A, Camerlingo M (1990) Clinical experience with cabergoline, a new ergoline derivative, in the treatment of Parkinson's disease. Adv Neurol 53: 539–543

Lera G, Vaamonde J, Muruzabal J, Obeso JA (1990) Cabergoline: a long-acting dopamine agonist in Parkinson's disease. Ann Neurol 28: 593–594

Lera G, Vaamonde J, Rodriguez M, Obeso JA (1993) Cabergoline in Parkinson's disease: long-term follow-up. Neurology 43: 2587–2590

Lieberman A, Imke S, Muenter M, Wheeler K, Ahlskog JE, Matsumoto JY, Maraganore DM, Wright KF, Schoenfelder J (1993) Multicenter study of cabergoline, a long-acting dopamine receptor agonist in Parkinson's disease patients with fluctuating responses to levodopa/carbidopa. Neurology 43: 1981–1984

Obeso JA, Luquin MR, Vaamonde J, Grandas F, Martinez-Lage JM (1987) Continuous dopaminergic stimulation for Parkinson's disease. Can J Neurol Sci 14: 488–492

Persiani S, Pianezzola E, Broutin F, Fonte G, Strolin Benedetti M (1992) Radioimmunoassay for the synthetic ergoline derivative in biological fluids. J Immunoassay 13: 457–476

Rabey JM, Schwartz M, Graff E, Harsat A, Vered Y (1991) The influence of bromocriptine on the pharmacokinetics of L-dopa in Parkinson's disease. Clin Neuropharmacol 14: 514–522

Rabey JM, Nissipeanu P, Inzelberg R, Korczyn AD (1994) Beneficial effect of cabergoline, new long-lasting D2 agonist in the treatment of Parkinson's disease. Clin Neuropharmacol 17: 286–293

Strolin Benedetti M, Pianezzola E, Persiani S, Grimaldi R, Obeso JA (1991) Evaluation of the linearity of cabergoline pharmacokinetics in parkinsonian patients. 10th International Symposium on Parkinson's disease, Tokyo, 1991 (Abstracts, p 240)

Sutton JP, Goetz CG, Buhrnfield C, Carvey PM (1990) The effect of bromocriptine cotherapy on L-dopa pharmacokinetics. Mov Disord 5 [Suppl 1]: 55

Authors' address: P. Del Dotto, MD, Institute of Clinical Neurology, University of Pisa, Via Roma, 67, I-56100 Pisa, Italy.

J Neural Transm (1995) [Suppl] 45: 267–270

Plasma levels of vitamin E in Parkinson's disease

A. Federico, C. Battisti, P. Formichi, and **M. T. Dotti**

Unit Neurometabolic diseases and Chair of Neurology (OPD), Institute of
Neurological Sciences, Medical School, University of Siena, and Associazione Anni
Verdi, Roma, Italy

Summary.   We report the analysis of plasma levels of vitamin E that has been
found normal in 20 italian patients with Parkinson's disease (PD) confirming
the previously reported results from other groups. We discuss the literature
data about the possible protective effect of antioxidant agents in the PD and
generally in the aging processes.

Introduction

The pathogenesis of the neuronal degeneration in substantia nigra-pars
compacta in Parkinson's disease (PD) is unknown. A variety of oxidative
mechanisms, involving the activity of monoamine oxidase and the formation
of free radicals, excessive lipid peroxidation promoted by free radicals and
reactive species (Dexter et al., 1989) have been hypothesized.

Vitamin E seems to play an important role as an antioxidant for unsatur-
ated lipids and in maintaining the integrity and stability of biological membranes. Its therapeutic role in movement disorders has been recently stressed
(Cadet, 1993). However the relationship between PD and vitamine E remain
controversial since vitamin E levels in PD serum (Fernandez-Calle et al.,
1993) and substantia nigra (Marsden, 1990; Adams et al., 1991) have been
reported as normal.

Here we report the results of the analysis of Vitamin E in the serum of an
italian population of PD patients compared with controls, confirming the
previously reported results from other groups.

Material and methods

Patients and controls. We measured the serum levels of vitamin E and Vitamin E/
Cholesterol ratio in 20 PD patients (12 men and 8 women, mean age 68 ± 2.5, mean age
of onset 60 ± 1.6 years). They fulfill the diagnostic criteria for PD. The control group is
comprehensive of 48 subjects without any neurological diseases, age matched, with the
same dietary habits. A previous article on changes of vitamin E serum levels during
development and aging has been reported by our group (Battisti et al., 1994). All patients
were under treatment with antiparkinsonian drugs alone or in combination, including

levodopa and anticholinergic drugs. The following exclusion criteria were applied including high ethanol intake, history of chronic hepathopathy or diseases causing malabsorption, history of systemic disease, atypical dietary habits; intake of drugs modifying lipid adsorption and vitamin therapy in the last 6 months.

Plasma tocopherol concentration was estimated blindly in non fasting samples of serum according with Muller et al. (1974).

Serum cholesterol concentrations were measured enzymatically using standard commercially available clinical chemistry kits. The results are expressed as Umoles/litres.

Results and discussion

The mean vitamin E serum levels of PD patients (24.8 ±7; range 16.7 to 38.8 Umoles/l) did not differ from controls of the same age group (24 ± 6.5, with a rage between 12 to 35 Umoles/l.) There was no significant difference in the vitamin E/ cholesterol ratio between the two groups (PD 0.48 ± 0.06; controls 0.50 ± 0.07).

The role of vitamin E in the pathogenesis of PD is controversial. Golbe et al. (1988, 1990) and Tanner et al. (1988) suggested that PD patients in early life may have eaten foods with lower vitamin E content that controls. Fahn (1989, 1992) reported that the use of high dose of vitamin E associated with Vitamin C may delay the need for levodopa by 2–6 years. Factor et al. (1990) reported that PD patients who were self administering high dose of Vitamin E show less parkinsonian abnormalities and less complications of drug therapy.

The concentration of vitamin E in substantia nigra (Adams et al., 1991; Dexter et al., 1989) and in serum (Fernandez Calle et al., 1992; The Parkinson's disease study Group, 1993) are similar in PD and controls. Similarly serum levels of other vitamins involved in the protective mechanisms against lipid peroxidation and free radical formations as vitamin A (Jimenez-Jimenez et al., 1992), ascorbic acid (Fernandez Calle et al., 1993), beta carotene and other carotenoids (Jimenez-Jimenez et al., 1993) have been reported normal in PD.

Contrarily to the negative evidence of serum levels of vitamin E in PD, other experimental data suggest that the nigrostriatal dopamine neurons are susceptible to the deficiency of Vitamin E. In fact Cartano et al. (1993) reported the increase of dopamine turnover in substantia nigra in rats under vitamin E deficient diet, while controversial data have been reported on the possible protective effect of pretreatment with vitamin E in the MPTP or 6-hydroxy-dopamine induced parkinsonism (Perry et al., 1985). In vitamin E deficient mice an increased susceptibility to MPTP-induced neurotoxicity in the substantia nigra has been showed by Odunze et al. (1990) and Adams et al. (1990). However, extrapyramidal signs has been never reported in cases with vitamin E deficiency in which cerebellum and peripheral nerve are mainly involved (Satya-Murti et al., 1986; Federico et al., 1991; Battisti et al., 1993).

All these evidences suggest that serum levels of vitamin E could not be expected to be useful in providing informations concerning vitamin E intake (Tangney et al., 1993).

The role, if any, of antioxidant agents in the pathogenesis of PD and generally of aging processes remains to be determined. The recent evidence reported by our group (Battisti et al., 1994) that in ultracentennaries the vitamin E plasma levels are higher than in the other ages appears of great interest, suggesting that this substance may play some role in the protection against death.

Acknowledgments

Research in part supported by a grant from CNR (Finalized project Aging) to AF.

References

Adams JR, Odunze IN, Sevanian A (1990) Induction by 1-methyl-4-phemyl-1,2,3,6-tetrahydropyridine of lipid peroxidation in vivo in vitamin deficient mice. Biochem Parmacol 39: R5–R8

Adams JD, Klaidman LK, Odunze IN, Shen HC, Miller CA (1991) Alzheimer's and Parkinson's disease: brain levels of glutathione, glutathione disulfide and vitamin E. Mol Chem Neuropathol 14: 213–226

Battisti C, Bonuccelli U, Dotti MT, Maremmani C, Muratorio A, Malandrini A, Federico A (1993) Late onset multisystem disorder associated with coeliac disease and vitamin E deficiency. Ital J Neurol Sci 14 (S7): 113

Battisti C, Dotti MT, Manneschi L, Federico A (1994) Increase of plasma levels of vitamin E during human aging: is it a protective factor against death? Arch Gerontol Geriat 17 (S1): 13–18

Castano A, Herrera AJ, Cano J, Machado A (1993) Effects of a short period of vitamin E-deficient diet in the turnover of different neurotransmitters in substantia nigra and striatum of the rat. Neuroscience 53: 179–185

Dexter DT, Carter CJ, Wells FR, Javoy-Agid F, Agid Y, Lees A, Jenner P, Marsden CD (1989) Basal lipid peroxidation in substantia nigra is increased in Parkinson's disease. J Neurochem 52: 381–389

Factor SA, Sachez-Ramos JR, Weiner WJ (1990) Vitamin E therapy in Parkinson's disease. Adv Neurol 53: 457–461

Fahn S (1989) The endogenous toxin hypothesis of the etiology of Parkinson's disease and a pilot trial of high dose antioxidant in attempt to slow the progress of the illness. Ann NY Acad Sci 570: 186–196

Fahn S (1992) A pilot trial of high dose alpha-tocopherol and ascorbate in early Parkinson's disease. Ann Neurol 32: S128–S132

Federico A, Battisti C, Eusebi MP, De Stefano N, Malandrini A, Mondelli M, Volpe N (1991) Vitamin E deficiency secondary to chronic intestinal malabsorption and effect of vitamin supplement: a case report. Eur Neurol 31: 365–375

Fernandez-Calle P, Molina JA, Jimenez FJ, Vazquez A, Pondal M, Garcia-Ruiz PJ, Urra DG, Domingo J, Codoceo R (1992) Serum levels of alpha tocopherol (Vitamin E) in Parkinson's disease. Neurology 42: 1064–1066

Fernandez-Calle P, Jimenez-Jimenez FJ, Molina JA, Cabrera-Valdinia F, Vazquez A, Urra DG, Bermejo F, Matallana MC, Codoceo R (1993) Serum levels of ascorbic acid (Vitamin C) in patients with Parkinson's disease. J Neurol Sci 118: 25–28

Golbe LI, Farell TM, Davis PH (1988) Case control study of early life dietary factors in Parkinson's disease. Arch Neurol 45: 1350–1353

Golbe LI, Farell TM, Davis PH (1990) Follow up study on early life protective and risk factors in Parkinson's disease. Mov Disord 5: 66–70

Jimenez-Jimenez FJ, Molina JA, Fernandez-Calle P, Vazquez A, Pondal M, del Ser T, Gomez Pastor A, Codoceo R (1992) Serum levels of vitamin A in Parkinson's disease. J Neurol Sci 111: 73–76

Jimenez-Jimenez FJ, Molina JA, Fernandez-Calle P, Vazquez A, Cabrera-Valdivia F, Catalan MJ, Garcia-Albea E, Bermejo F, Codoceo R (1993) Serum levels of beta-carotene and other carotenoids in Parkinson's disease. Neurosci Lett 157: 103–106

Marsden CD (1990) Parkinson's disease. Lancet 335: 948–952

Muller DPR, Harries JT, Lloyd JK (1974) The relative importance of the factors involved in the absorption of vitamin E in children. Gut 15: 966–971

Odunze IN, Klaidman L, Adams JD (1990) MPTP toxicity in the mouse brain and vitamin E. Neurosci Lett 108: 346–349

Perry TL, Yong VW, Clavier RM, Jones K, Wright JM, Foulks JG, Wall RA (1985) Partial protection from the dopaminergic neurotoxin N-methyl-4-phenyl-1,2,3,6-tetrahydropyridine by four different antioxidants in the mouse. Neurosci Lett 60: 109–114

Tangney CC, Tanner CM (1993) Vitamin E and PD. Neurology 43: 634–635

Tanner CM, Cohen JA, Summerville BC, Goetz CG (1988) Vitamin use and Parkinson's disease. Ann Neurol 24: 182

The Parkinson study group (1993) Effects of tocopherol and deprenyl on the progression of disability in early Parkinson's disease. N Engl J Med 328: 176–183

Authors' address: Prof. A. Federico, Unit Neurometabolic diseases, Institute of Neurological Sciences, Medical School, University, Viale Bracci, I-53100 Siena, Italy.

J Neural Transm (1995) [Suppl] 45: 271–279

Interaction of neuroprotective substances with human brain superoxide dismutase. An in vitro study

W. Gsell[1], **N. Reichert**[1], **M. B. H. Youdim**[2], and **P. Riederer**[1]

[1] Department of Psychiatry, Clinical Neurochemistry, University of Würzburg, Federal Republic of Germany
[2] Technion, Department of Pharmacology, Haifa, Israel

Summary. Human brain total superoxide dismutase activity (SOD) was assayed in the presence of increasing concentrations of neuroprotectives. Superoxide-dependent nitrobluetetrazolium (NBT) reduction served as control for direct radical interaction of these substances. High concentrations of the dopamimetic substances L-DOPA slightly and the monoamine oxidase B inhibitor selegiline more effectively inhibit SOD activity. The MAO-B inhibitor RO 16-6491 (N-(2-aminoethyl)-4-chlorobenzamide hydrochloride) has no effect on SOD enzyme activity. Reduced glutathione stimulates SOD activity. Moreover it exhibits slight activity in scavenging radicals in vitro. Oxidized glutathione and vitamin E are unable to do so. Ascorbic acid mimics the activity of reduced glutathione, but directly interacts with NBT reduction. Thioctic acid shows no effect on SOD activity but stimulates superoxide-dependent NBT reduction. The Ginkgo biloba extract EGb 761 is highly active in inhibiting superoxide-dependent NBT reduction as well as SOD activity.

Introduction

Free oxygen radical mechanisms in neurodegenerative processes have first been adopted by Harmon (1981) for theory of aging. The discovery that the neurotoxin 1-methyl-4-phenyl-1,2,3,6-tetrahydrophyridine (MPTP) induces neuropathological and neurochemical alterations as well as clinical signs very similar to those of Parkinson's disease suggests that a similar chemical compound may cause Parkinson's disease (Ballard et al., 1985; Burns et al., 1985). The first concept on MPTP action proposes that excess formation of free radicals occurs as a result of toxin action. MPTP expresses its toxicity as a consequence of its oxidation to the 1-methyl-4-phenyl-pyridinium ion (MPP$^+$) by monoamine oxidase type B (MAO-B) (Chiba et al., 1984; Salach et al., 1984; Heikkila et al., 1985). Inhibition of the oxidation of MPTP to MPP$^+$ by MAO-B inhibtors such as selegiline and pargyline prevents the neurotoxic effects in animal models (Cohen et al., 1984; Heikkila et al., 1984; Langston et al., 1984). As Parkinson's disease is widespread throughout the world, chronic intoxication by selective exposure to a specific environmental toxin that contributes to the etiology of Parkinson's disease is unlikely. Endogenous compounds with neurotoxic actions similar to those of MPTP, like tetrahydroisoquinolines (Saitoh et al., 1988) and β-carbolines (Drucker et al., 1990; Bringmann et al., 1992) are discussed. For the neurotoxin 6-hydroxydopamine (6-OHDA) a similar radical action is proposed, as retrograde degeneration of nigrostriatal dopaminergic neurons after intrastriatal injection of 6-OHDA is potentiated by coinjection with iron or by simultaneous depletion of reduced glutathione (GSH) with l-buthionine sulfoximine (Pileblad et al., 1989). 6-OHDA toxicity is reduced by intranasogastral supplementation of DL-α-tocopherol (Cadet et al., 1989) or intrastriatal desferrioxamin (Ben-Shachar et al., 1991).

The metabolism of dopamine itself is related to oxidation reactions and free radical formation in the pathogenesis of Parkinson's disease. Both auto-oxidation of dopamine (Rosengren et al., 1985), forming neuromelanin by polymerization of auto-oxidative products, and oxidative deamination by MAO-B result in formation of hydrogen peroxide. Hydrogen peroxide is metabolized either by glutathione peroxidase reaction, where reduced glutathione (GSH) is oxidized (GSSG), or by catalase reaction. In the presence of iron, hydrogen peroxide can be reduced to form the toxic hydroxyl radical (Halliwell and Gutteridge, 1984). MAO activity in the brain increases with aging (Fowler et al., 1980), is higher in brains of patients with dementia of Alzheimer type (DAT) (Adolfsson et al., 1980), higher in platelets of patients with DAT (Danielczyk et al., 1988). MAO activation may lead to an increase in hydrogen peroxide formation. This is more pronounced the more metabolizing reactions via the glutathione system and catalase reaction are reduced. Reduction in the glutathione system in Parkinson's disease has been found by Perry and coworkers (1982), Riederer and coworkers (1989), Cohen (1990), Sofic et al. (1992) and in Alzheimer's disease by Adams and coworkers (1991). Reduction in catalase activity was demonstrated in Parkinson's disease (Ambani et al., 1975) and in dementia of Alzheimer type (Gsell et al., 1995). Thus hydrogen peroxide is insufficiently cleared, leading to increased hydroxyl radical formation, facilitated either by substantially increased iron content in Parkinsonian substantia nigra (Riederer et al., 1989; Dexter et al., 1987; Jellinger et al., 1990; Sofic et al., 1991) or by aluminium-potentiated iron toxicity (Aruoma et al., 1989) in dementia of Alzheimer type.

In the present study we investigated the activity of the superoxide radical detoxifying enzyme SOD in relation to neuroprotectives mentioned above. SOD is the first step of the oxygen free radical detoxication chain, leading to the formation of hydrogen peroxide. Direct interaction of neuroprotectives with SOD as inhibitor of initiation or propagation of neurodegenerative processes is still unclear. Interaction of SOD with neuroprotectives as therapeutical target is in discussion. It is known that SOD activity is increased in vivo by dopamimetics (Clow et al., 1991, 1992; Carrillo et al., 1991). Its role as neuroprotective agent or enhancer of the neurodegenerative process is discussed.

Material and methods

Chemicals and media

Organic and biochemical substances were supplied from Sigma (Munich, Germany), inorganic substances were supplied by Merck (Darmstadt, Germany) and neuroprotectives were supplied by RBI (Natick, MA, U.S.A.) respectively at highest grade available. The homogenization medium contained 250 mM sucrose, 50 mM sodium phosphate buffer, 0.1 mM EDTA, pH 7.0. SOD assay buffer contained 100 mM sodium phosphate buffer, pH 8.6.

Postmortem brain tissue

The brain from a 19 year old man, dying from suffocation by accident, was handled according to a standard protocol (Gsell et al., 1993). Postmortem time of tissue was 48 hours, storage time of tissue was at least 36 months. 65 g of frontal cortex was allowed to plunge frozen in a potter into the threefold volume (w/v) of homogenization medium. Then it was grinded with a pistil for about 5 minutes. Thereafter the crude homogenate was centrifuged in a microfuge (Hettich, Mikroliter, Germany, 15,000 rpm) for 3 minutes. The supernatant was immediately frozen in 1 ml aliquots at $-80°C$ prior to enzymic analyses.

Biochemical examinations

Superoxide was produced via xanthine oxidase/hypoxanthine reaction according to McCord and Fridovich (1969) and superoxide was detected by nitrobluetetrazolium reduction (NBT) (Beauchamp and Fridovich, 1971). Superoxide-dependent NBT reduction served as control for direct radical interaction of the substances tested. SOD activity was measured as competitive reaction to NBT reduction. One unit of SOD is then arbitrarily defined by that amount that causes a 50% inhibition of the NBT reduction (Fridovich, 1986). SOD activity was then corrected to that amount of superoxide radical that has been present in the assay, irrespective its interaction with the different substances. Protein was determined according to Bradford (1976) using bovine serum albumin as reference. The mean protein concentration was 6.8 µg protein/µl homogenate (n = 10).

Calculations

Each point in the figures represents the mean of three measurements with standard deviation. Where no standard deviation is shown, it lies within the mark.

Results

Influence of neuroprotectives on superoxide-dependent NBT reduction (Fig. 1)

While vitamin E and oxidated glutathione show no influence on NBT reduction, increasing thioctic acid levels stimulate NBT reduction by about 35%.

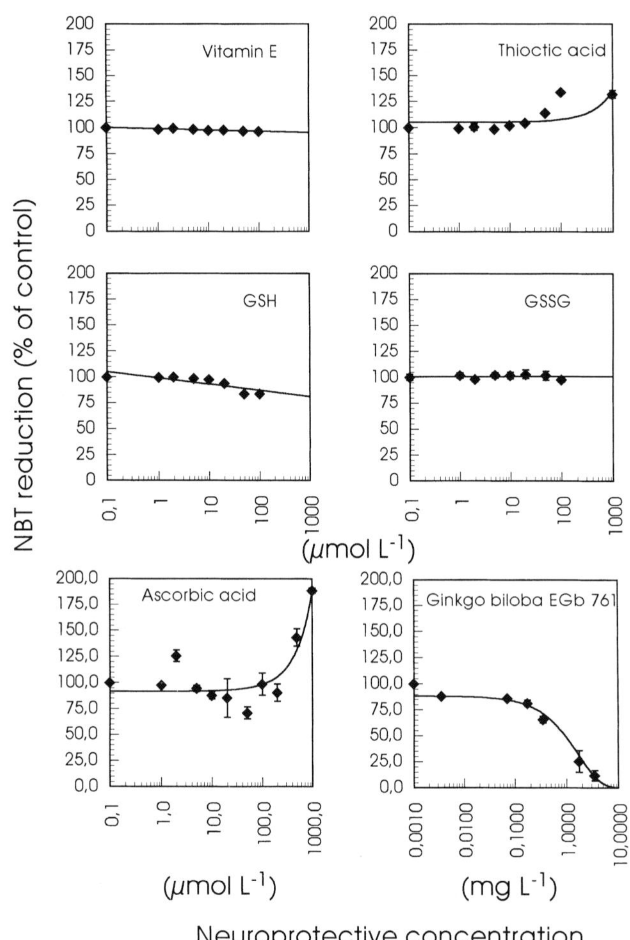

Fig. 1. Interaction of neuroprotective substances with NBT reduction

Increasing levels of reduced glutathione however reduce NBT reduction by about 20%. At increasing concentrations of ascorbic acid NBT reduction increases progessively and reaches up to 185% of control value. NBT reduction is inhibited by 50% by a Ginkgo biloba concentration of about 0.8 mg L⁻¹.

Influence of neuroprotectives on SOD activity (Fig. 2)

Human brain SOD acitivity is stimulated in vitro by about 25% by reduced glutathione, while the Ginkgo biloba extract EGb 761 inhibits the enzyme activity at a concentration of about 2 mg L⁻¹ by about 50%. Vitamin E, thioctic acid and oxidized glutathione were ineffective in influencing SOD activity. In contrast, ascorbic acid seems to have a strong stimulating effect on enzyme activity in vitro.

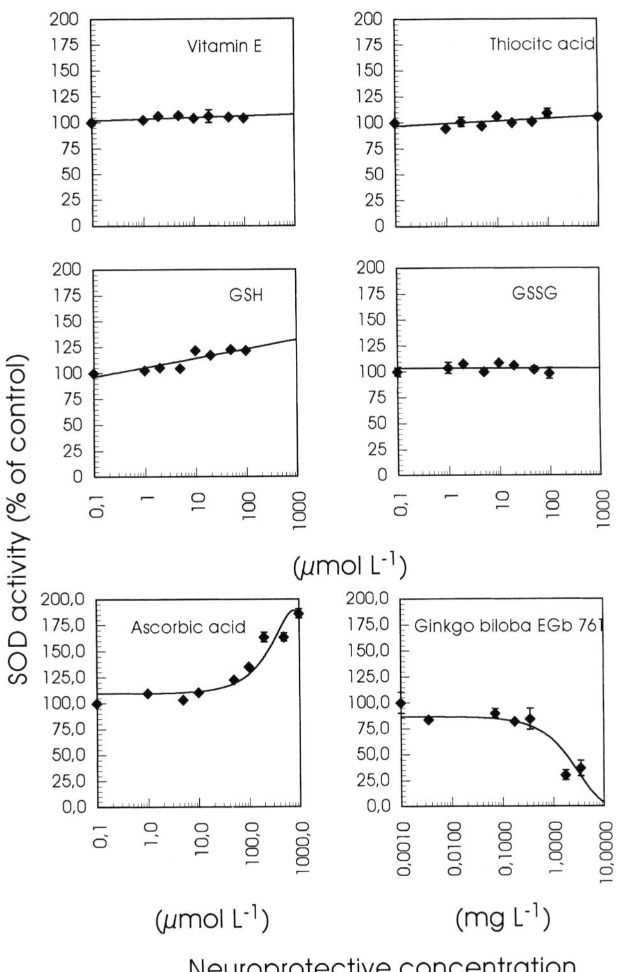

Fig. 2. Interaction of neuroprotective substances with SOD activity

Influence of dopamimetics on superoxide-dependent NBT reduction
(Fig. 3 left side)

L-DOPA is highly capable of scavenging superoxide radicals and thus inhib
its NBT reduction by 50% at a concentration of about $200\,\mu mol\,L^{-1}$.
The MAO-B inhibitors selegiline and RO 16-6491 have no effect on NBT
reduction.

Influence of dopamimetics on SOD activity (Fig. 3 right side)

L-DOPA as well as the MAO-B inhibitor selegiline slighty inhibit SOD
activity at higher concentrations by about 20 to 25% (trend to significance),
while the MAO-B inhibitor RO 16-6491 shows no such effect.

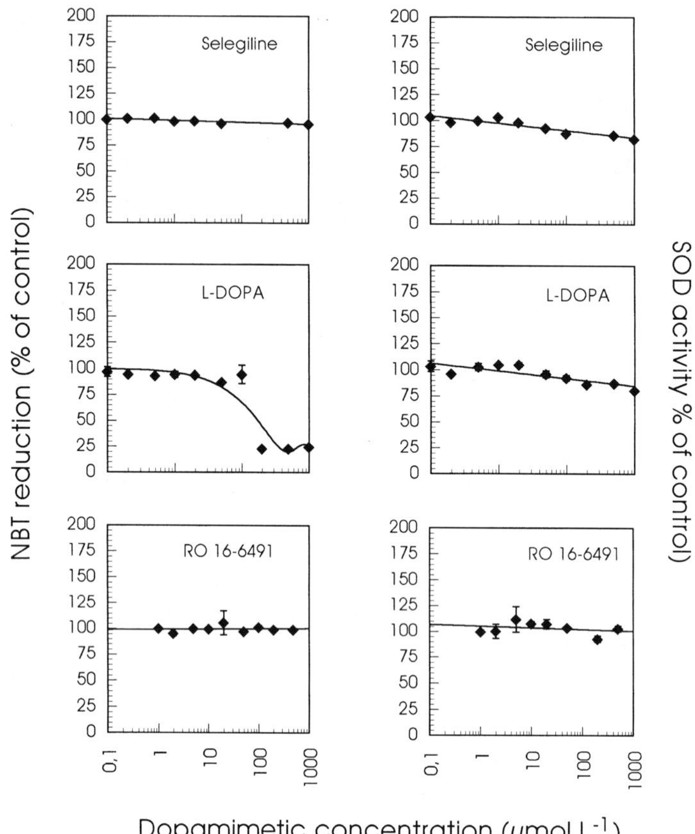

Fig. 3. Interaction of dopamimetic substances with NBT reduction (left side) and SOD activity (right side)

Discussion

Human brain superoxide dismutase is influenced by neuroprotective substances in vitro in multiple ways. Information on SOD activity in human brain in different neurodegenerative disorders is less or provides conflicting results however. Within the substantia nigra pars compacta, CuZn-SOD gene is preferentially expressed in the neuromelanin-pigmented neurons and its mRNA seems to increase in Parkinson's disease (Ceballos et al., 1990). Marttila et al. (1988) reported an increased CuZn-SOD activity in temporal cortex, red nucleus, thalamus, substantia nigra and basal nucleus of Meynert, while Saggu et al. (1989) found an increase only in mitochondrial Mn-SOD in the substantia nigra, but not in the cerebellum. Inreased SOD has been suggested to be an adaptive increase to excess formation superoxide radicals via mitochondrial respiratory chain and various enzymes, e.g. xanthine oxidase (Jenner et al., 1992). In Alzheimer's disease, an increase of SOD was found by Marklund et al. (1985) and Gsell et al. (1995), but it did not reach the level of significance in both cases.

The dopamimetic substances L-DOPA and the MAO-B inhibitor selegiline are beneficial to Parkinson's disease therapy without a direct effect to SOD activity (Fig. 3, right side). From Clow et al. (1991) there is evidence that selegiline treatment to rats can induce SOD activity in vivo. Whether this is an adaptive increase to excess formation of superoxide or other oxygen radicals, is still unclear. Scavenging of superoxide radicals by L-DOPA (Fig. 3, left side) may indicate the starting of a radical propagation mechanism.

The beneficial effects of reduced glutathione in radical scavenging (Fig. 1) as well as in stimulating SOD activity (Fig. 2) might be mediated by glutathione stimulation of glutathione peroxidase reaction. As oxidized glutathione inhibits glutathione peroxidase reaction, no effect on radical scavenging and SOD acivity can be observed.

Ascorbic acid directly interacted with nitroblue tetrazolium in a control experiment. Thus clear information of radical scavening or SOD stimulating abilities is not available with this test system.

The beneficial effect of Ginkgo biloba extract EGb 761 in scavenging superoxide radicals at a k_i of about $0.8 \, mg \, L^{-1}$ (Fig. 1), also observed by other authors (Chatterjee and Gabard, 1981) may be counteracted by its inhibition of SOD at a k_i of about $2 \, mg \, L^{-1}$.

In summary, the beneficial effects of dopamimetic substances in Parkinson's disease do not emerge from a direct effect on human brain SOD. Despite of reduced glutathione, no stimulating substance was found, although this substance acts on human brain SOD in an indirect way.

Acknowledgement

This study was supported by the German Bundesministerium für Forschung und Technologie, grant number 01KL91010.

References

Adams JD Jr, Klaidman LK, Odunze IN, Shen HC, Miller CA (1991) Alzheimer's and Parkinson's disease. Brain levels of glutathione, glutathione disulfide, and vitamin E. Mol Chem Neuropathol 14: 213–226

Adolfsson R, Gottfries CG, Oreland L, Wiberg A, Winblad B (1980) Increased activity of brain and platelets monoamine oxidase in dementia of Alzheimer type. Life Sci 27: 1029–1034

Ambani LM, Van Woert MH, Murphy S (1975) Brain peroxidase and catalase in Parkinson's disease. Arch Neurol 32: 114–118

Aruoma OI, Halliwell B, Laughton MJ, Quinlan GJ, Gutteridge JMC (1989) The mechanism of initiation of lipid peroxidation. Evidence against a requirement for an iron (II)-iron (III) complex. Biochem J 258: 617–620

Ballard PA, Tetrud JW, Langston JW (1985) Permanent human parkinsonism due to MPTP. Neurology 35: 969–976

Beauchamp C, Fridovich I (1971) Superoxide dismutase: improved assays and an assay applicable to acrylamide gels. Anal Biochem 44: 276–287

Ben-Shachar D, Eshel G, Finberg JPM, Youdim MBH (1991) The iron chelator desferrioxamine (Desferal) retards 6-hydroxydopamine-induced degeneration of nigrostriatal dopamine neurons. J Neurochem 56: 1441–1444

Bradford MM (1976) A rapid and sensitive method for the quantitation of microgram quantities of protein utilizing the principle of protein-dye binding. Anal Biochem 72: 248–254

Bringmann G, Friedrich H, Feineis D (1992) Trichloroharmanes as potential endogenously formed inducers of Morbus Parkinson: synthesis, analytics, and first in vivo-investigations. J Neural Transm [Suppl 38]: 15–26

Burns RS, Le Witt P, Ebert MH, Pakkenberg H, Kopin IJ (1985) The clinical syndrome of striatal dopamine deficiency: parkinsonism induced by MPTP. N Engl J Med 312: 1418–1421

Cadet JL, Katz M, Jackson-Lewis V, Fahn S (1989) Vitamin E attenuates the toxic effects of intrastriatal injection of 6-hydroxydopamine (6-OHDA) in rats: behavioral and biochemical evidence. Brain Res 476: 10–15

Carrillo MC, Kanai S, Nokubo M, Kitani K (1991) (-) selegiline induces activities of both SOD and catalase but not of glutathione peroxide in the striatum of young male rats. Life Sci 48: 517–521

Ceballos I, Lafon M, Javoy-Agid F, Hirsch EC, Nicole A, Sinet PM, Agid Y (1990) Superoxide dismutase and Parkinson's disease. Lancet 335: 1035–1036

Chatterjee SS, Gabard B (1981) Protective effect of an extract of Ginkgo biloba and other hydroxyl radical scavengers against hypoxia. 8th International Congress of Pharmacology, Tokyo

Chiba K, Trevor A, Castagnoli N Jr (1984) Metabolism of the neurotoxic tertiary amine, MPTP, by brain monoamine oxidase. Biochem Biophys Res Comm 120: 574–578

Clow A, Hussain T, Glover V, Sandler M, Dexter DT, Walker M (1991) (-)-selegiline can induce soluble SOD in rat striata. J Neural Transm 86: 77–80

Clow A, Hussain T, Glover V, Sandler M, Walker M, Dexter D (1992) Pergolide can induce solulbe SOD in rat striata. J Neural Transm [GenSect] 90: 27–31

Cohen G (1990) Monoamine oxidase and oxidative stress at dopaminergic synapsis. J Neural Transm [Suppl 32]: 229–238

Cohen G, Pasik P, Cohen B, et al (1984) Pargyline and selegiline prevent the neurotoxicity of 1-methyl-4-phenyl-1,2,3,6-tetraphydrophyridine (MPTP) in monkeys. Eur J Pharmacol 101: 209–210

Danielczyk W, Streifler M, Konradi C, Riederer P, Moll G (1988) Platelet MAO-B activity and the psychopathology of Parkinson's disease, senile dementia and multi-infarct dementia. Acta Psychiatr Scand 78: 730–736

Dexter DT, Wells FR, Agid F, Agid Y, Lees AJ, Jenner P, Marsden CD (1987) Increased nigral iron content in postmortem Parkinsonian brain. Lancet ii: 1219–1220

Drucker G, Raikoff R, Neafsey EJ, Collins MA (1990) Dopamine uptake inhibitory capacities of β-carboline analogs of N-methyl-4-phenyl-1,2,3,6-tetrahydropyridine (MPTP) oxidation products. Brain Res 509: 125–133

Fowler CJ, Wiberg A, Oreland L, Marcusson J, Winblad B (1980) The effect of age on the activity and molecular properties of human brain monoamine oxidase. J Neural Transm 49: 1–20

Fridovich I (1986) Superoxide dismutase. Adv Enzymol 58: 61–97

Gsell W, Lange KW, Pfeuffer R, Heckers H, Heinsen H, Senitz D, Jellinger K, Ransmayr G, Wichart I, Vock R, Beckmann H, Riederer P (1993) How to run a brain bank. A report from the Austro-German brain bank. J Neural Transm [Suppl 39]: 31–70

Gsell W, Conrad R, Hickethier M, Sofic E, Frölich L, Wichart I, Jellinger K, Moll G, Ransmayr G, Beckmann H, Riederer P (1995) Decreased catalase activity but unchanged SOD activity in brains of patients with dementia of Alzheimer type. J Neurochem 64: 1216–1223

Halliwell B, Gutteridge JMC (1984) Oxygen toxicity, oxygen radicals, transition metals and disease. Biochem J 219: 1–14

Harmon D (1981) The aging process. Proc Natl Acad Sci USA 78: 7124–7128

Heikkila RE, Manzino L, Duvoisin RC, Cabbat FS (1984) Protection against the dopaminergic neurotoxicity of 1-methyl-4-phenyl-1,2,3,6-tetrahydropyridine by monoamine oxidase inhibitors. Nature 311: 467–469

Heikkila RE, Manzino L, Cabbat FS, Duvoisin RC (1985) Studies on the oxidation of the dopaminergic neurotoxin 1-methyl-4-phenyl-1,2,3,6-tetrahydropyridine by monoamine oxidase B. J Neurochem 45: 1049–1054

Hornykiewicz O, Kish SJ (1986) Biochemical pathophysiology of Parkinson's disease. Adv Neurol 45: 19–34

Jellinger K, Paulus W, Grundke-lqbal I, Riederer P, Youdim MBH (1990) Histochemical demonstration of increased iron and ferritin in parkinsonian substantia nigra. J Neural Transm [P-D Sect] 2: 327–340

Jenner P, Dexter DT, Sian J, Schapira AHV, Marsden CD (1992) Oxidative stress as a cause of nigral cell death in Parkinson's disease and incidental Lewy body disease. Ann Neurol [Suppl] 32: 82–87

Langston JW, Irwin I, Langston EP, Forno LS (1984) Pargyline prevents MPTP-induced parkinsonism in primates. Science 225: 1480–1482

Marklund SL, Adolfsson R, Gottfries CG, Winblad B (1985) Superoxide isoenzymes in normal brains and in brains from patients with dementia of Alzheimer type. J Neurol Sci 67: 319–325

Marttila RJ, Lorentz H, Rinne UK (1988) Oxygen toxicity protecting enzymes in Parkinson's disease. Increase of SOD-like activity in the substantia nigra and basal nucleus. J Neurol Sci 86: 321–331

McCord JM, Fridovich I (1969) Superoxide dismutase. An enyzmatic function for erythrocuprein (hemocuprein). J Biol Chem 244: 6049–6055

Perry TL, Godin DV, Hansen S (1982) Parkinson's disease: a disorder due to nigral glutathione deficiency? Neurosci Lett 33: 305–310

Pileblad E, Magnusson T, Fornstedt B (1989) Reduction of brain glutathione by L-buthionine sulfoximine potentiates the dopamine-depleting action of 6-hydroxydopamine in rat striatum. J Neurochem 52: 978–980

Riederer P, Sofic E, Rausch W-D, Schmidt B, Reynolds GP, Jellinger K, Riederer P (1989) Transition metals, ferritin, glutathione, and ascorbic acid in Parkinsonian brains. J Neurochem 52: 515–520

Rosengren E, Linder-Eliasson E, Carlsson A (1985) Detection of 5-cysteinyldopamine in human brain. J Neural Transm 63: 247–253

Saggu H, Cooksey J, Dexter DT, Wells FR, Lees A, Jenner P, Marsden CD (1989) A selective increase in particulate SOD activity in parkinsonian substantia nigra. J Neurochem 53: 692–697

Saitoh T, Mizuno Y, Nagatsu T, Yoshida M (1988) Effect of long-term administration of 1,2,3,4-tetrahydroisoquinoline (TIQ) on striatal dopamine and 3,4-dihydroxyphenylacetic acid (DOPAC) content in mice. Neurosci Lett 92: 321–324

Salach JI, Singer TKP, Castagnoli N Jr, Trevor A (1984) Oxidation of the neurotoxic amine 1-methyl-4-phenyl-1,2,3,6-tetrahydropyridine (MPTP) by monoamine oxidases A and B and suicide inactivation of the enzymes of MPTP. Biochem Biophys Res Comm 125: 831–835

Sofic E, Paulus W, Jellinger K, Riederer P, Youdim MBH (1991) Selective increase of iron in substantia nigra zona compacta of parkinsonian brains. J Neurochem 56: 978–982

Sofic E, Lange KW, Jellinger K, Riederer P (1992) Reduced and oxidized glutathione in the substantia nigra of patients with Parkinson's disease. Neurosci Lett 142: 128–130

Authors' address: Prof. Dr. P. Riederer, Department of Psychiatry, Clinical Neurochemistry, Füchsleinstrasse 15, D-97080 Würzburg, Federal Republic of Germany.

J Neural Transm (1995) [Suppl] 45: 281–285
© Springer-Verlag 1995

Effects of acute n-hexane and 2,5-hexanedione treatment on the striatal dopaminergic system in mice

C. Masotto[1], **C. Bisiani**[1], **C. Camisasca**[1], **R. Fusi**[1], **S. Ricciardi**[1], **N. Fonzi**[3], **L. Perbellini**[2], **M. Scatturin**[1], **C. B. Mariani**[3], **M. Canesi**[3], and **G. Pezzoli**[3]

[1] Zambon Group, Bresso Milan, [2] Institute of Occupational Medicine, University of Verona, and [3] Ospedale Maggiore Policlinico, Institute of Neurology, University of Milan, Milan, Italy

Summary. In order to investigate the effect of n-hexane and its metabolites on the Central Nervous System (CNS), we treated mice with n-hexane and 2,5-hexanedione (2,5-HD) by intraperitoneal (i.p.) administration. Gas-cromatographic mass spectrometric (GCMS) analyses of striatum and cerebellum revealed a consistent increase of 2,5-HD concentration at 0.5 and 2 hours after treatment and a decline to baseline levels at 24 hours. Traces of 2,5-HD were detected in the brain of control animals. Biochemical analyses revealed a precocious, short lasting, significant increase of striatal dopamine (DA) and homovanillic acid (HVA) levels. A significant increase of striatal synaptosomal DA uptake, suggesting a DA releasing effect on the dopaminergic terminals, was also observed. These results support the hypothesis of a possible role of n-hexane and its metabolites in inducing parkinsonism in humans and animals.

n-Hexane is an aliphatic hydrocarbon, found in petroleum ether and gasoline, it is commonly used in industrial solvents, glues, paints, lacquers, and printing ink. In several species, n-hexane is converted by oxidative metabolic processes, cytochrome P-450 dependent, to 2-hexanol, forming methyl n-butyl ketone and 2,5-HD, the most neurotoxic derivative, which is also used as a biological monitor for occupational exposure to n-hexane (Ahonen et al., 1988; Governa et al., 1987) Perbellini et al., 1980). Recent findings have revealed that 2,5-HD is also a metabolite of endogenous origin, normally found in the human and animal body (Perbellini et al., 1993) and lipid peroxidation has been suggested as a possible source of these endogenous hydrocarbons (Fedtke and Bolt, 1986; Gutteridge and Halliwell, 1990). The neurotoxicity of n-hexane and its metabolites on the Peripheral Nervous System in occupational exposed subjects has been largely documented (Cavender et al., 1984; Change, 1987; Passero et al., 1983; Pezzoli et al., 1990; Spencer and Schaumburg, 1980). Some authors have demonstrated the toxic effect of 2,5-HD on rat CNS, particularly on the neocortical neurons (Strange et al., 1991) and cholinergic fibers (Di Patre and Butcher, 1991). It has been shown that this compound induces alteration of neuronal and glial intermediate filaments (Karlsson et al., 1991) and of the neuronal axonal flow (Hammond-Tooke, 1992). A neurotoxic selective effect of n-hexane and similar hydrocarbons, on the nigro-striatal dopaminergic pathway, has been demonstrated on experimental animals (Ikeda et al., 1986; Pezzoli et al., 1990) and suggested in humans (Pezzoli et al., 1989; Spencer et al., 1980; Tetrud et al., 1990). The purpose of the present study was to investigate the effects of n-hexane and 2,5-HD acute i.p. treatment on the dopaminergic system, and the accumulation and persistance of these substances in the brain.

Adult male white VCD-1(ICR)BR mice were used for this experiment. The animals were housed under controlled environmental conditions. Three experiments were carried out by treating animals i.p., at a dose of 1 g/kg, with n-hexane (ACS Merck, 99%), or 2,5-HD (Aldrich-Chemie, 97%), or saline solution.

In the first experiment animals were treated with 2,5-HD, or n-hexane or normal saline solution. After treatment the animals were sacrificed by decapitation at 0.5, 2 and 24 hours, the brain dissected and the nucleus striatum collected for biochemical analysis. The 2,5-HD contents were measured by a GCMS method. Samples were heated at 100°C for 45 minutes; the extraction of 2,5-HD was carried out by using cartridges prewashed by methanol and acid water. 2,5-HD was eluted with a 5% acetonitrile/water solution and was extracted using dichloromethane. The ricovered solvent was evaporated and used for the analysis (Perbelli et al., 1990). A drastic increase of 2,5-HD content in the striatum and cerebellum of the 2,5-HD treated animals was observed at 0.5 and 2 hours after treatment, whereas at 24 hours 2,5-HD content declined to control values (Fig. 1). A mild increase of 2,5-HD (5.63 ± 0.4 μg/g) was observed in the striatum of the n-hexane treated animals at 1 hour after treatment. In control animals 2,5-HD concentration was approximately 2–3 μg/g of tissue revealing the physiological presence of 2,5-HD in the cerebral tissue of mice.

In the second experiment animals were treated as for the first experiment and sacrificed at 0.5, 1, 2, 4, 6, 8, 24 hours, the brain dissected and the nucleus

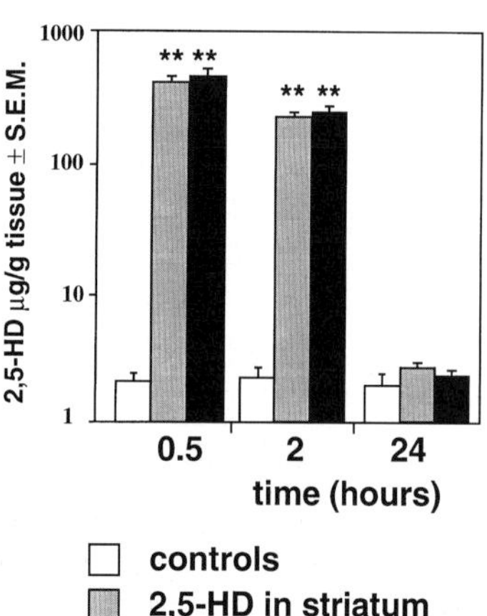

Fig. 1. 2,5-hexanedione content in striatum and cerebellum of 2,5-hexanedione treated mice. **p < 0.01 versus normal saline treated mice, one way ANOVA

striatum collected for biochemical analysis. The striatal contents of DA, HVA, and 3,4-dihydroxyphenylacetic acid (DOPAC) were measured by HPLC with electrochemical detector. Samples were prepared and analysed as previously described (Achilli et al., 1985). Compared to controls higher levels of DA and HVA were found in the striatum of treated mice at 0.5 and 1 hours after 2,5-HD treatment (Fig. 2A), whereas DOPAC levels remained unmodified at any time. A mild increase of DA and HVA content at 1 hour was observed in n-hexane treated animals (data not shown).

In the third experiment the effect of n-hexane and 2,5-HD on the striatal DA uptake, was investigated. Animals were treated as in the first and the second experiment and decapitated at 0.5 and 1 hours. DA uptake was measured in the striatum following a previously described method (Boulton et al., 1989). Striatal synaptosomal DA uptake was significantly higher, at 0.5 and 1 hours, after n-hexane and 2,5-HD treatment compared to controls (Fig. 2B).

The high concentration of 2,5-HD observed in the striatum and cerebellum in treated animals clearly indicates that this compound can cross the blood brain barrier. Since, in normal circumstances, only unconjugated 2,5-HD can cross the blood brain barrier, we assume that, in this experiment, the high dose of 2,5-HD administered, might have partially circumvented the liver

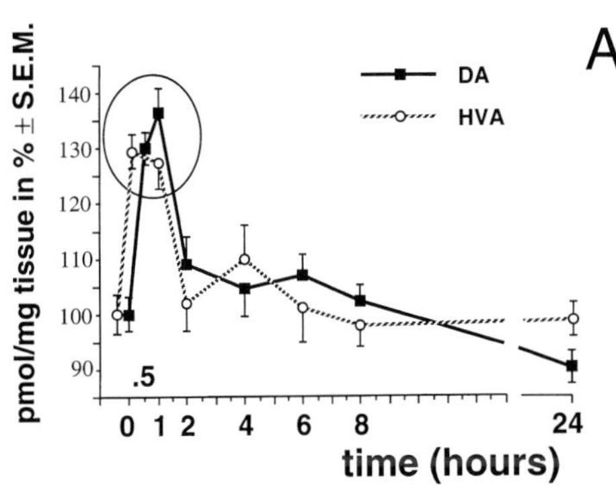

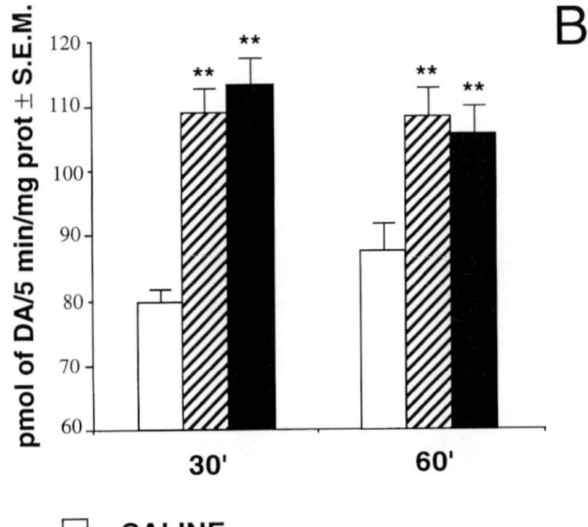

Fig. 2. A DA and HVA contents in murine striatum after 2,5-hexanedione treatment (1 g/kg) at time 0. Circled area: p < 0.01 versus time 0, one way ANOVA. **B** Striatal synaptosomal DA uptake in mice treated with n-hexane or 2,5-hexanedione (1 g/kg), 30 or 60 minutes prior to sacrifice. **p < 0.01 versus saline treated animals, one way ANOVA

conjugation. The peak of 2,5-HD and that of DA and HVA levels in the striatum occurred concurrently at 30 minutes after treatment, but the decrease of DA and HVA levels to baseline condition was more rapid than that of 2,5-HD. The decline of 2,5-HD contents at 24 hours after the treatment was probably due to the rapid systemic diffusion and the subsequent conjugation in the liver, and/or to a possible CNS specific scavenging mechanism capable of eliminating this toxic compound. The increase of striatal DA, its extracellular metabolite HVA, and the unmodified DOPAC level, observed in the treated animals suggest a DA stimulating and releasing effect exerted by n-hexane and 2,5-HD on the nigro-striatal dopaminergic terminals. Previous data had revealed a drastic reduction of the nigro-striatal DA and HVA contents ($\approx -40\%$) after chronic n-hexane and 2,5-HD treatment in rats, suggesting a consistent loss of the cellular function probably due to chronic overstimulation. The findings of the present study can better explain the biochemical mechanism by which a chronic exposure to these hydrocarbons may lead to the exhaustion of the nigrostriatal dopaminergic pathway. On the bases of these data we assume that parkinsonian patients (or subjects in a preclinical state of parkinsonism) are more vulnerable to these hydrocarbons, than healthy subjects.

The presence of 2,5-HD in the CNS of control animals confirms that this compound is not only an industrial and environmental contaminant but also an endogenous product of metabolic systems.

This observation requires further investigations in order to verify the physiological and/or pathological role of 2,5-HD in the CNS.

References

Achilli G, Perego C, Ponzio F (1985) Application of the dual-cell coulometric detector: a method for assaying monoamines and their metabolites. Anal Biochem 148: 1–9

Ahonen I, Schimberg RW (1988) 2,5-Hexanedione excretion after occupational exposure to n-hexane. Br J Ind Med 45: 133–136

Boulton AA, Baker GB, Juorio AV (1989) Drugs as tools in neurotransmitter research. Neuromethods, vol 12. Humana Press, Clifton New Jersey, p 351

Cavender FL, Casey HW, Salem H, Graham DG, Swenberg JA, Gralla EJ (1984) A 13-week vapor inhalation study of n-hexane in rats with emphasis on neurotoxic effects. Fundam Appl Toxicol 4: 191–201

Change YC (1987) Neurotoxic effects of n-hexane on the human central nervous system: evoked potential abnormalities in n-hexane polyneuropathy. J Neurol Neurosurg Psychiatry 50: 269–274

Di Patre PL, Butcher LL (1991) Cholinergic fiber perturbations and neuritic outgrowth produced by intrafimbrial infusion of the neurofilament-disrupting agent 2,5-hexanedione. Brain Res 539: 126–132

Fedtke N, Bolt HM (1986) Detection of 2,5-hexanedione in the urine of persons not exposed to n-hexane. Int Arch Occup Environ Health 57: 143–148

Governa M, Calisti R, Coppa G, Tagliavento G, Colombi A, Troni W (1987) Urinary excretion of 2,5-hexanedione and peripheral polyneuropathies workers exposed to hexane. J Toxicol Environ Health 20: 219–228

Gutteridge JM, Halliwell B (1990) The measurement and mechanism of lipid peroxidation in biological systems. Trends Biochem Sci 15: 129–135

Hammond-Tooke GD (1992) Slow axonal transport is impaired by intrathecal 2,5-hexanedione. Exp Neurol 116: 210–217

Ikeda M, Koizumi A, Kasahara M, Fujita H (1986) Combined effects of n-hexane and toluene on norepinephrine and dopamine levels in rat brain tissues after long-term exposures. Bull Environ Contam Toxicol 36: 510–517

Karlsson JE, Rosengren LE, Haglid KG (1991) Quantitative and qualitative alterations of neuronal and glial intermediate filaments in rat nervous system after exposure to 2,5-hexanedione. J Neurochem 57: 1437–1444

Passero S, Battistini N, Cioni R, Giannini F, Paradiso C, Battista F, Carboncini F, Sartorelli E (1983) Toxic polyneuropathy in shoe workers in Italy. Ital J Neurol Sci 4: 463–472

Perbellini L, Brugnone F, Pavan I (1980) Identification of the metabolites of n-hexane, cyclohexane, and their isomers in men's urine. Toxicol Appl Pharmacol 53: 220–229

Perbellini L, Marhuenda Amoros DM, Cardora Llorens AC, Giuliari C, Brugnone F (1990) An improved method of analysing 2,5-hexanedione in urine. Br J Int Med 47: 421–424

Perbellini L, Pezzoli G, Brugnone F, Canesi M (1993) Biochemical and physiological aspects of 2,5-hyxanedione: endogenous or exogenous product? Int Arch Occup Environ Health 65: 49–52

Pezzoli G, Barbieri S, Ferrante C, Zecchinelli A, Foa' V (1989) Parkinsonism due to n-hexane exposure. Lancet ii: 874

Pezzoli G, Ricciardi S, Masotto C, Mariani CB, Carenzi A (1990) n-hexane induces parkinsonism in rodents. Brain Res 531: 355–357

Spencer PS, Schaumburg HH (1980) Experimental and clinical neurotoxicology. Williams and Wilkins, Baltimore, p 456

Spencer PS, Schaumburg HH, Sabri MI, Veronesi B (1980) The enlarging view of hexacarbon neurotoxicity. CRC Crit Rev Toxicol 7: 279–356

Strange P, Moller A, Ladefoged O, Lam HR, Larsen JJ, Arlien-Soborg P (1991) Total number and mean cell volume of neocortical neurons in rats exposed to 2,5-hexanedione with and without acetone. Neurotoxicol Teratol 13: 401–406

Tetrud JW, Langston JW, Irwin I, Snow B (1990) Acute and persistent parkinsonism associated with ingestion of petroleum product mixture. Ann Neurol 28: 296

Authors' address: G. Pezzoli, Ospedale Maggiore Policlinico, Pad. Ponti, Via F. Sforza 35, I-20122 Milan, Italy.

J Neural Transm (1995) [Suppl] 45: 287–296

Molecules with neurotrophic effects on the human developing mesencephalic dopaminergic neurons

V. Silani[1], S. Bernasconi[1], A. Pizzuti[1], A. Sampietro[1], A. Brioschi[1], M. Buscaglia[2], and G. Scarlato[1]

[1] The Institute of Neurology and "Dino Ferrari" Center, University of Milan Medical School, Milan, and [2] Department of Obstetrics and Gynecology, University of Milan Medical School, San Paolo Hospital, Milan, Italy

Summary. Parkinson's disease (PD) is characterized by the degeneration of the mesencephalic dopaminergic (mesDA) neurons innervating the striatum. Neurotrophic factor(s) that prevents the degeneration and increases the functional activity of the remaining mesDA neurons are of substantial clinical interest. The origin and development of mesDA neurons were characterized in the human mesencephalon from 5.0 to 12 Postconception (PC) weeks. Tyrosine Hydroxylase (TH) immunoreactive cells were first demonstrated at 5.5 PC weeks next to the ventricular zone. In primary culture, TH immunoreactive neurons represent 3 to 5% of the total cells at days *7 in vitro* and basic Fibroblast growth factor (bFGF) was demonstrated to induce a significant increase of both TH immunoreactive cell number and TH enzymatic activity. This effect was mediated by proliferating glial fibrillary acidic protein immunoreactive cells. Nerve growth factor treatment did not have any appreciable effect. The effect of bFGF on TH positive cells described in this human bioassay is only a preliminary evidence that, if confirmed by experiments *in vivo*, may provide a starting rationale for investigating alternative strategies in the treatment of PD.

Introduction

Parkinson's disease (PD) is characterized by the degeneration of the mesencephalic dopaminergic (mesDA) neurons innervating the striatum. The main focus in current clinical treatment is the pharmacological increase of the striatal dopamine. This approach does not prevent the mesDA neuron degeneration that represents the pathological basis of PD. Neurotrophic factors have been shown to be essential not only for development, but also for maintenance of the mature Central Nervous System (CNS) normal function. They promote the neural cell regeneration after injury and degenerative processes. Therefore, neurotrophic molecules may be therapeutically useful to specifically prevent the neuronal degeneration and increase the functional activity of the remaining mesDA neurons in PD (Lindsay et al., 1993).

Development and regeneration of afferent mesDA neurons to the striatum appear to be regulated by release of a specific striatal DA trophic molecule(s) that has not been characterized yet (Carvey et al., 1991, 1993). Identification of this molecule(s) may open new prospectives for a definitive treatment of extrapyramidal disorders. In the last few years, several molecules able to spur neuronal development and repair in the CNS were isolated (Thoenen, 1991). Nerve growth factor (NGF), Brain derived neurotrophic factor (BDNF), neurotrophin-3 (NT-3), and neurotrophin 4/5 (NT-4/5) are among them (Snider and Johnson, 1990). The first demonstration of the striatal DA neuroptrophic effect on the afferent mesDA neurons dates back to 1979, when Prochiantz et al. showed that mouse embryonic co-cultures of substantia nigra and striatum were responsible for a few fold increase in dopamine uptake (Prochiantz et al., 1979, 1981; Di Porzio et al., 1980). Some molecules were subsequently demonstrated effective on afferent DA neurons during development and after lesion of the nigro-striatal pathway (Denis-Donini et al., 1983, 1984; Tomozawa and Appel, 1986; Hyman et al., 1991, 1994). In particular ghial derived neurotrophic petor (GDNF), which was recently discovered, must be considered the most specific dopaminergic neurotrophic molecule so far defined at molecular level (Lin et al., 1993; Strömberg et al., 1993). One of the main limitation in neurotrophic factor research is the *in vivo* reproducibility of the *in vitro* effect. Furthermore, different species may respond in different ways to the same neurotoxin agent (MPTP is the best example), and the same may be true also for neurotrophic molecules.

The availability of recombinant molecules in such amounts to be therapeutically useful gives the chance to test neurotrophic molecules in PD. Testing the efficacy and toxicity of such molecules in humans may take advantage of the use of simple and reproducible cellular models such as neuronal tissue culture. In order to characterize such a model, we grew *in vitro* mesDA neuronal cells from different species including human mesencephalic neurons (Silani et al., 1992). Primary cultures offer a sensitive assay to test, in a controlled environment, neurotrophic-mediated cellular effects and neuro-glial interactions that are specific to the mesencephalic area.

In this study, two neurotrophic factors, NGF and basic Fibroblast growth factor (bFGF), were added to human nigral primary cultures. Effects on survival, differentiation of mesDA neurons, and proliferation of glial cells were monitored. bFGF was previously reported to reverse deficits in the nigrostriatal system of the lesioned mice (Dorte and Unsicker, 1990) and to be present in mesDA neurons (Cintra et al., 1991).

Material and methods

Human embryonic CNS tissues were obtained after therapeutical abortion according to the current Italian regulations. The age of the embryos was determinated by preoperative ultrasound scanning, which allowed a good estimation of embryonic crown-rump length (CRL) and staging before abortion. For PC age, donors were staged by CRL as determined ultrasonically in utero (Drumm and O'Rahilly, 1977). Sonographic measurements are able to predict the gestational age with accuracy of $\pm$ 4 days (Robinson and Fleming, 1975; Robinson, 1993). The age of the embryos was estimated by a combination of the above features and expressed as a PC week, according to CAPIT that reached the group consensus to use the term "postconception age" as the standard way of referring to fetal age (Langston et al., 1992). PC weeks and days were derived from CRL values as previously reported (Robinson, 1993).

To demonstrate the development of the mesDA neurons, specimens were immediately immersion-fixed for 12 to 24 hours in 4% paraformaldehyde, rinsed, cryoprotected in increasing sucrose concentration (7 to 15%), and frozen in dry ice reduced to powder. Frozen 16-μm coronal or horizontal sections (Top Cryo-E, Pabisch) were treated immediately for immunohistochemical studies. Sets of sections, 16 μm thick through the mesencephalon, were processed by fluorescence analysis. TH-immunoreactivity was used as a marker for mesDA neurons. Two commercial antibodies against TH (monoclonal from Incstar and polyclonal from Eugene Tech) (1:100 to 500 dilution, respectively) were used. All the sections were collected, added with primary antisera, and freshly diluted in 0.2% TRITON X-100 + 1% goat serum. Sections were then incubated overnight in diluted antisera at 4°C. After incubation, sections were rinsed in PBS (3 washes of at least 60 sec. each) at room temperature. The last rinse was replaced with goat anti-mouse or anti-rabbit IgG-fluorescein (FITC)-conjugated (1:100), freshly diluted in PBS, for 1 hour. Sections were then immediately mounted in oil. In negative controls, the first antibody was omitted or replaced by normal mouse or rabbit serum. Sections were examined on a Zeiss transmitted-light photomicroscope III equipped with epi-fluorescence condenser.

For tissue culture of mesDA neurons, fifteen specimens from PC week 6.0 to 11.0 were collected in sterile Hank's balanced salt solution, pH 7.4 (Gibco), additioned with antibiotics and 10% heat inactivated fetal calf serum (FCS-Gibco) and immediately processed for tissue culture as previously described (Silani et al., 1994). CNS was dissected using sterile technique, under an inverted microscope. After careful dissection of the nervous tissue from meninges, vessels and any other contaminant, the ventral mesencephalon was isolated and immediately dissected in pieces using scissors. The tissue was then added with DMEM (Gibco) and antibiotics, supplemented with glucose (5 mg/liter), in presence of 10% heat inactivated FCS, and gently dissociated by trituration with Pasteur pipettes of progressively smaller bore size. Trypsin (II, Sigma) at very low concentration (0.08%, v/v) was used for specific specimens (older than PC Week 9.5 specimens): in this case, tissue was incubated for 15 to 20 min, trypsin blocked with excess of serum (FCS), dispersed cells centrifuged (500 $\times$ g for 10 min), and the supernatant discarded. Dispersed cells were resuspended in DMEM/FCS and plated. The mean number of viable cells obtained from a single mesencephalon was 0.8 to 2 $\times$ 10^7. 0.75 to 0.85 $\times$ 10^6 cells were plated in 35-mm Falcon dishes that were pre-coated overnight with poly-L-lysine. For TH biochemical microassay (see below), cells were plated at a 2 $\times$ 10^5 cells/well density in a volume of 200 μl (96 microwell culture plate). Cultures were incubated at 36.5°C in a humidified atmosphere of 5.5 CO_2. Every 2-3 day half of the medium was removed from each well and replaced with an equal volume of fresh medium (DMEM/FCS). Cultures were fed every other day and daily observed with inverted microscope (Leitz Diavert).

For NGF and bFGF treatment, cells were additionated with 7 or 2.5 S NGF (Sigma) or bFGF (human recombinant, Boehringer) after 24 hours in culture in DMEM/FCS at 50 ng/ml final concentration.

To demonstrate neuronal specific enolase (NSE) and TH in primary cultures, mesencephalic cells were fixed with 4% paraformaldehyde for 1 hour and permeabilized with 0.1% Triton X-100 for 30 min. After adding goat serum, cultures were incubated with the anti-NSE serum diluted 1:100 (Incstar) and subsequently with goat FITC conjugated anti-rabbit IgG 1:100 (Bio-Yeda). MesDA neurons were identified using anti-TH monoclonal or polyclonal antibody, as previously mentioned (1:100 and 1:500 dilution, respectively) and with goat FITC conjugated anti-mouse IgG (1:100) (bio-Yeda). Astrocytes

290 V. Silani et al.

were demonstrated, after fixation and permeabilization, with a monoclonal antibody against GFAP diluted 1:100 overnight at 4 °C (BioMakor bm) and lastly with goat FITC anti-mouse diluted 1:100 for 1 hour at 4 °C. Primary and secondary antibodies were both diluted in PBS + 0.1% Triton X-100 + 1% goat serum. Cells were examined on a Zeiss transmitted-light photomicroscope III equipped with epi-fluorescence condenser. For NSE or TH positive cell counting, approximately 2.5% of the total surface of the 35 mm tissue culture dishes was evaluated.

For TH enzymatic determination, the assay was adapted for microwells as previously described (Bostwick and Le, 1991). Cells were grown on a 96 microwell culture plate and homogenized at the moment of the assay in the plate. This microradiometric assay can detect the production of 5 pmol of $^{14}CO_2$ (coupled nonenzymatic decarboxylation of L-$^{[14C]}$Dopa). Assays were run in triplicate, at day 8 to 10 in vitro, and were duplicated for each week of the donor.

Results

Twenty-three specimens were obtained for histological analysis and tissue culture experiments. The gestational age of the samples ranged between PC week 5.0 and 12.0. The ventral mesencephalon was recognizable in all the specimens (Fig. 1). Surface landmarks (tuberculum of Hochstetter and fasciculus retroflexus) were identified in the mesencephalic region of the intact CNS containing the developing substantia nigra (Fig. 2).

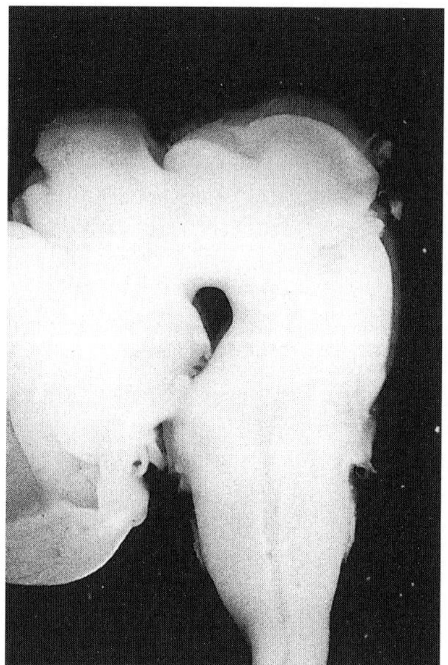

Fig. 1. Microscopic photograph of the developing human brain, PC week 8.0. Accurate anatomical dissection is a pre-requisite to obtain high recovery of TH positive neurons. The suction abortion technique we developed, under ultrasound scanning, maintains intact midbrain and forebrain structures, facilitating dissection of different anatomical regions (substantia nigra, corpus striatum, etc.). Two anatomical landmarks are particularly useful for identifying the anatomical region of developing dopaminergic neurons, i.e. the tuberculum of Hochstetter and the fasciculus retroflexus (80× magnification)

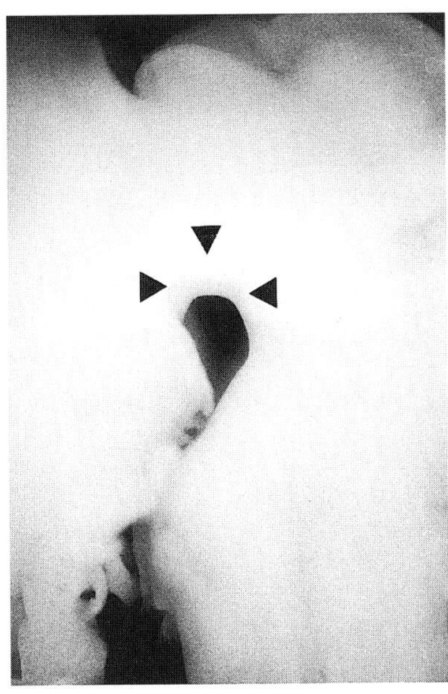

Fig. 2. High magnification of the anatomical region of the human mesencephalon we dissected to obtain high percentage of dopaminergic neurons. Arrows define the dissection line (100× magnification)

Mesencephalic TH immunoreactivity was first observed at PC week 5.5 next to the ventricular zone in the caudal mesencephalic tegmentum. No TH staining was observed within the ventricular zone of the PC week 11.1 specimens (complete dopaminergic neuronal cell migration).

MesDA neuronal development

At PC week 5.5, a few TH immunoreactive neurons were localized in the medial ventral mesencephalon adjacent to the ventricular zone. At a later date TH-immunoreactive neurons were also observed adjacent to the ventral surface of the mesencephalon. By 7.3 weeks, TH-immunoreactive neurons were found in a crescentic band in the middle third of the mesencephalic width. Subsequently, only a few TH immunoreactive neurons were demonstrated adjacent to the ventricular zone (diminishing mesDA neurogenesis) and three samples at PC Week 11.1, 11.5 and 12.0 did not display positive cells in this zone. MesDA cells showed neuritic extensions at PC week 7.5 and the mesostriatal pathway was first observed at PC week 8.3. TH immunoreactive cells were visualized using both monoclonal and polyclonal antibodies (Table 1).

MesDA neurons in primary cultures

MesDA neurons were obtained from specimens of PC 6.0 to 11.0 weeks. The total cellular yield from the mesencephalic region was dependent on accurate examination of the anatomical landmarks on dissection, but independent from the age of the tissue. We obtained 2.0 to 8.5 × 10^7 cells from a single

Table 1. Ontogeny of the human nigrostriatal system

Embryonic age (Postconception Weeks)	Development event
5.5	TH-immunoreactivity first seen in the mesencephalic ventricular zone
8.5	TH$^+$ neurons localized in a crescentic band in the middle third of mesencephalon (coronal sections)
9.0	Dopaminergic innervation of the striatum starts in the putamen
11.2	All TH$^+$ neurons have migrated ventrally. A large number of neuron possess neuritic extensions.

mesencephalon. At the time of plating, cells were completely dissociated and uniformly distributed throughout petri dishes. Cell attachment was obtained in a few hours (1 to 2) on poly-L-lysine pre-coated dishes. Most cells appeared spherical and some of them exhibited rudimentary neurites or residual proximal neuritic stems. Neurite outgrowth started at hour 4th to 7th *in vitro*. NSE and GFAP immunoreactivity were used to identify neuronal and astroglial cells, respectively. NSE positive neuronal cells tended to grow in close contact with glial cells and to send processes toward them, forming cell microaggregates (Fig. 3). GFAP immunoreactive cells were shown after 24 to 36 hrs *in vitro*, bearing different morphologies. They tended to proliferate in clones. Monolayers of proliferating cells were obtained from single elements (Fig. 4).

TH immunoreactive neurons were identified after staining both with monoclonal or polyclonal antibodies. In all the ages examined, the percentage of the TH immunoreactive cells in the total cell population was 3.2 ± 1.5 SEM at day 5 to 7, depending upon accurate anatomical dissection of the middle two thirds of the mesencephalon. One feature of TH positive neurons was the ability to grow long neurites in tissue culture even without a specific target (e.g. striatum) (Fig. 5).

TH enzymatic activity was determined using the TH microassay as described (Bostwick and Le, 1991). 10^5 cells were plated in a 96 microwell plate and the TH activity assayed at day 6 to 10. TH enzymatic activity per well did not show significant variations at the different gestational ages.

In DMEM/FCS growing medium, NGF did not effect either TH positive cell survival or TH enzymatic activity. NSE negative or GFAP positive cells were equally unaffected (no proliferative or differentiative effects). On the contrary, treatment of mesencephalic primary cultures with bFGF (50 ng/ml) significantly increased both the number of surviving TH positive neurons and TH enzymatic activity after 7 to 10 days *in vitro*. Furthermore, bFGF induced a significant proliferation of glial NSE negative cells. In defined medium bFGF did not affect survival and TH activity of dopaminergic neurons. The number of surviving NSE negative cells was minimally affected by bFGF (no significant proliferative effect) under these experimental conditions (Table 2).

Table 2. Effects of bFGF and NGF treatment on TH immunoreactive cells

	% TH$^+$ cells	TH activity*	% of NSE$^-$ cells
Controls	3.2 ± 1.5%	1.660 ± 250 dpm/well/20 min	51 ± 7
+ bFGF (50 ng/ml)	5.3 ± 1.8%	4.850 ± 350 dpm/well/20 min	78 ± 4
+ NGF (50 ng/ml)	3.4 ± 1.6%	1.750 ± 178 dpm/well/20 min	52 ± 5

* Assays were run in triplicate, at day 8 to 10 in culture. Data were duplicated for each weak of gestational ages and expressed as mean ± SEM. bFGF effect was statistically significant on TH positive cell percentage in vitro (p < 0.01; Student's t-test), TH activity (p < 0.001) and % of NSE$^-$ cells (p < 0.001). Percentage of TH positive or NSE positive cells was determined after analysis of 3% of the total surface of 35-mm tissue culture dishes in triplicate experiments

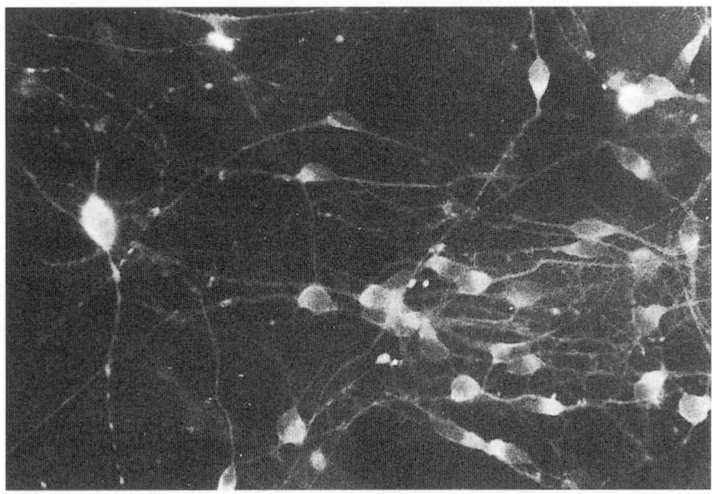

Fig. 3. Phase-contrast photomicrograph of human fetal mesencephalic neurons at day 10 *in vitro*. After dissociation, cells were grown in DMEM medium containing serum (10% heat inactivated fetal calf serum) on poly-L-lysine pre-treated dishes. Neuronal cells were demonstrated by anti-Neuronal-specific enolase (NSE) antibody (rabbit anti-NSE antibody — 1:100 dilution). NSE positive cells tend to grow on and to send neurites towards NSE negative /GFAP positive glial cells (200×)

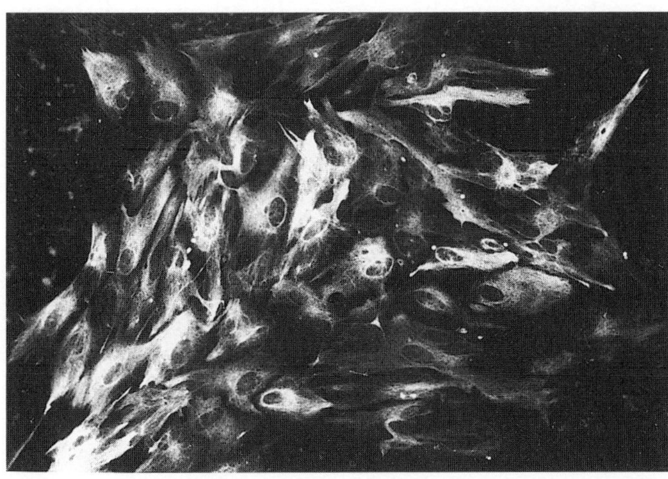

Fig. 4. Cultured GFAP positive cells were obtained from the human mesencephalon. Astroglial cells show different morphologies and tend to grow in clusters (170×)

294 V. Silani et al.

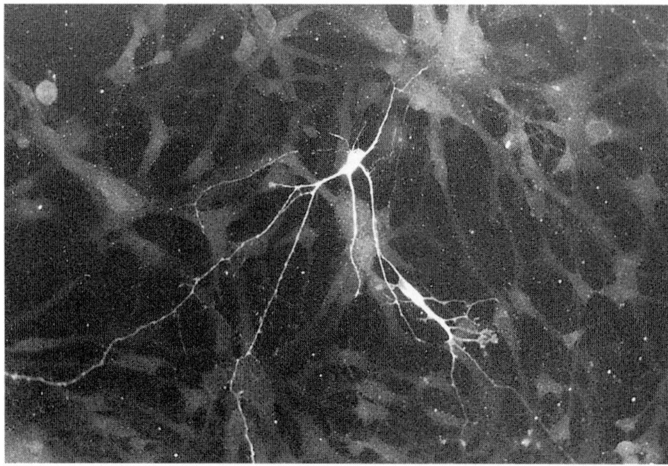

Fig. 5. TH positive neurons represented with serum in the growing medium, about 3.2 ± 1.5% SEM of the total cells (neurons and glia) at day 5 to 7 in culture. They showed long neurites also in absence of the specific striatal target (200×)

Discussion

The present study investigates the developmental stages of the human mesDA neurons and their early appearance in the human mesencephalon at PC week 5.5. This data complements previous observations: TH immunoreactivity was previously reported in the human mesencephalon at PC week 5.0 (Verney et al., 1991), and 6.5 (Freeman et al., 1991). The age of the specimens we analyzed corresponds to the developmental time when mesDA neurons establish synaptic connection with the striatal target. Theoretically, this is the age when mesDA neurons become most selectively dependent for survival on trophic molecule(s) produced by the target. The analysis of the neuronal characteristics and of the cell perturbation induced by candidate molecules at this age can contribute significantly to the identification of molecules with specific activity on the substantia nigra.

bFGF, previously shown to be active in rodents (Ferrari et al., 1989), is also active on human nigral cells, at least *in vitro*. Data obtained from our series of experiments agrees with previous observations by others on different species. Mediators of the response appear to be non neuronal cells. Actually, cultures grown in a chemically defined medium with a reduced number of astroglial cells were unable to significantly increase TH activity after bFGF treatment (Silani et al., 1994).

Human primary cultures appear a useful tool to obtain preliminary biological information before therapeutical trials on PD patients. The possibility to cryopreserve human neuronal cells for unlimited periods (Silani et al., 1988), to grow primary cultures from the human adult CNS in PD patients (Silani et al., 1988), and to obtain unlimited passages of EGF-dependent human progenitor cells (Silani et al., 1994) may open new perspectives in defining the role of genetic and epigenetic influences on the growth and regeneration fate of mesDA neurons, severely affected in PD.

Acknowledgments

The authors gratefully acknowledge the support of this research by the "Associazione Amici Centro Dino Ferrari" for Neuromuscular and Neurodegenerative Diseases of the University of Milan Medical School.

References

Bostwick RJ, Le WD (1991) A tyrosine hydroxylase assay in microwells using coupled nonenzymatic decarboxylation of Dopa. Anal Biochem 192: 125–130

Carvey PM, Ptak LR, Lo ES, Lin D, Buhrfield CM, Goetz CG, Klawans HL (1991) Levodopa reduces the growth promoting effects of striatal extracts on rostral mesencephalic tegmentum cultures. Exp Neurol 114: 28–34

Carvey PM, Ptak LR, Nath ST, Sierens DK, Mufson EJ, Goetz CG, Klawans HL (1993) Striatal extracts from patients with Parkinson's disease promote dopamine neuron growth in mesencephalic cultures. Exp Neurol 120: 149–152

Cintra A, Cao Y, Oelling C, Tinner B, Bortolotti F, Goldstein M, Pettersson RF, Fuxe K (1991) Basic FGF is present in dopaminergic neurons of the ventral midbrain of the rat. 2: 597–600

Denis-Donini S, Glowinski J, Prochiantz A (1983) Specific influence of striatal target neurons on the *in vitro* outgrowth of mesencephalic dopaminergic neurites: a morphological quantitative study. J Neurosci 3: 2292–2299

Denis-Donini S, Glowinski J, Prochiantz A (1984) Glial heterogeneity may define the three-dimensional shape of mouse mesencephalic dopaminergic neurones. Nature 307: 641–643

Di Porzio U, Daguet MC, Glowinski J, Prochiantz A (1980) Effect of striatal cells on *in vitro* maturation of mesencephalic dopaminergic neurones grown in serum-free conditions. Nature 288: 370–373

Dorte O, Unsicker K (1990) Basic FGF reverses chemical and morphological deficits in the nigrostriatal system of MPTP-treated mice. J Neurosci 10: 1912–1921

Drumm J F, O' Rahilly R (1977) The assessment of prenatal age from the crown-rump length determined ultrasonically. Am J Anat 148: 550–560

Ferrari G, Minozzi MC, Toffano G, Leon A, Skaper AD (1989) Basic fibroblast growth factor promotes the survival and development of mesencephalic neurons in culture. Dev Biol 133: 140–147

Freeman TB, Spence MS, Boss BD, Spector DH, Strecker RE, Olanow CW, Kordower JH (1991) Development of dopaminergic neurons in the human substantia nigra. Exp Neurol 113: 344–353

Hyman C, Hofer M, Barde YA, Juhasz M, Yancopoulos GD, Squinto SP, Lindsay RM (1991) BDNF is a neurotrophic factor for dopaminergic neurons of the substantia nigra. Nature 350: 230–233

Hyman C, Juhasz M, Jackson C, Wright P, Ip NY, Lindsay RM (1994) Overlapping and distinct actions of the neurotrophins BDNF, NT-3, and NT-4/5 on cultured dopaminergic and GABAergic neurons of the ventral mesencephalon. J Neurosci 14: 335–347

Langston JW, Widner H, Goetz GC (1992) Core assessment program for intracerebral transplantation (CAPIT). Mov Disord 7: 2–13

Lin LFH, Doherty DH, Lile JD, Bektesh S, Collins F (1993) GDNF: a glial cell linederived neurotrophic factor for midbrain dopaminergic neurons. Science 260: 1130–1132

Lindsay RM, Altar CA, Cedarbaum JM, Hyman C, Wiegand SJ (1993) The therapeutic potential of neurotrophic factors in the treatment of Parkinson's disease. Exp Neurol 124: 103–108

Prochiantz A, Daguet MC, Herbet A, Glowinski J (1981) Specific stimulation of *in vitro* maturation of mesencephalic dopaminergic neurons by striatal membranes. Nature 293: 570–572

Prochiantz A, di Porzio U, Kato A, Berger B, Glowinski J (1979) *In vitro* maturation of mesencephalic dopaminergic neurons from mouse embryos is enhanced in presence of their striatal target cells. Proc Natl Acad Sci USA 76: 5387–5391

Robinson HP (1993) Gestational age determination: first trimester. In: Chervenak FA, Isaacson GC, Campbell S (eds) Ultrasound in obstetrics and gynecology. Little, Brown and Company, Boston, pp 295–304

Robinson HP, Fleming J EE (1975) A critical evaluation of sonar "crown-rump length" measurements. Br J Obstet Gynaecol 82: 702–710

Silani V, Borasio GD, Zhou FC, Bernasconi S, Pizzuti A, Sampietro A, Scarlato G (1994) NGF-response of EGF-dependent progenitor cells obtained from human sympathetic ganglia. NeuroReport 5: 2085–2089

Silani V, Mariani D, Donato MF, Ghezzi C, Mazzucchelli F, Buscaglia M, Pardi G, Scarlato G (1994) Development of dopaminergic neurons in the human mesencephalon and *in vitro* effects of basic fibroblast growth factor treatment. Exp Neurol 128: 59–76

Silani V, Mariani D, Donato MF, Mazzucchelli F, Buscaglia M, Pardi G, Scarlato G (1992) *In vivo* and *in vitro* development of human mesencephalic dopaminergic neuron. J Neur Transplant Plast 3: 255–256

Silani V, Pezzoli G, Motti E, Falini A, Pizzuti A, Ferrante C, Zecchinelli A, Marossero F, Scarlato G (1988) Primary cultures of human caudate nucleus. Appl Neurophysiol 51: 10–20

Silani V, Pizzuti A, Strada O, Falini A, Buscaglia M, Scarlato G (1988) Human neuronal cell viability demonstrated in culture after cryopreservation. Brain Res 473: 169–174

Snider WD and Johnson EM (1990) Neurotrophic molecules. Ann Neurol 26: 489–506

Strömberg I, Björklund L, Johansson M, Tomac A, Collins F, Olson L, Hoffer B, Humpel C (1993) Glial cell line-derived neurotrophic factor is expressed in the developing but not adult striatum and stimulates developing dopamine neurons *in vivo*. Exp Neurol 124: 401–412

Thoenen H (1991) The changing scene of neurotrophic factors. Trends Neurosci 5: 165–170

Tomozawa Y, Appel SH (1986) Soluble striatal extract enhances development of mesencephalic dopaminergic neurons *in vitro*. Brain Res 399: 111–124

Verney C, Zecevic N, Nikolic B, Alvarez C, Berger B (1991) Early evidence of catecholaminergic cell groups in 5- and 6-week-old human embryos using tyrosine hydroxylase and dopamine-β-hydroxylase immunocytochemistry. Neurosci Lett 131: 121–124

Authors' address: V. Silani, M.D., The Institute of Neurology, University of Milan Medical School, Via F. Sforza 35, I-20122 Milan, Italy.

J Neural Transm (1995) [Suppl] 45: 297–305
© Springer-Verlag 1995

The inhibition of peroxide formation as a possible substrate for the neuroprotective action of dihydroergocryptine

A. Favit[1], M. A. Sortino[1], G. Aleppo[1], U. Scapagnini[1], and P. L. Canonico[2]

[1] Institute of Pharmacology, University of Catania School of Medicine, Catania, and
[2] Chair of Pharmacology, University of Pavia School of Dentistry, Pavia, Italy

Summary.   Dihydroergocryptine is an ergot alkaloid endowed with pharmacological actions mainly related to its dopaminomimetic activity. Free radical formation and subsequent lipid peroxidation had been postulated to partecipate broadly to the pathogenesis of tissue injury, including the brain injury induced by hypoxia, ischemia or trauma, as well as in the physiopathology of chronic neurodegenerative diseases, such as Parkinson's disease. Here we report that dihydroergocryptine protects cultured rat cerebellar granule cells against age-dependent and glutamate-induced neurotoxicity. Dihydroergocryptine antagonizes in fact both the neuronal death produced by acute exposure to a toxic glutamate concentration as well as the normal age-dependent degeneration in culture, presumably by exerting a scavenger action. This effect does not seem mediated entirely by interactions with the dopamine D_2 receptors. The neuroprotective action of dihydroergocryptine suggests a potential usefulness in halting the acute and chronic neurodegenerative diseases related to excitotoxic damage and free radical formation, including Parkinson's disease.

Introduction

In the central nervous system, a homeostatic control exists over oxidant and antioxidant agents that regulate the energetic levels of the neuronal cells (Sohal et al., 1985). The formation of oxygen free radicals and related activated oxygen species, such as superoxide radical, hydrogen peroxide, hydroxyl radical, is regulated through the activation of an enzymatic system particularly consisting of superoxide dismutase, glutathione peroxidase, glutathione reductase and glucose-6-phosphate dehydrogenase. An altered turnover due to an excessive production or an inadequate defence against reactive oxygen species results in a modification of the lipidic components of the neuronal membrane, with an increased lipid peroxidation and promotion of extensive cellular damage.

Abnormal free radical formation is involved in the neurodegenerative processes occurring in aging (Benzi et al., 1988a,b; Gorini et al., 1988) as well as in several neurological diseases, including Parkinson's disease (Graham, 1978, 1984; Cohen, 1983, 1985; see also Riederer, this volume). Experimental studies on the 1-methyl-4-phenyl-1,2,3,6-tetrahydropyridine (MPTP)-induced Parkinsonism in monkey brain areas have confirmed the involvement of reactive oxygen species in neurodegeneration through an oxidative deamination of monoamines and particularly of nigro-striatal dopamine (Graham, 1978; Burns et al., 1983; Langstone et al., 1984; Johannessen et al., 1985). Interestingly, MPTP, the selective neurotoxin that distroys the dopaminergic nigrostriatal pathways and results in a parkinsonian syndrome, increases the rate of apoptosis and kills cerebellar granule cells in culture via induction of programmed cell death (Dipasquale et al., 1991).

It is now well established that glutamate-induced neuronal damage may contribute importantly to neuronal death in several neurological diseases, including cerebral hypoxia-ischemia and chronic degenerative diseases (e.g. Huntington's disease, amyotrophic lateral sclerosis, Alzheimer's disease). The molecular mechanisms responsible for the glutamate-induced neuronal degeneration are complex and apparently involve multiple stages. Formation of free radicals represents the final mediator of cellular destruction, a process that also includes the activation of other mechanisms such as Ca^{2+} mobilization and triggering of Ca^{2+}-dependent enzymes (Choi, 1990).

Dihydroergocryptine and neuronal degeneration

In physiological conditions, oxidative stress is balanced by a variety of reducing agents such as cysteine, α-tocoferol, glutathione (Miyamoto et al., 1989); during the excitotoxin-induced neuronal degeneration that occurs in different neurodegenerative diseases this equilibrium is modified, mainly due to an increased production of oxygen free radicals (reviewed in Choi, 1990). Thus, a novel therapeutical approach to neurodegenerative processes is represented by agents which inhibit free radical formation and/or antagonize their effects.

Dihydroergocryptine is an ergot alkaloids (Berde and Schild, 1978) endowed mainly with a potent dopamine D_2 receptor agonist activity (Berde and Schild, 1978; Caron et al., 1978; Fiore et al., 1978). For this reason, dihydroergocryptine is widely used for the treatment of parkinsonian patients (see other reports in this volume). Dihydroergocryptine has been recently reported to modify cerebral antioxidant enzyme activities (i.e. superoxide dismutase, glutathione reductase or oxidase) in different brain areas, and to increase the content of reduced glutathione in rat forebrain during aging (Benzi et al., 1988a,b; Gorini et al., 1988). In addition, dihydroergocryptine attenuates the reduction of striatal dopamine produced by MPTP in mice and improves the parkinsonian symptoms induced by MPTP treatment in Cynomolgus monkeys. Hence, dihydroergocryptine has a potential interest as a new agent against neurotoxin-induced neuronal degeneration. To investigate this potential neuroprotective effect we have used primary cultures of cerebellar granule cells. Cultured rat cerebellar granule cells represent a suitable model to study the mechanisms underlying glutamate-induced neurotoxicity (Novelli et al., 1988; Manev et al., 1990). These cultures comprise of a rather pure and homogeneous population of glutamatergic neurons (the granule cells), which express different subtypes of excitatory amino acid receptors and degenerate spontaneously within 12–15 days of incubation in vitro (DIV). In our experiments cell viability was determined by exposing the cells to fluorescein diacetate (FDA) and propidium iodide (PI) (Manev et al., 1990). Neuronal injury curtails FDA staining (Rotman and Papermaster, 1966), but allows permeation by PI through the interaction with nuclear DNA (Krishan, 1975).

As a first step, we have examined the effects of dihydroergocryptine on the age-related neuronal degeneration. In cultures at 14 DIV more than 90% of neuronal population was degenerated or dead. Daily addition of dihydroergocryptine (once a day from the 2nd day in culture) partially protected the cerebellar granule cells against age-related degeneration. The neuroprotective action of dihydroergocryptine was significant ($p < 0.01$) at concentrations ranging between 100 nM and 1 µM (Fig. 1). At these concentrations, dihydroergocryptine rescued 50–60% of granule cells when the viability was estimated by comparing the number of intact FDA-positive cells to the number of degenerating PI-positive cells after 14 DIV. The effect of dihydroergocryptine declined progressively at concentrations greater than 1 µM (Fig. 1). The reasons for this decline are unclear, but a similar pharmacological profile has been reported for dihydroergocryptine in relation to the reduced glutathione concentrations in the forebrain of 10-month-old rats (Gorini et al., 1988). A possible explanation would be the metabolic degradation of dihydroergocryptine, yielding a neurotoxic amino acid as e.g. proline (Nadler et al., 1988; Cordero et al., 1991).

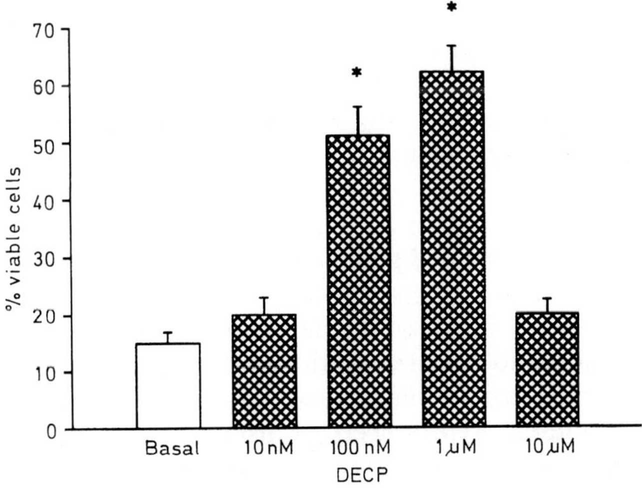

Fig. 1. Effect of a daily treatment with dihydroergocryptine on spontaneous neuronal degeneration occurring in cultured cerebellar granule cells at 14 DIV. Results (mean ± SEM of three separate experiments) are expressed as percentage of surviving neurons; viability was estimated by intravital staining of the culture. * $p < 0.01$ if compared to basal values

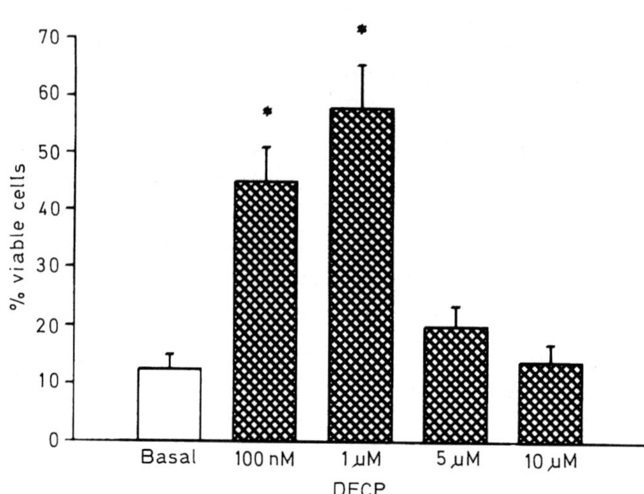

Fig. 2. Concentration-dependent effect of dihydroergocryptine (added daily from the 2nd DIV; last addition 3 hrs before glutamate) against glutamate-induced cytotoxicity. Cultures were exposed to toxic concentrations (100 μM) of glutamate for 30 min. Results represent the mean ± SEM of three different experiments performed in quadruplicate. *p < 0.01 if compared to basal values

One of the proposed mechanisms for this "age-related" degeneration is that the progressive depletion of energetic substrates from the culture medium allows the toxic action of the endogenously released glutamate (Novelli et al., 1988). For this reason we have evaluated the effects of dihydroergocryptine on the glutamate-induced neurotoxicity. In cultured granule cells, a 30-min exposure of the neurons to toxic concentrations (100 μM) of glutamate in Mg^{2+}-free buffer led to a delayed degeneration of granule cells. Chronic treatment (once a day from the 2nd DIV, last addition 3 h before the glutamate pulse) with dihydroergocryptine at concentrations ranging between 100 nM and 1 μM protected cerebellar granule cells against the toxic action of glutamate (Fig. 2), while greater concentrations were devoid of any neuroprotective effect.

Dihydroergocryptine and glutamate-induced peroxide formation

The neurodegenerative processes promoted by an increased free radical-induced damage in pathological conditions may be due to either a decline of antioxidant enzymatic and non-enzymatic defenses or to an increased production of oxygen free radicals (produced for instance by the excitotoxic action of glutamate). In physiological conditions, neurons are protected by an effective network of antioxidant mechanisms and the reduced glutathione (GSH) plays a pivotal role in protecting cells from oxidative stress by the intervention of enzyme scavengers, such as peroxide dismutase and glutathione peroxidase. The modification of the cerebral glutathione system with age (Benzi et al., 1988a) or the depletion of glutathione levels in specific brain areas due to neurodegenerative pathologies is likely to be responsible for the increased vulnerability of the brain to free radicals and peroxidation (Bannon et al., 1984; Choi, 1990).

Thus, the neuroprotective activity of dihydroergocryptine may be mediated by removal of free radicals and/or inhibition of lipid peroxidation. In vivo studies show that a chronic treatment with dihydroergocryptine in aged rats induces a significant increase in the concentrations of reduced glutathione in the forebrain (Benzi et al., 1988a) and modifies cerebral antiperoxidative enzyme activities in different brain areas in aged rats under chronic oxidative stress conditions (Benzi et al., 1988b). In addition, chronic pretreatment with dihydroergocryptine partially counteracts the GSH depletion induced in the forebrain of 15-month-old-rats by the intraperitoneal injection of the prooxidant electrophilic agents cycloexene-1-one and cycloheptene-1-one (Benzi et al., 1991).

In line with these findings, dihydroergocryptine antagonized glutamate-induced peroxide formation in vitro. In cultured cerebellar granule cells peroxide formation was assessed by using the fluorescent probe 2,7-dichlorofluorescin diacetate. Glutamate caused a significant increase in the percentage of fluorescent cells after a 6-h exposure. The increase in the number of fluorescent cells after exposure to 100 μM glutamate was markedly suppressed (by 40–50%) by chronic dihydroergocryptine treatment (added daily starting from the 2nd DIV and throughout the glutamate exposure). The dose-response analysis showed that the effect was maximal between 100 nM and 1 μM; at greater concentrations, the action of dihydroergocryptine progressively declined (data not shown). In addition, also a single treatment with 1 μM dihydroergocryptine 1 h or 30 min before glutamate significantly reduced (by about 30%) the rise in intracellular peroxides induced by a single pulse of glutamate (Fig. 3). Conversely, when added 3 h before or 30 min after the glutamate pulse, dihydroergocryptine was ineffective. Thus, it is tempting to hypothesize that the reduction of peroxide formation by dihydroergocryptine is responsible for its neuroprotective action. However, we cannot exclude that dihydroergocryptine inhibitory effect on peroxide formation may be an indirect consequence of cell protection.

Interestingly, the protective effect of dihydroergocryptine against glutamate-induced peroxide formation does not seem to be mediated entirely by interaction with dopamine D$_2$ receptor. In fact, dopamine addition was unable to modify the peroxide formation induced by glutamate in granule cells, and, under basal conditions, produced a slight, but not significant, increase of intracellular peroxides (Fig. 4). However, the failure of dopamine to inhibit peroxide formation may be also interpreted as direct toxicity of dopamine (Tanaka et al., 1991). As a matter of fact two D$_2$ receptors antagonists, haloperidol and sulpiride, only partially counteracted dihydroergocryptine effect suggesting that at least part of the neuroprotective effect of dihydroergocryptine is independent of its interaction with the D$_2$ receptor (Fig. 5). Accordingly, Van Muiswinkel et al. (1993) reported that chronic D$_2$ receptor stimulation did not influence the survival and differentiation of cultured dopaminergic neurons. Dihydroergocryptine does however also in-

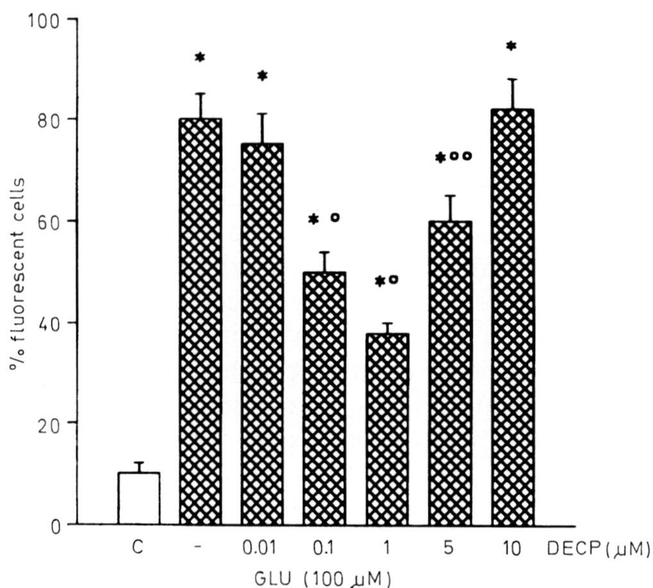

Fig. 3. Peroxide scavenging action of a single pulse of 1 µM dihydroergocryptine at different times on glutamate-induced peroxide formation in cerebellar granule cells in primary cultures. −3, −1, −0.5, +0.5 = 3 h, 1 h, 30 min before, and 30 min after glutamate (GLU), respectively. Values represent the mean ± SEM of 4 determinations for each group. Representative of 2 separate experiments which gave similar results. *p < 0.01 versus control (C); °p < 0.01 versus glutamate alone

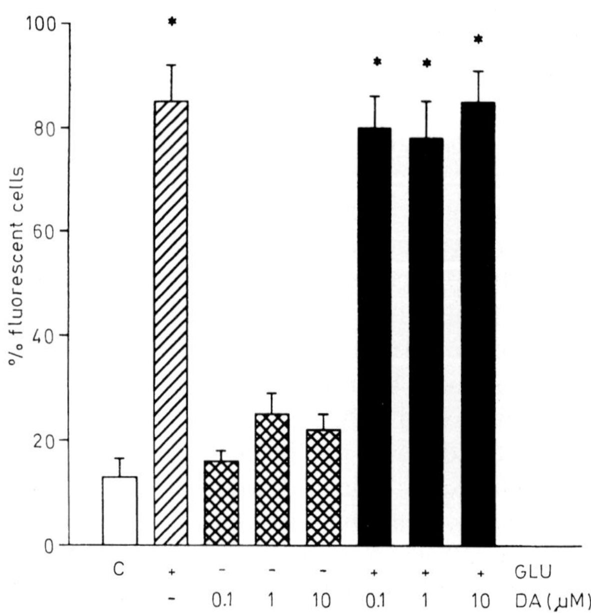

Fig. 4. Effect of dopamine on basal and glutamate-stimulated peroxide formation in cerebellar granule cells in primary cultures. Values represent the mean ± SEM of 4 determinations for each group. Representative of 2 separate experiments which gave similar results. *p < 0.01 versus control (C)

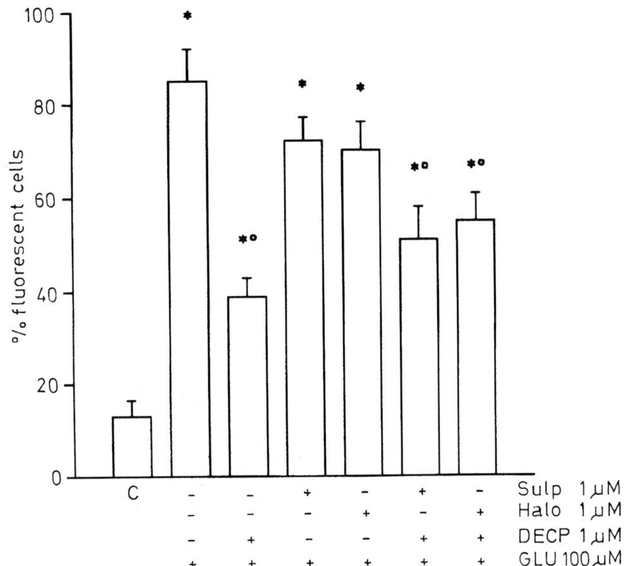

Fig. 5. Effect of haloperidol (Halo) and sulpiride (Sulp) on glutamate (GLU)-stimulated peroxide formation in cerebellar granule cells in primary culture. Values represent the mean ± SEM of 4 determinations for each group. Representative of 2 separate experiments which gave similar results. *p < 0.01 versus control (C); °p < 0.01 versus glutamate alone

teract with other neurotransmitter receptors, including the dopamine D_1 receptor (Berde and Schild, 1978; Groppetti et al., 1989), and interestingly dopamine D_1/D_2-receptor antagonists have been reported to potentiate the neuroprotective action of the noncompetitive NMDA receptor antagonist MK-801 (Nurse et al., 1991).

Conclusions

In conclusion, the neuroprotective activity of dihydroergocryptine may be mediated by removal of free radicals and inhibition of lipid peroxidation. This is consistent with the neuroprotective activity of a variety of reducing agents such as cysteine, α-tocopherol, glutathione, idebenone (Miyamoto et al., 1989) and 21-aminosteroids (which inhibit oxygen free radical-induced lipid peroxidase) (Braughler et al., 1987) in relation to exposure to toxic concentrations of glutamate. The precise mechanisms of these effects of dihydroergocryptine remain to be elucidated. Besides a possible "scavenger action", dihydroergocryptine may also influence positively the glutathione turnover, thus increasing the reduced cellular charge and decreasing lipoperoxidative cellular degeneration. Whatever the mechanism(s), dihydroergocryptine has a great potential as a neuroprotective agent in the therapy and/or the prevention of chronic neurodegenerative diseases, including Parkinson's disease.

                                  A. Favit et al.

Acknowledgments

This work was supported in part by a grant from Poli Industria Chimica S.p.A., Milano.

References

Bannon MJ, Goedert M, Williams B (1984) The possible relation of glutathione, melanine and N-methyl-4-phenyl-1,2,3,6-tetrahydro-pyridine (MPTP) to Parkinson's disease. Biochem Pharmacol 33: 2697–2698

Benzi G, Pastoris O, Marzatico F, Villa RF (1988a) Influence of aging and drug treatment on cerebral glutathione system. Neurobiol Aging 9: 371–375

Benzi G, Pastoris O, Villa RF (1988b) Changes induced by aging and drug treatment on cerebral enzymatic antioxidant system. Neurochem Res 13: 467–478

Benzi G, Pastoris O, Gorini A, Marzatico F, Villa RF, Curti D (1991) Influence of aging on the acute depletion of reduced glutathione induced by electrophilic agents. Neurobiol Aging 12: 227–231

Berde B, Schild O (1978) Ergot alkaloids and related compounds. Springer, Berlin Heidelberg New York

Braughler JN, Pregenzer JF, Chase RL, Duncan LA, Jacobsen AJ, McCall JM (1987) Novel 21-aminosteroids as potent inhibitors of iron-dependent lipid peroxidation. J Biol Chem 262: 10438–10440

Burns RS, Chiueh CC, Markey SP, Ebert MH, Jacobowitz DM, Kopin IJ (1983) A primate model of parkinsonism: selective destruction of dopaminergic neurons in the pars-compacta of the substantia nigra by N-methyl-4-phenyl-1,2,3,6-tetrahydropyridine. Proc Natl Acad Sci USA 80: 4546–4550

Caron MG, Beaulieu M, Raymond V, Gagnè B, Drouin J, Lefkowitz J, Labrie F (1978) Dopaminergic receptors in the anterior pituitary gland. Correlation of ^{3}H-dihydroergocryptine binding with the dopaminergic control of prolactin release. J Biol Chem 253: 2244–2253

Choi DW (1990) Methods for antagonizing glutamate-induced neurotoxicity. Cerebrovasc Brain Metab Rev 2: 105–147

Cohen G (1983) The pathobiology of Parkinson's disease: biochemical aspects of dopamine neuron senescence. J Neural Transm [Suppl] 19: 89–103

Cohen G (1985) Oxidative stress in the nervous system. In: Sies H (ed) Oxidative stress. Academic Press, London, pp 383–402

Cordero ML, Negron AE, Ortiz JC, Blanco C, Santiago G (1991) Inhibition of high-affinity [^{3}H]L-proline binding to rat brain membranes by 2-amino-7-phosphonoheptanoic acid. Eur J Pharmacol 208: 179–181

Dipasquale B, Marini AM, Youle RJ (1991) Apoptosis and DNA degradation induced by 1-methyl-4-phenilpyridinium in neurons. Biochem Biophys Res Commun 181: 1442–1448

Fiore L, Scapagnini U, Canonico PL (1987) Effect of dihydroergocryptine and dihydroergocristine on cyclic AMP accumulation and prolactin release in vitro: evidence for a dopaminomimetic action. Horm Res 25: 171–177

Gorini A, Arnaboldi R, Vercesi L, Dossena M (1988) Influence of some ergot alkaloids on the cerebral reduced glutathione. Il Farmaco 11: 887–890

Graham DG (1978) Oxidative pathways for catecholamines in the genesis of neuromelanine and cytotoxic quinones. Mol Pharmacol 14: 633–634

Graham DG (1984) Catecholamines toxicity: a proposal for the molecular pathogenesis of manganese neurotoxicity and Parkinson's disease. Neurotoxicology 5: 83–96

Groppetti A, Ceresoli G, Del Monaco S, Parenti M (1989) Diidroergocriptina: studio degli effetti sui recettori dopaminergici striatali. Giornale di Psiconeurofarmacologia XI: 10–15

Johannessen JN, Chiueh CC, Burns RS, Markey SP (1985) Differences in the metabolism of MPTP in the rodent and primate parallel differences in sensitivity to its neurotoxic effects. Life Sci 36: 219–224

Krishan A (1975) Rapid flow cytofluorometric analysis of mammalian cell cycle by propidium iodide staining. Cell Biol 66: 188–193

Langstone JW, Forno LS, Rebert CS, Irwin I (1984) Selective nigral toxicity after systemic administration of 1-methyl-4-phenyl-1,2,3,6-tetrahydropyridine (MPTP) in the squirrel monkey. Brain Res 292: 390–394

Manev H, Favaron M, Vicini S, Guidotti S, Costa E (1990) Glutamate-induced neuronal death in primary cultures of cerebellar granule cells: protection by synthetic derivatives of endogenous sphingolipids. J Pharmacol Exp Ther 252: 419–427

Miyamoto M, Murphy TH, Schnaar RL, Coyle JT (1989) Antioxidants protect against glutamate-induced cytotoxicity in a neuronal cell line. J Pharmacol Exp Ther 250: 1132–1140

Nadler JV, Wang A, Hakim A (1988) Toxicity of L-proline toward rat hippocampal neurons. Brain Res 456: 168–172

Novelli A, Reilly JA, Lysko PG, Henneberry RC (1988) Glutamate becomes neurotoxic via the N-methyl-D-aspartate receptor when intracellular energy levels are reduced. Brain Res 451: 205–212

Nurse SM, Corbett D, Evans SJ (1991) Combined treatment with MK-801 and a D1/D2 dopamine antagonist reduces cerebral ischemic damage. Soc Neurosci 17: Abs 501.7

Rotman B, Papermaster BW (1966) Membrane properties of living mammalian cells as studied by enzymatic hydrolysis of fluorogenic esters. Proc Natl Acad Sci USA 55: 134–141

Sohal RS, Allen RG, Farmer KJ, Newton RK, Toy PL (1985) Effects of exogenous antioxidants on the level of endogenous antioxidants, lipid-soluble fluorescent material and life-span in the housefly, Musca domestica. Mech Ageing Dev 31: 329–336

Tanaka M, Sotomatsu A, Kanai H, Hirai S (1991) DOPA and dopamine cause cultured neuronal death in the presence of iron. J Neurol Sci 101: 198–203

Van Muiswinkel FL, Drukarch B, Steinbusch HWM, Stoof JC (1993) Chronic dopamine D_2 receptor activation does not affect survival and differentiation of cultured dopaminergic neurons: morfological and neurochemical observations. J Neurochem 60: 83–92

Authors' address: A. Favit, M.D., Instite of Pharmacology, University of Catania School of Medicine, Viale A. Doria 6, I-95125 Catania, Italy.

J Neural Transm (1995) [Suppl] 45: 307–317
© Springer-Verlag 1995

Neuroprotective activity of α-dihydroergocryptine in animal models

G. Coppi

Research Centre, Poli Indutria Chimica, Rozzano, Milan, Italy

Summary. α-Dihydroergocryptine (α-DHEC) is a well known dopaminergic agent successfully employed in the treatment of Parkinson's disease. α-DHEC showed a neuroprotective activity against total cerebral ischemia induced by $MgCl_2$ in mice and histocytic anoxia by NaCN in mice and rats. Moreover the drug promoted the recovery of locomotor activity in rats after cerebral ischemic damage and protected mice against convulsions induced by intracerebroventricular injections of NMDA and glutamate. α-DHEC showed a protective activity on neuronal degeneration induced by MPTP in monkeys, as evaluated through animal's behaviour and morphological-cytochemical changes in the *substantia nigra*, suggesting a preservative effect on neuronal morphology and brain architecture. In the MPTP-treated monkeys, the α-DHEC administration induced a restoration of the unstimulated MDA values to control levels. The neuroprotective activity of α-DHEC is related to its peculiar activity on antioxidative enzymes of GSH system and to reduction of lipid-peroxide-induced cellular degeneration.

Introduction

α-Dihydroergocryptine (α-DHEC) is a new anti-Parkinson drug which shows affinity for both D_1 and D_2 dopamine receptors; it is an antagonist of D_1 and a strong agonist of D_2. The efficacy of α-DHEC in the treatment of Parkinson's disease has been verified in many clinical trials. In double-blind studies versus bromocriptine and lisuride, α-DHEC showed no statistically significant differences in therapeutic activity, but very low frequency of side-effects and drop-outs. α-DHEC has also been shown to be effective in lowering prolactin levels in blood (Coppi, 1991).

In this paper we report a neuroprotective activity of α-DHEC in some animal models. The protective effects of α-DHEC are tested against total cerebral ischemia induced by $MgCl_2$ in mice, histocytic anoxia produced by NaCN in mice and rats, locomotor activity in rats 24 hours after cerebral ischemia induced by occlusion of bilateral common carotid arteries for 3 hours, convulsions induced by i.c.v. injection of glutamate and NMDA in mice and on Parkinson disease-like syndrome induced by 1-methyl-4-phenyl-1,2,3,6-tetrahydropyridine (MPTP) in monkeys.

Material and methods

Total cerebral ischemia induced by $MgCl_2$ in mice

The method of Berga et al. (1986) was followed with minor changes. Male Crl: CD-1(ICR)BR mice, weighing 20–25 g were used. Animals were allowed food and water "ad libitum" and randomly divided into different treatment groups of 20–30 mice. The animals received the treatments reported in Table 1 before inducing cardiac arrest and complete global cerebral ischemia by the intravenous injection of $MgCl_2$ (100 mg/Kg/10 ml). The interval between the $MgCl_2$ injection and the last observable inspiratory movement in each mouse was recorded and taken as survival time.

Histocytic anoxia induced by NaCN in mice and rats

The method of Berga et al. (1986) was followed with minor changes. Male Crl: CD-1(ICR)BR mice, (20–25 g) and male Crl: CD(SD)BR rats (75–100 g) were used. Animals were allowed food and water "ad libitum" and randomly divided into different treatment groups (12–30 mice; 8–17 rats). The rapid intravenous injection of 2 mg/Kg/10 ml or 2.5 mg/Kg/5 ml of NaCN was given to mice or rats respectively, after pretreatment with α-DHEC according to dosage and route described in Table 2. The interval between the NaCN injection and the death of each animal was taken as survival time.

Table 1. Effects of α-DHEC on total cerebral ischemia induced by $MgCl_2$ in mice

Dose (mg/Kg)	Route	Time before $MgCl_2$ (min)	Mice (no)	Survival time (sec) (mean ± S.E.)	Variation (%)
—	iv	—	30	26.57 ± 0.40	—
30	ip	15	20	32.35* ± 0.70	+21.75
10	iv	2	20	30.05* ± 0.47	+13.10

*p < 0.01 (Dunnett's t test)

Table 2. Effects of α-DHEC on histocytic anoxia induced by NaCN in mice and rats

Animal	Dose (mg/Kg)	Route	Time before NaCN (min)	Animals (no)	Survival time (sec) (mean ± S.E.)	Variation (%)
Mouse	—	iv	—	30	53.67 ± 1.30	—
	30	ip	15	12	72.42* ± 2.79	+34.94
	10	iv	2	12	73.50* ± 1.52	+36.95
Rat	—	iv	—	17	91.53 ± 1.14	—
	30	ip	15	8	109.51 ± 4.66	+19.63
	10	iv	2	8	206.57* ± 35.54	+125.47

*p < 0.01 (Dunnett's t test)

Locomotor activity after cerebral ischemic damage in rats

Male Crl: CD(SD)BR rats of 200 g were used. Cerebral ischemia was induced by occlusion of bilateral common carotid arteries for 3 hours and blood reperfusion was allowed for 24 hours. Animals with cerebral ischemic damage showed a reduced locomotor activity after 24 hours; they were randomly divided into different treatment groups as reported in Table 3. The animals (3/cage) were placed in a Basile apparatus (Comerio, Varese, Italy) and the horizontal locomotion activity was checked for 4 hours at 1 hour interval (Coppi and Falcone, 1989).

Convulsions induced by intracerebroventricular injection
of glutamate and NMDA in mice

The method of Beani et al. (1990) was followed with minor changes. Male Crl: CD-1(ICR)BR mice of 22–25 g were cannulated 24 hours before the experiment. Under ether anaesthesia an incision was made along the mid-line of the skull and the bones were cleaned of connective tissue. Using an intramuscular needle with a sharp end, a small hole was made in the skull at the following coordinates: 3.7 mm anterior to the lamba and 1.5 mm lateral to the interhemispheric suture. Here a polyethylene cannula (PE-10, Becton Dickinson, USA) was fixed on the skull with a little amount of acrylic dental cement. After an overnight recovery, L-glutamate (C.Erba, Italy) or N-methyl-D-aspartate (NMDA) (Sigma, USA) were administered through the cannula into the lateral ventricle (depth: 2.1 mm from the cortical surface) with a Hamilton syringe. 2 μl of saline solution containing 1 μmol of glutamate or 0.6 nmol of NMDA were injected in unanaesthetized animals and the onset of convulsions in the first minute after i.c.v. injection was scored as a positive response. α-DHEC was administered i.p. or i.v. before the excitatory aminoacids injections at the times and doses showed in Tables 4 and 5; valproic acid (Sigma, USA) and diazepam (Roche, Swiss) were used as reference compounds. Anticonvulsant effect was expressed as percent of animals without seizures in each group.

Parkinson disease-like syndrome induced by MPTP in monkeys

In this study 18 male *Macaca fascicularis* (Cynomolgus monkeys, C.River, UK) of 3.5–5.5 Kg were used. The animals were randomly allocated to three groups and treated as described.

Group 1 was given as a first phase 2 ml/Kg deionized water orally, twice a day (6-h interval), for 5 days. The Parkinson disease-like syndrome was induced in his group in a second phase by intravenous injections of 0.3 mg/Kg per day of MPTP base (0.25 ml/Kg)

Table 3. Effects of α-DHEC on locomotor activity after cerebral ischemic damage in rats

Treatment	Exp. (no)	Rats (no)	Horizontal locomotor activity (0–4 h) (total counts) (mean ± S.E.)	Variation (%)
—	10	30	889 ± 68	—
α-DHEC	5	15	2766* ± 538	+211.14

*p < 0.01 (Student's t test). α-DHEC was given intraperitoneally (30 mg/Kg) just before the analysis of motor activity

Table 4. Anticonvulsant effects of α-DHEC against seizures induced in mice by icv injection of glutamate (1 μmol/mouse)

Drug/Dose (mg/Kg)	Route	Pre-treatment times (min)	No of convulsant animals	Protection (%)
—	iv	−30	20	0
α-DHEC	iv	−90	18	10
10		−60	16	20
		−30	12	40**
		−15	14	30*
—	ip	−30	20	0
α-DHEC	ip	−120	20	0
30		−90	16	20
		−60	16	20
		−30	13	35*
		−15	10	50**
Diazepam 5	ip	−30	0	100**
Valproic acid 200	ip	−30	0	100**

*$p < 0.05$; **$p < 0.01$ X^2 test vs. respective control group

Table 5. Anticonvulsant effects of α-DHEC against seizures induced in mice by icv injection of NMDA (0.6 nmol/mouse)

Drug/Dose (mg/Kg)	Route	Pre-treatment times (min)	No of convulsant animals	Protection (%)
—	iv	−30	20	0
α-DHEC	iv	−90	20	0
10		−60	14	30*
		−30	16	20
		−15	16	20
—	ip	−30	20	0
α-DHEC	ip	−120	18	10
30		−90	14	30*
		−60	12	40**
		−30	16	20
		−15	16	20
Diazepam 5	ip	−30	0	100**
Valproic acid 200	ip	−30	2	100**

*$p < 0.05$; **$p < 0.01$ X^2 test vs. respective control group

for 5 consecutive days. In this phase 2 ml/Kg deionized water was given orally, just before and at about 6 h after each MPTP injection. In a third phase group 1 was given 2 ml/Kg deionized water, twice a day (6-h interval), for an additional 5 days.

Group 2 was given as a first phase 6 mg/Kg α-DHEC orally, twice a day (6-h interval), for 5 days. Animals were then treated with 6 mg/kg of α-DHEC orally, just before and 6 h after each MPTP injection (as described above) for 5 consecutive days. In a third phase, animals received 6 mg/Kg α-DHEC orally, twice a day (6-h interval) for additional 5 days.

Group 3 was given 2 ml/Kg deionized water orally, twice a day (6-h interval), for 5 days. The group was then injected with saline (0.25 ml/Kg per day) for 5 consecutive days and was given 2 ml/Kg deionized water orally, twice a day, just before and 6 h after each saline injection. In the last phase the animals received 2 ml/Kg deionized water, twice a day (6-h interval), for 5 days.

The animals were killed 18 days after the beginning of the experiment under sodium pentobarbital (50 mg/Kg i.v.) anaesthesia. Animals were bled to death through the femoral arteries and the brains were removed.

During the experiments five treated monkeys died (three MPTP-treated and two α-DHEC and MPTP-treated).

Behaviour and clinical conditions of the animals were checked daily by a veterinarian 1 h after the first oral administration (deionized water or α-DHEC), 1 and 4 h after MPTP or saline injection, and 1 h after the second oral administration (deionized water or α-DHEC). The posture, tremor twitching, motor activity and sedation behaviour was checked and scored according to the following scale. Posture: 0 = normal, erect posture; 1 = frequently sitting; 2 = continuously sitting; 3 = occasionally supine or prone; 4 = continuously supine or prone. Tremor/twitching: 0 = none; 1 = mild; 2 = moderate; 3 = severe. Motor activity: 0 = normal; 1 = slightly reduced; 2 = moderately reduced; 3 = markedly reduced. Sedation: 0 = absent; 1 = mild; 2 = moderate; 3 = marked.

Two 1-cm-thick sections of right hemiencephalon, including *substantia nigra*, were fixed by immersion in Bouin solution for 6 h in 4% formaldehyde for 5 days. After washing in 70% ethanol or in running tap water, the sections were dehydrated, cleared in xylene and embedded in paraffin. Sections of embedded tissue, 8 μm thick, were used for staining with hematoxylin-eosin, after fixation with either Bouin or formaldehyde and for immunocytochemistry for neurofilament protein (NF) and glial fibrillary acid protein (GFAP) as follows. The immunocyochemical staining for NF was done on Bouin-fixed sections by the peroxidase-antiperoxidase (PAP) method of Sternberger et al. (1970). The immunocytochemistry of GFAP was performed on formaldehyde-fixed sections according to Bernocchi et al. (1992).

Immediately after death the left hemiencephalon of each monkey was immersed in an ice isotonic sucrose medium (0.32 M sucrose and 1 mM EDTA) for 3 minutes. The tissue samples were obtained, washed in isotonic saline solution, frozen in dry ice and stored at −80°C until the biochemical analysis was performed (Marzatico et al., 1993).

Basal and stimulated MDA formation tissue homogenate was assayed by a spectrophotometric technique. The tissue samples were homogenized with 20 volumes of ice cold 50 mM Tris-HCl buffer (pH 7.6). An aliquot of 100 μl of homogenate was added to 200 μl of sodium dodecyl sulphate (8.1% wt/v) to solubilize the tissue, 1.5 ml of 20% acetic acid at pH 3.5, and 1.5 ml of 0.8% (wt/v) thiobarbituric acid (Ohkawa et al., 1979). Lipid peroxidation (MDA production) was stimulated by incubating aliquots of tissue homogenate (100 μl) with 200 μl of 0.01 mM $FeSO_4$ plus 0.25 mM ascorbic acid in a final volume of 4 ml with distilled water. The samples were boiled for 30 minutes, cooled with ice and centrifuged at 4°C for 10 minutes at 4000 r.p.m. and the absorbance of the resultant solutions was measured at 532 nm with a Beckman 35 spectrophotometer. The basal and stimulated MDA levels were calculated using a molar extinction coefficient of 1.54×10^5 and were expressed as nmoles of MDA for milligram of protein. Protein concentration was determined by a spectrophotometric tecnique with albumine bovine as standard (Lowry et al., 1951).

Statistical analysis

Statistical analysis was carried out by ANOVA followed by Dunnett's t test, Student's test, χ^2 test and Mann-Whitney test for comparisons with controls and by Scheffe F test for multiple comparisons.

Results

α-Dihydroergocryptine caused a significant increase of survival time in mice submitted to total cerebral ischemia induced by $MgCl_2$. This neuroprotective activity was observed after both intravenous and intramuscular administration (Table 1).

A clearcut neuroprotective effect of α-DHEC on histocytic anoxia induced by NaCN in mice and rats has been obtained. On the basis of the survival time, α-DHEC elicited a significant activity both by i.v. and i.p. administration in mice, while the activity was high only after intravenous administration (4 animals survived more than 300 sec) in rats (Table 2).

α-Dihydroergocryptine proved to be very effective in improving the locomotor behaviour altered in rats after the ischemic damage resulting from bilateral occlusion of common carotid arteries. In fact, α-DHEC increased dramatically the motor activity after intraperitoneal injection (Table 3).

Results reported in Table 4 show that α-DHEC is able to protect mice from glutamate-induced seizures. The protective activity was significant when the drug was administered, either ip or iv, 15 or 30 minutes before the i.c.v. injection of glutamate. Similary, α-DHEC protected mice form NMDA-induced seizures. The effect was significant when α-DHEC was injected ip 60 or 90 min or iv 60 min before NMDA administration (Table 5). As expected, reference compounds displayed a complete anticonvulsivant activity, while all the control animals showed convulsion after i.c.v. injection of excitatory aminoacids (E.A.A.).

The Parkinson-like symptomatology raised in MPTP-treated monkeys consisted of abnormal posture, tremors and twitchings, motor activity and sedation: this behaviour was marked in all MPTP-treated monkeys after the 3rd/4th injection. A progressive worsening of clinical conditions was observed in the animals of group 1 after the 5-day MPTP treatment cycle. In the monkeys from group 2, the overall score of syndrome represented always a lower degree of health impairment (Fig. 1). The score of control group was always 0.

The number of neurons in the *substantia nigra* was calculated on hematoxylin-eosin-stained sections. After treatment with MPTP (group 1), there was severe loss (74%) of neurons in comparison with controls (Fig. 2) (Table 6). In treated monkeys, most of the surviving neurons showed clear signs of degeneration (Fig. 3); they were very shrunken or swollen. After treatment with α-DHEC and MPTP (group 2), the decrease in the number of neurons was 20% on the average and the differences versus controls were not significant (Table 6). The surviving population has some shrunken neurons only (Fig. 4).

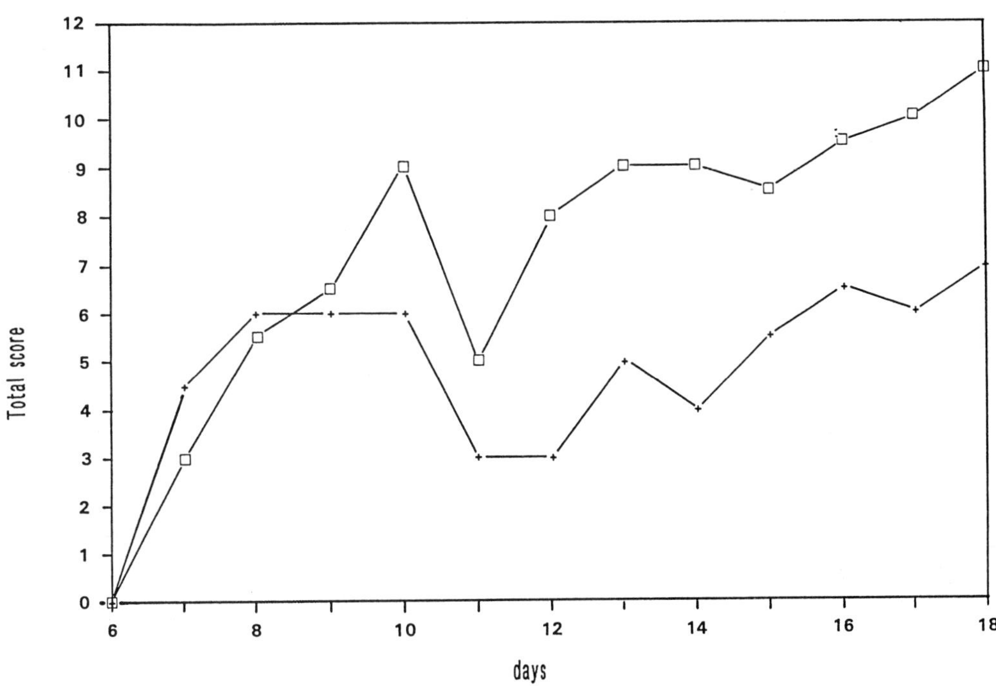

Fig. 1. Effects of α-DHEC on behaviour of MPTP-treated monkeys. MPTP group
(□——□); α-DHEC + MPTP group (+——+)

Table 6. Effects of α-DHEC on neurons in the "substantia nigra" of MPTP-treated
monkeys

Groups	Treatment	Animals (no)	Number of neurons (mean ± S.D.)	Variation (%)
1	MPTP	3	10 ± 2.65	−74
2	α-DHEC+MPTP	4	31 ± 11.62	−20
3	Control	6	39 ± 4.51	—

The number represent the counts made in 4 to 6 fields of vision (objective magnification
× 25) in four sections per animal (16 to 24 fields). Differences between group 1 and 2 or
3 are significant ($p < 0.05$). Difference between group 2 and 3 is not significant (Mann-
Whitney test)

Table 7. Effects of α-DHEC on basal and stimulated MDA production in "caudate
putamen" and "substantia nigra" of MPTP treated monkeys

Brain areas	Treatment	Animals (no)	Basal MDA[a] levels (mean ± S.E.)	Stimulated MDA[a] levels (mean ± S.E.)	Basal and stimulated MDA ratio
Caudate/ putamen	MPTP	3	6.35 ± 0.79*	13.9 ± 1.06	2.2
	α-DHEC+MPTP	4	4.00 ± 0.39	14.5 ± 1.35	3.6
	Control	6	4.77 ± 0.29	15.3 ± 0.87	3.2
Substantia nigra	MPTP	3	3.83 ± 0.42	9.3 ± 1.24**	2.4
	α-DHEC+MPTP	4	3.35 ± 0.46	10.3 ± 0.54	3.1
	Control	6	2.88 ± 0.39	13.5 ± 0.70	4.7

[a]The levels of MDA are expressed as mmol/mg protein. *$p < 0.02$; **$p < 0.01$ (ANOVA and
Scheffe F test)

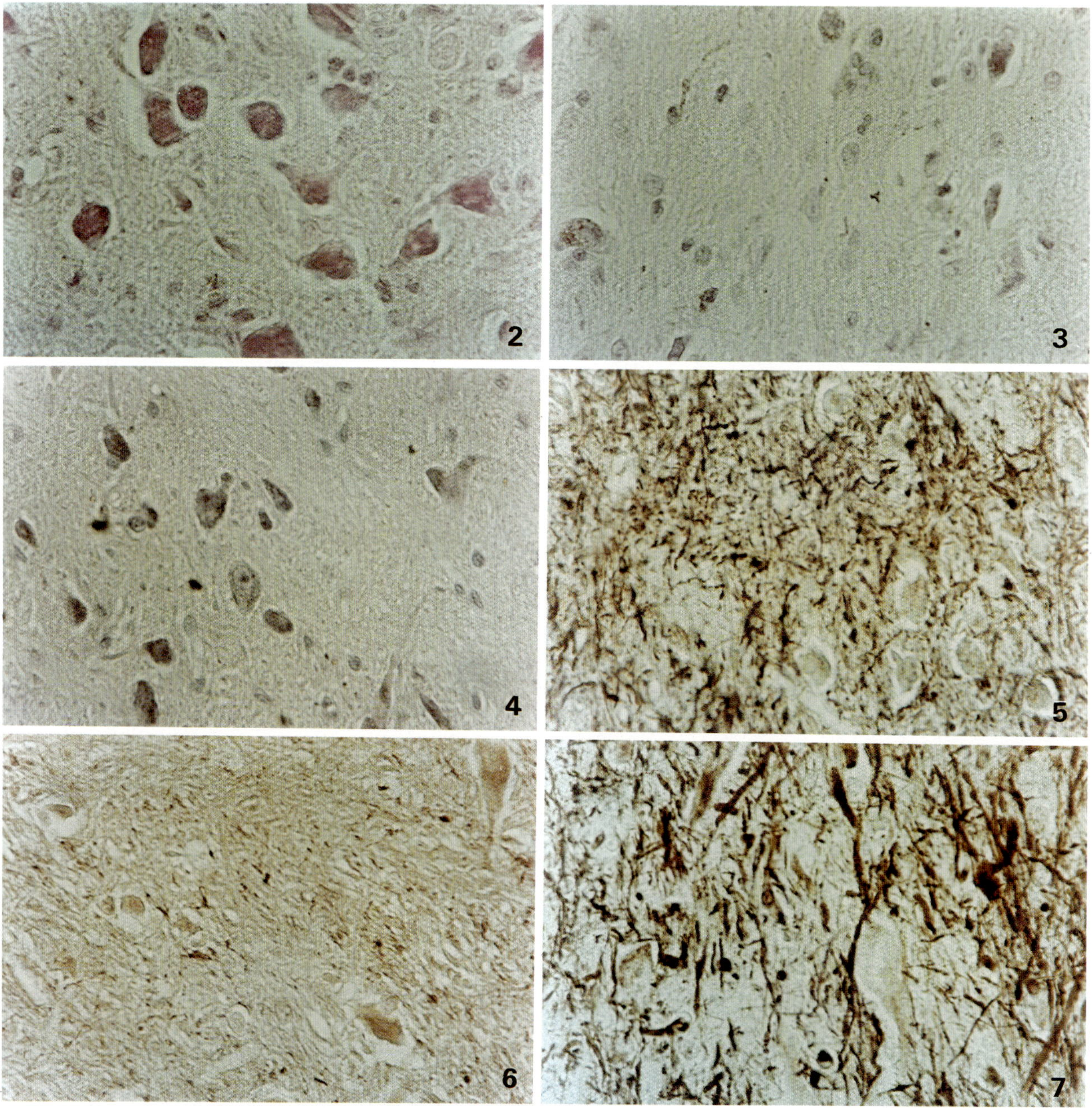

After immunocytochemical reaction phosphorilated neurofilaments (NF) in the *substantia nigra* of control monkey were found exclusively in the axons (Fig. 5). After treatment with MPTP, the immunopositive filamentous structures (axons) were markedly decreased in comparison with controls (Fig. 6). After treatment with α-DHEC and MPTP, there were several immunopositive filamentous structure (axons). Some of those axons showed enlarged caliber and strong reactivity (Fig. 7) and their highest density was at the more peripheral areas of the pars compacta.

Immunocytochemical reaction with anti-GFAP, which detected mainly astrocytes, revealed only few immunopositive glials cells in the *substantia nigra* of control animals. After treatment with MPTP the number of GFAP-immunopositive cells increased by 60% and after α-DHEC and MPTP the increase was 76%.

The basal levels of MDA were different in the *caudate putamen* and *substantia nigra*. The MPTP treatment increased about 30% the basal MDA in both areas, reaching the statistical significance in *caudate putamen*. The stimulated production of MDA, in presence of $FeSO_4$ plus ascorbic acid, was lower in MPTP treated monkeys, mainly in the *substantia nigra* (Table 7). The administration of α-DHEC counteracted the significant enhancement of basal MDA levels in *caudate putament* but improved only slightly the changes occurred in *substantia nigra*.

Discussion

α-DHEC elicits in acute pharmacological experiments an interesting neuroprotective activity. This effectiveness is evident in total cerebral ischemia induced by $MgCl_2$ in mice, in histocytic anoxia induced by NaCN in mice and rats and in locomotor activity after cerebral ischemic damage in rats. Moreover, α-DHEC protects experimental animals against convulsions induced by i.c.v. administration of glutamate and NMDA. This result, obtained in *in vivo* animal models, indicate that α-DHEC interacts with EAA systems producing a neuroprotective activity against massive introduction into CNS of glutamate and NMDA. Our data are in agreement with other experimental results (Favit et al., 1993) showing interaction between α-DHEC and EAA systems.

Fig. 2. Hematoxilin-eosin staining in brains of control monkeys after fixation by immersion in 4% formaldeyde. Neurons of the pars compacta ×16

Fig. 3. Hematoxilin-eosin staining in brains of MPTP-treated monkeys after fixation by immersion in 4% formaldeyde. Neurons of the pars compacta ×16. There are few neurons and they show signs of dark or light degeneration

Fig. 4. Hematoxilin-eosin staining in brains of α-DHEC and MPTP-treated monkeys after fixation by immersion in 4% formaldeyde. Neurons of the pars compacta ×16. The surviving neurons are numerous; only some neurons show degeneration

Fig. 5. Immuocytochemistry with an anti-200 kDa neurofilament (NF) antibody, control monkeys. In the pars compacta there are immunopositive axons ×40

Fig. 6. Immunocytochemistry with an anti-200 kDa neurofilament (NF) antibody, MPTP-treated monkeys. There is a drastic decrease of immunopositive axons in the pars compacta ×40

Fig. 7. Immunocytochemistry with an anti-200 kDa neurofilament (NF) antibody, α-DHEC and MPTP treated monkey. There are immunopositive axons in the pars compacta ×40; some axons are increased in caliber and reactivity

MPTP causes behavioural deficits, biochemical changes and neuropathological alterations in primates similar to those observed in humans with idiopathic Parkinson's disease (Burns et al., 1986). The behavioural observations recorded in this study demonstrate a clear anti-Parkinson activity of α-DHEC.

As described in the literature (Burns et al., 1983; Crossman et al., 1987; Langston et al., 1984; Ricaurte et al., 1987; Seniuk et al., 1990) MPTP treatment causes death of neuronal population of the *pars compacta*. We found a percentage loss of neurons in the range of those reported by Pakkenberg and Brody (1965) and Pakkenberg et al. (1991) in patients with Parkinson's disease. The disappearance of neurons was accompanied by a great degeneration of axons, of which only a few in the neuropil of the SN remained. The dominant aspect after MPTP treatment was the strong degeneration of the SN neuronal bodies and processes.

The addition of α-DHEC to MPTP treatment seems to lower the health impairment and to prevent the dramatic neuronal death. The surviving nerve cells were better preserved in number and morphology and the glial reaction was greater after α-DHEC than after treatment with MPTP alone. It must be taken into account that a moderate activation of astrocytes is important for promoting restoration of neuronal function by enhancing neuron survival and axon growth in the injured areas (Muller et al., 1991). In fact, after α-DHEC, in addition to a mild glial reaction, there was a large number of axon intensively immunoreactive for NF. Thus, α-DHEC is neuroprotective against MPTP-induced damages, in terms of preservation of neuronal morphology of the brain architecture. In addition, the presence of several axons in the pars compacta does not exclude an axonal sprouting and remodelling.

The major metabolite of MPTP *in vivo* (Markey et al., 1984) is the positively charged ion 1-methyl-4-phenylpyridinium (MPP+) that seems to exert its toxicity interferring with the functions of mitochondria (Vyas et al., 1986), increasing the possibility of the reactive oxygen species to throw a leakage of electrons from the normal electron flow of the respiratory chain (Nohl, 1986).

The oxidative deamination of monoamine and particularly of nigrastriatal dopamine, results in the formation of hydrogen peroxide and other potentially toxic products such as hydroxyl radicals, superoxide and hydroxyquinones (Cohen, 1983; Graham, 1984) so that some role of the radical species in the pathogenesis of Parkinson's disease is accepted.

The increases basal levels of MDA in parkinsonian *substantia nigra* and *caudate putamen* of the monkeys indicate that the model utilized in this study was rather severe, since the peroxidative pattern in the *caudate putamen* seems not to be affected in parkinsonian brain (Dexter et al., 1989).

α-DHEC treatment has been recently demonstrated to interfere positively with the glutathione cycle and with some antioxidant enzymatic activities. The chronic treatment with α-DHEC induced an increase of glutathione peroxidase activity in the *caudate putamen* of the aged rat brain and an increase of reduced glutathione and glutathione redox index in aged and oxidatively stressed rat brain (Benzi et al., 1988, 1989).

The data of this study confirm the cerebroprotective activity of α-DHEC in a severe Parkinson-like syndrome, possibly through the influence of the lipoperoxidative damage in *substantia nigra* and *caudate putamen*. The biochemical data are strenghtened by immunocytochemical data showing an improvement of the nerve cells number and morphology, and by behavioural observations demonstrating a sharp amelioration of the Parkinson-like symptoms.

Our data suggest that the α-DHEC administration could display its role as neuroprotective agent, particularly in Parkinson-like syndrome, in different ways: a) as D_2 agonist agent, like bromocriptine; b) by interaction with EAA systems; c) positively influencing the glutathione turnover, improving cellular energy metabolism and d) decreasing the lipoperoxidative cellular degeneration.

References

Beani L, Bianchi C, Baraldi PG, Manfredini S, Pollini GP (1990) Protection by pyroglutamic acid and some of its newly synthesized derivatives against glutamate-induced seizures in mice. Arzneimittelforschung/Drug Res 40: 1187–1191

Benzi G, Pastoris O, Marzatico F, Villa RF (1988) Influence of aging and drug treatment on the cerebral glutathione system. Neurobiol Aging 9: 371–375

Benzi G, Pastoris O, Villa RF (1988) Changes induced by aging and drug treatment on cerebral enzymatic antioxidant system. Neurochem Res 13: 467–478

Benzi G, Pastoris O, Marzatico F, Villa RF (1989) Age-related effect induced by oxidative stress on the cerebral glutathione system. Neurochem Res 14: 473–481

Berga P, Beckett PR, Roberts DJ, Llenas J, Missingham R (1986) Synergistic interactions between piracetam and dihydroergocristine in some animal models of cerebral hypoxia and ischaemia. Arzneimittelforschung/Drug Res 36: 1314–1320

Bernocchi G, Gerzeli G, Scherini E, Vignola C (1992) Neuroprotective effects of α-Dihydroergocryptine against damages in the *substantia nigra* caused by severe treatment with 1-methyl-4-phenyl-1,2,3,6-tetrahydropyridine. Acta Neuropathol 85: 404–413

Burns RS, Chiueh CC, Markey SP, Ebert MH, Jacobowitz DM, Kopin IJ (1983) A primate model of parkinsonism: selective destruction of dopaminergic neurons in the *pars compacta* of the *substantia nigra* by N-methyl-4-phenyl-1,2,3,6-tetrahydropyridine. Proc Natl Acad Sci USA 80: 4546–4550

Burns RS, Chiueh CC, Parisi J, Markey S, Kopin IJ (1986) Biochemical and pathological effects of MPTP in the Rhesus monkey. In: Fahn S, et al (eds) Recent developments in Parkinson's disease. Raven Press, New York, pp 127–136

Cohen G (1983) The pathology of Parkinson's disease: biochemical aspects of dopamine neurone senescence. J Neural Transm [Suppl] 19: 89–103

Coppi G (1991) Dihydroergocryptine, a new anti-Parkinson drug: a pharmacological and clinical review. Arch Gerontol Geriatr [Suppl] 2: 185–190

Coppi G, Falcone A (1989) Effects of α-Dihydroergocryptine on locomotor activity of normal and supersensitive mice. 6th Capo Boi Conference on Neuroscience, 4–9 June, p 175

Crossman AR, Clarke CE, Boyce S, Robertson RG, Sambrook MA (1987) MPTP-induced Parkinsonism in the monkey: neurochemical pathology, complications of treatment and pathophysiological mechanisms. Can J Neurol Sci 14: 428–435

Dexter DT, Carter CJ, Wells FR, Javoy-Agid F, Agid Y, Lees A, Jenner P, Marsden CD (1989) Basal lipid peroxidation in *substantia nigra* is increased in Parkinson's disease. J Neurochem 52: 381–389

Favit A, Sortino A, Aleppo G, Scapagnini U, Canonico PL (1993) Protection by dihydroergocryptine of glutamate-induced neurotoxicity. Pharmacol Toxicol 73: 224–228

Graham DG (1984) Catecholamine toxicity: a proposal for the molecular pathogenesis of manganese neurotoxicity and Parkinson's disease. Neurotoxicol 5: 83–96

Langston JW, Forno LS, Rebert CS, Irwin I (1984) Selective nigral toxicity after systemic administration of 1-methyl-4-phenyl-1,2,3,6-tetrahydropyridine (MPTP) in the squirrel monkey. Brain Res 292: 390–394

Lowry OH, Rosenbrough NJ, Farr AL, Randall RJ (1951) Protein measurement with the Folin phenol reagent. J Biol Chem 193: 265–275

Markey SP, Johannessen JN, Chiueh CC, Burns RS, Herkenham MA (1984) Intraneuronal generation of a pyridinium metabolite may cause drug induced parkinsonism. Nature 311: 464–467

Marzatico F, Cafè C, Taborelli M, Benzi G (1993) Experimental Parkinson's disease in monkeys. Effect of ergot alkaloid derivative on lipid peroxidation in different brain areas. Neurochem Res 18: 1101–1106

Muller HW, Matthiessen HP, Schmalenbach C, Schroeder WO (1991) Glial support of CNS neuronal survival, neurite growth and regeneration. Restor Neurol Neurosci 2: 229–232

Nohl H (1986) Oxygen radical release in mitochondria: influence of age. In: Free radicals, aging and degenerative diseases. Alan R Liss, New York, pp 77–97

Ohkawa H, Ohisi N (1979) Assay for lipid peroxides in animal tissue by thiobarbituric acid reaction. Anal Biochem 95: 351–358

Pakkenberg H, Brody H (1965) The number of nerve cells in the *substantia nigra* in paralysis agitans. Acta Neuropathol (Berl) 5: 320–324

Pakkenberg B, Moller A, Gundersen HJG, Mouritzen Dam A, Pakkenberg H (1991) The absolute number of nerve cells in *substantia nigra* in normal subjects and in patients with Parkinson's disease estimated with an unbiased stereological method. J Neurol Neurosurg Psychiatry 54: 30–33

Ricaurte GA, Irwin I, Forno LS, DeLanney LE, Langston E, Langston JW (1987) Aging and 1-methyl-4-phenyl-1,2,3,6-tetrahydropyridine-induced degeneration of dopaminergic neurons in the *substantia nigra*. Brain Res 403: 43–51

Seniuk NA, Tatton WG, Greenwood CE (1990) Dose dependent destruction of the coeruleus-cortical and nigral-striatal projections by MPTP. Brain Res 527: 7–20

Sternberger LA, Hardy PH, Cuculis JJ, Meyer JD (1970) The unlabeled antibody-enzyme method of immunocytochemistry. Preparation and properties of soluble antigen antibody comples (HRP-anti-HRP) and its use in identification of spirochetes. J Histochem Cytochem 10: 315–328

Vyas I, Heikkila RE, Nicklas WJ (1986) Studies on the neurotoxicity of 1-methyl-4-phenyl-1,2,3,6 tetrahydropyridine: inhibition of NAD-linked substrate oxidation by its metabolite, 1-methyl-4-phenyl pyridinium. J Neurochem 46: 1501–1507

Authors' address: Prof. G. Coppi, Research Centre, Poli Industria Chimica, Via Volturno no. 48, I-20089 Rozzano, Milan, Italy.

Subject Index